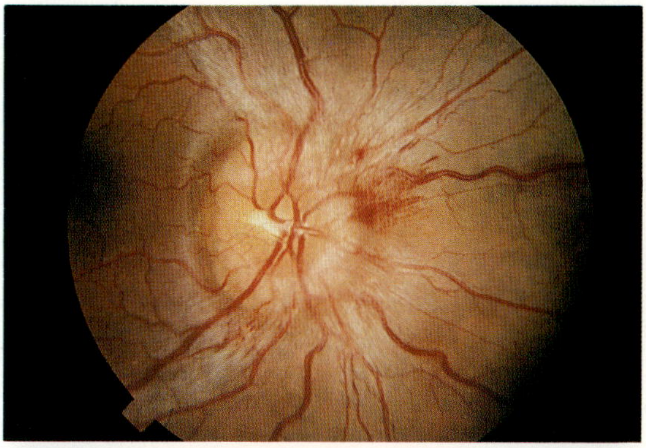

Plate 1 Acute optic disc swelling in a patient with idiopathic intracranial hypertension. 1

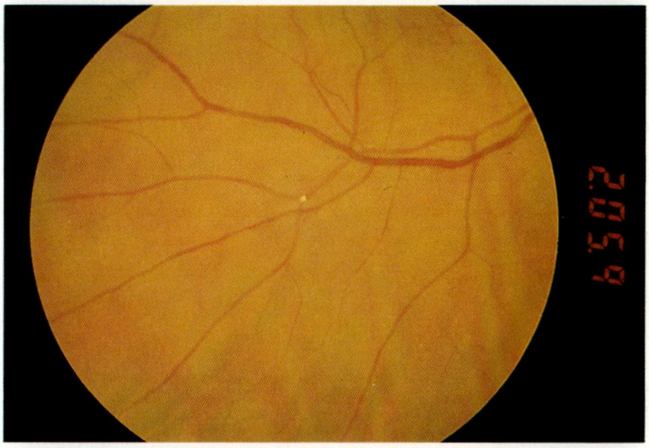

Plate 2 Cholesterol embolus (Hollenhorst plaque) at a third order retinal artery bifurcation. 2

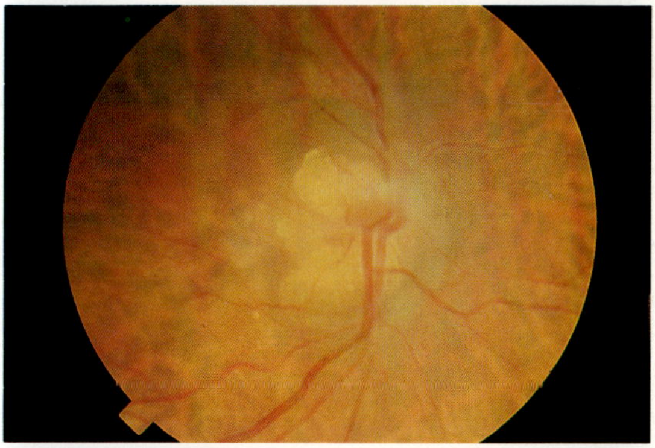

Plate 3 Florid optic disc drusen. 3

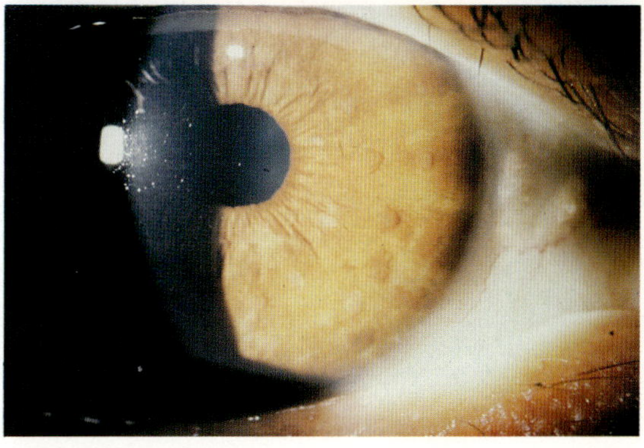

Plate 4 Iris hamartomas (Lisch nodules) in a patient with neurofibromatosis 1. 4

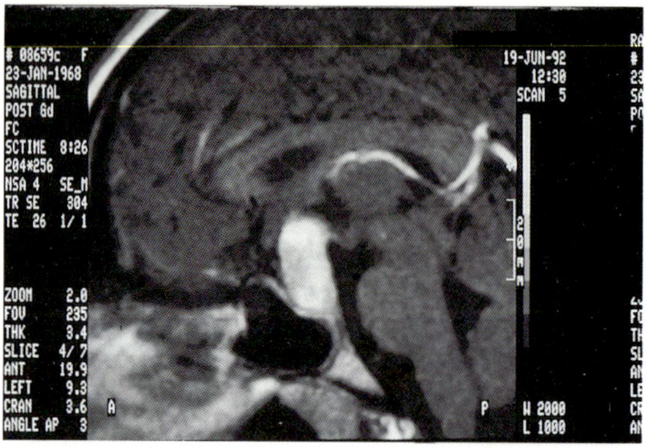

5

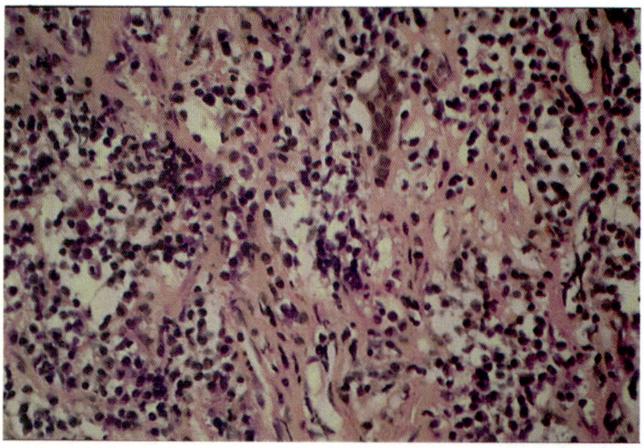

6

Plates 5 and 6 Sagittal MRI brain scan showing a large mass arising in the pituitary fossa with suprasellar extension resulting in visual failure. Histology shows a chronic inflammatory infiltrate in the anterior pituitary gland. This patient had post-partum lymphocyctic adenohypophysitis.

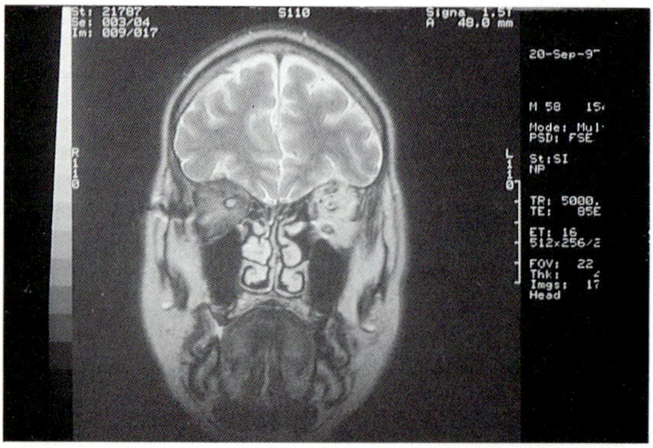

7

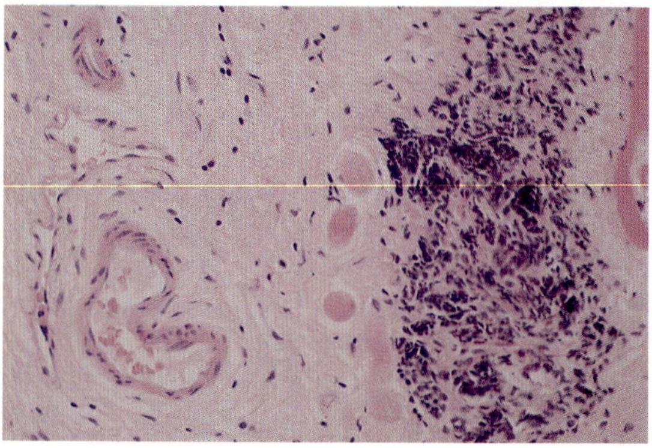

8

Plates 7 and 8 Coronal MRI orbital scan showing diffuse signal change in the right orbital fat, extraocular muscles and optic nerve sheath. Histology shows lymphoid aggregates and dense bands of fibrous tissue. This patient had sclerosing idiopathic orbital inflammatory disease (orbital pseudotumour).

COMMON PROBLEMS IN NEURO-OPHTHALMOLOGY

Volume 32 in the Series

Major Problems in Neurology
PROFESSOR CP WARLOW, BA, MB, BChir, MD, FRCP
PROFESSOR J VAN GIJN, MD, FRCPE
Consulting Editors

OTHER MONOGRAPHS IN THE SERIES

Barnett, Foster and Hudgson: **Syringomyelia**
Dubowitz and Brooke: **Muscle Biopsy: A Modern Approach**
Pallis and Lewis: **The Neurology of Gastrointestinal Disease**
Hutchinson and Acheson: **Strokes**
Gubbay: **The Clumsy Child**
Hankinson and Banna: **Pituitary and Parapituitary Tumours**
Behan and Currie: **Clinical Neuroimmunology**
Cartlidge and Shaw: **Head Injury**
Lisak and Barchi: **Myasthenia Gravis**
Johnson, Lambie and Spalding: **Neurocardiology: The Interrelationships between Dysfunction in the Nervous and Cardiovascular Systems**
Parkes: **Sleep and its Disorders**
Hopkins: **Headache Problems in Diagnosis and Management**
Wood and Anderson: **Neurological Infections**
Critchley: **Neurological Emergencies**
Ross: **Syncope**
Donaldson: **Neurology of Pregnancy** SECOND EDITION
Porter: **Epilepsy: 100 Elementary Principles** SECOND EDITION
Harper: **Myotonic Dystrophy** SECOND EDITION
Sjaastad: **Cluster Headache Syndrome**
Hodges: **Transient Amnesia: Clinical and Neuropsychological Aspects**
Vermeulen, Lindsay and Van Gijn: **Subarachnoid Haemorrhage**
Bauer and Hanefeld: **Multiple Sclerosis**
Hankey and Warlow: **Transient Ischaemic Attacks of the Brain and Eye**
Zakrzewska: **Trigeminal Neuralgia**
Hilton-Jones, Squier, Taylor and Matthews: **Metabolic Myopathies**
Hoogenraad: **Wilson's Disease**
Harper: **Huntington's Disease** SECOND EDITION

COMMON PROBLEMS IN NEURO-OPHTHALMOLOGY

JAMES F. ACHESON MRCP FRCS FCOphth
Consultant Ophthalmologist
Department of Neuro-Ophthalmology
The National Hospital for Neurology and Neurosurgery
Queen Square, London

MICHAEL D. SANDERS FRCP FRCS FCOphth
Consultant Ophthalmologist
Department of Neuro-Ophthalmology
The National Hospital for Neurology and Neurosurgery
Queen Square, London

W. B. Saunders Company Ltd
London · Philadelphia · Toronto · Sydney · Tokyo

W. B. Saunders Company Ltd
24–28 Oval Road
London NW1 7DX, UK

The Curtis Center
Independence Square West
Philadelphia, PA 19106–3399, USA

Harcourt Brace & Company
55 Horner Avenue
Toronto, Ontario M8Z 4X6, Canada

Harcourt Brace & Company, Australia
30–52 Smidmore Street
Marrickville, NSW 2204, Australia

Harcourt Brace & Company, Japan
Ichibancho Central Building, 22–1 Ichibancho
Chiyoda-ku, Tokyo 102, Japan

A catalogue record for this book is available from the British Library

ISBN 0–7020–1879–1

This book is printed on acid-free paper

Typeset by Phoenix Photosetting, Chatham, Kent
Printed and bound in Great Britain by The University Press, Cambridge

Contents

To Lesley and Esmé
from whom the time was taken

Foreword

Too often ophthalmologists and neurologists approach the eye and its function in widely differing ways. For ophthalmologists the eye may represent a world in itself, limited only by the bony walls of the orbit. For neurologists, vision and eye movements, as well as the outer and inner appearance of the eye, merely represent a single fragment of a greater whole: the nervous system. Each approach has its limitations: failure to see underlying relationships on the one hand, and lack of attention to detail on the other (for example, when neurologists have 'a look at the retina' they simply peer through a keyhole at the optic disc). Neuro-ophthalmology has emerged as a subdiscipline to fill this vacuum and, traditionally, its practitioners have been trained initially as ophthalmologists – apparently it is easier to acquire expertise in neurology for eye specialists than vice versa. The two authors of this monograph are no exception. Both are distinguished consultants from the National Hospital for Neurology and Neurosurgery in London; their scientific work includes studies on optic nerve sheath decompression to relieve raised pressure on the cerebrospinal fluid, and optic nerve involvement in hereditary disorders of the central nervous system (with the late Professor Anita Harding). For someone who has profited personally from the didactic skills of one of the authors, the erudition and clinical expertise demonstrated in this monograph come as no surprise. The comprehensive, yet succinct chapters will help readers greatly in bridging the gaps between neurology and ophthalmology. They will be even more pleasantly surprised by the inclusion of chapters on disorders of the facial nerve and on headaches, by which the authors once more prove their firm grounding in neurology. I wish this concise monograph the success it deserves amidst the more weighty tomes in the field.

J. VAN GIJN

Preface

Clinical neuro-ophthalmology encompasses a wide range of topics within vision science, neurology and ophthalmology. In addition, there are overlaps with neuro-radiology, neurosurgery, and neurophysiology as well as radiotherapy, neuro-otology and head and neck surgery. However, the fundamental clinical skills remain based on the accurate and informed assessment of visual symptoms, and it is from an ophthalmic perspective that we have prepared this review monograph. The topics have been selected to reflect the pattern of referrals to both the Department of Neuro-Ophthalmology at the National Hospital for Neurology and Neurosurgery, London, and the Medical Eye Unit at St Thomas' Hospital, London where the requirement for adequate multidisciplinary consideration of each patient's problems has always been considered a high priority.

In the 1990s the practice of clinical neuro-ophthalmology is hard to imagine without day-to-day access to the teaching and publications of many authors from both sides of the Atlantic. In particular we freely acknowledge our debt to Dr Neil Miller and Dr Joel Glaser for their wonderfully written, edited and produced texts which have made our task so much easier, and to Dr Frank Walsh and Professor Bill Hoyt who have defined and taught the speciality as we know it. The bibliography in our text is highly selective with an emphasis on recent contributions and the interested reader is referred to the following key texts for more comprehensive reviews of the literature: Neil Miller's encyclopaedic 4th edition of *Walsh and Hoyt's Clinical Neuro-Ophthalmology* (Williams & Wilkins, Baltimore/London, 1982–1994); the 2nd edition of *Glaser's Neuro-Ophthalmology* (Lippincott, Philadelphia, 1990), and the 2nd edition of *Leigh and Zee's Neurology of Eye Movements* (Davis, Philadelphia, 1992).

JAMES F. ACHESON
MICHAEL D. SANDERS

1

Synopsis of anatomy and physiology of the visual sensory system

THE ORGANIZATION OF THE HUMAN VISUAL SENSORY SYSTEM – PARALLEL PROCESSING AND RETINOTOPY

The elucidation of the central visual pathways in humans is a task very much to the forefront of contemporary neurobiology, as the physical basis of certain perceptual functions is unravelled. Contemporary clinical concepts involve the convergence of a wide range of methodologies, ranging from cognitive psychology and computer science (artificial intelligence) to human lesion studies based on imaging, neuropathology, psychophysics and electrophysiology, through to single cell physiology in the animal model. Recently, the advent of functional imaging of the human brain has allowed the non-invasive study of the normal workings of the cerebral cortex — including the visual system — and these techiques may also be applicable to certain abnormalities of visual perception (Rademacher *et al.*, 1992; Zeki *et al.*, 1991; Belliveau *et al.*, 1991).

PARALLEL PROCESSING

The concept of parallel processing is helpful to an overview of the organization of the visual system. It is evident that distinct classes of neurons process visual information from retina to cortex in parallel streams; that primarily dealing with colour vision, high spatial resolution and fine static stereopsis is referred to as parvocellular (referring to the relatively small size of the retinal ganglion cells — P cells) and that dealing primarily with motion detection, low spatial resolution and coarse motion stereopsis is referred to as magnocellular (relatively large retinal ganglion cells — M cells). In the retina, the macula is composed primarily of P cells whereas in the peripheral retina, P cells only slightly outnumber M cells. Parvocellular and magnocellular neurons are also morphologically distinct in the lateral geniculate ganglion and cortex, and further subsystems may also exist. The parvocellular stream can be further segregated into two substreams, parvo-blob and parvo-interblob. Blobs are clusters of cells in the primary visual cortex that stain intensely for cytochrome oxidase indicating high metabolic activity. The parvo-interblob stream appears to be involved with fine spatial acuity and the parvo-blob in colour discrimination. Although these parallel streams characterize the organization of the visual system, the picture is complicated by the fact that there are extensive interactions between the subsystems at a cortical level and oversimplification may be misleading. Nonetheless,

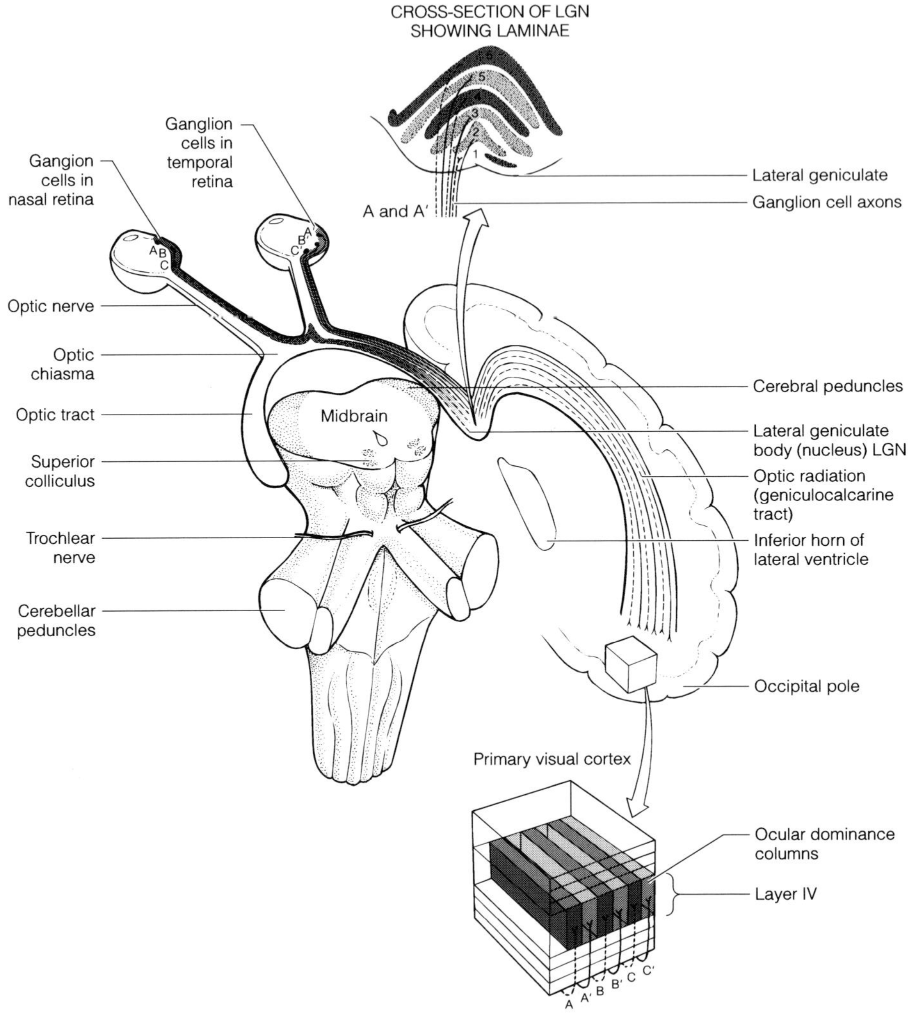

Figure 1.1 Overall scheme of the visual pathways. The manner of retinotopic projection to the lateral geniculate nucleus (LGN) and the ocular dominance columns in the primary visual cortex from left and right eyes is illustrated by three imaginary points or images (A, B, C) from the left visual field (not shown) falling on the right half of each retina (A, B, C in left eye and A′, B′, C′ in right eye).

an appreciation of these arrangements is helpful in the understanding of a variety of pathological processes including cerebral achromatopsia, motion blindness, blindsight and statokinetic dissociation (see below) (Sadun, 1986; Maunsell, 1992; Merigan, 1993).

RETINOTOPY

The retinal ganglion cells project to the brain according to the principle of retinotopy. This refers to the fact that the point-by-point correspondence of the representation of visual space on the retina is preserved in the visual pathways all the way from each eye to both cortical hemispheres. In this way the superior visual field is transmitted by the inferior retina and is mediated by inferior axons in the optic nerve, chiasm, optic tract, radiations and cortex. The retinal nerve fibre layer in the temporal retina is divided about a horizontal raphé with axons originating from the superior retina arching over the fovea to reach the superior optic nerve head, and fibres from the inferior retina arching beneath the fovea.

This division of retinal nerve fibres reflects the displacement of all retinal elements except the photoreceptors away from the fovea, and defines the horizontal meridian of the visual field throughout the visual system. As a result, ganglion cells adjacent to each other in the temporal retina send projections to remote parts of the optic nerve. Nearly a third of all axons in the optic nerve serve the central 5 degrees of visual field. Near the globe these are clustered in the central and temporal portion of the optic nerve (papillo-macular bundle) but more proximally they become intermingled with fibres serving peripheral vision throughout the nerve. Approaching the chiasm, fibres destined to decussate, shift into progressively more nasal positions in the posterior optic nerve. At the chiasm, fibres from the ganglion cells nasal to the fovea cross to merge with non-crossing fibres from the temporal retina of the contralateral eye. As a result fibres from each eye representing common points in the visual field come to be aligned together in the optic tract. The precision of this alignment increases towards the cortex, while in the lateral geniculate ganglion the retinotopic map is rotated through 90 degrees. The interpretation of visual field defects rests heavily on an appreciation of the principle of retinotopy, as the clinician seeks to determine whether bilateral field loss derives from the anterior or from the posterior (post-chiasmal) visual pathways (Horton, 1992).

THE ANTERIOR VISUAL PATHWAYS: RETINA, OPTIC NERVE AND CHIASM

RETINA

The retina contains the initial neural substrate for the transmission of visual information from the eye to cortex. Vision in the retina is served at three neuronal levels: the photoreceptor, the bipolar cell and the ganglion cell which projects to the lateral geniculate ganglion. In embryogenesis the neural retina is a derivative of the diencephalon and therefore the retina can be regarded as a part of the brain. As the optic vesicle becomes invaginated to form the optic cup, two tissue layers are formed, with a potential space between them which is referred to as the subretinal space which forms the cleavage plane in retinal detachment. The outer wall nearest the brain becomes a one cell thick layer — the retinal pigment epithelium. Outside the retina lies the choroid, a highly vascular tunic of tissue which is served by 90% of the total ocular blood flow. The capillary bed of the choroid — the choriocapillaris — maintains fenestrations facing towards the basement membrane and the retina. The basement membrane of the choriocapillaris and the basement membrane of the retinal pigment epithelium fuse to form Bruch's membrane, and the outer blood retinal barrier is provided by tight junctions across the apices of the retinal pigment epithelial cells. The retinal pigment epithelium transfers and provides nutrients from the choroidal circulation to the photoceptors and removes products of photoreceptor function by active transport and phagocytosis.

The inner layer, nearest the vitreous cavity, differentiates to form the remaining

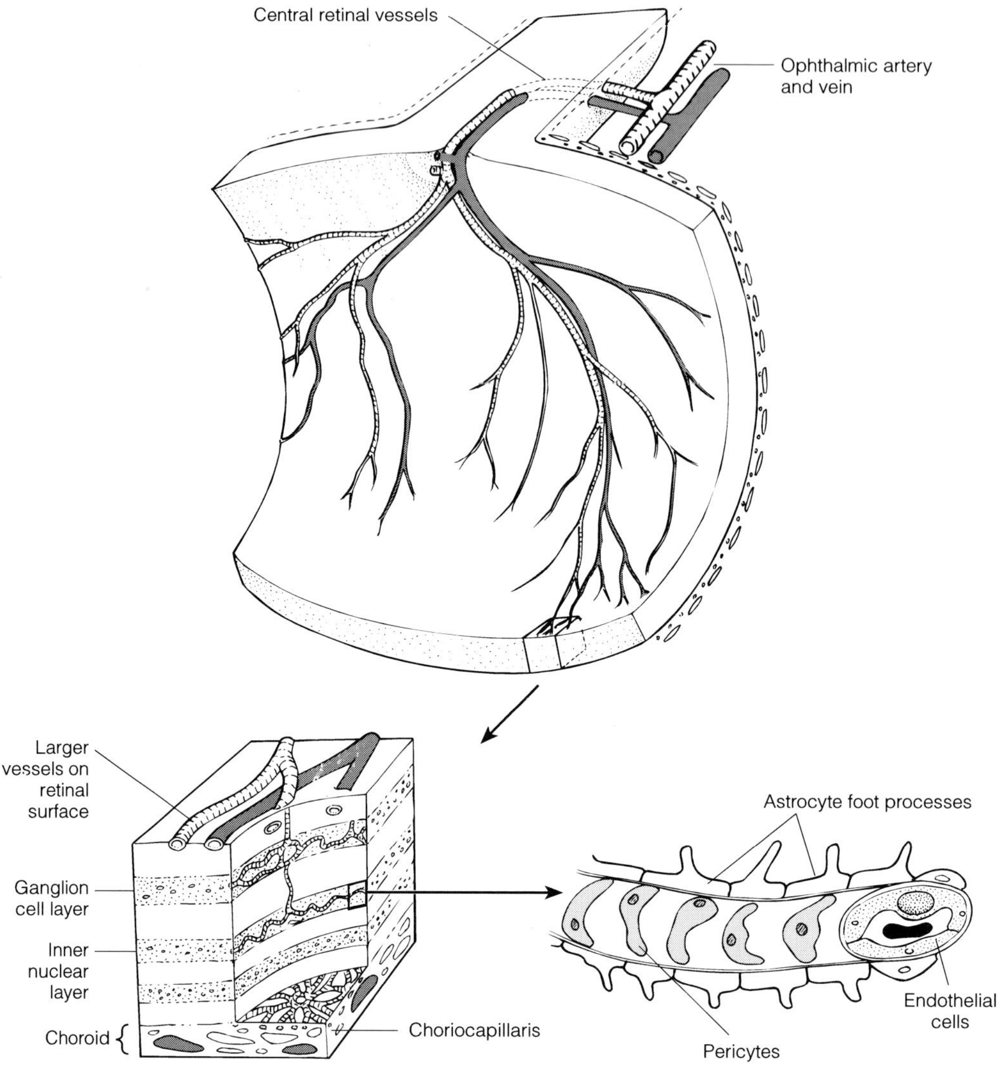
Central retinal vessels
Ophthalmic artery and vein
Larger vessels on retinal surface
Ganglion cell layer
Inner nuclear layer
Choroid
Choriocapillaris
Astrocyte foot processes
Endothelial cells
Pericytes

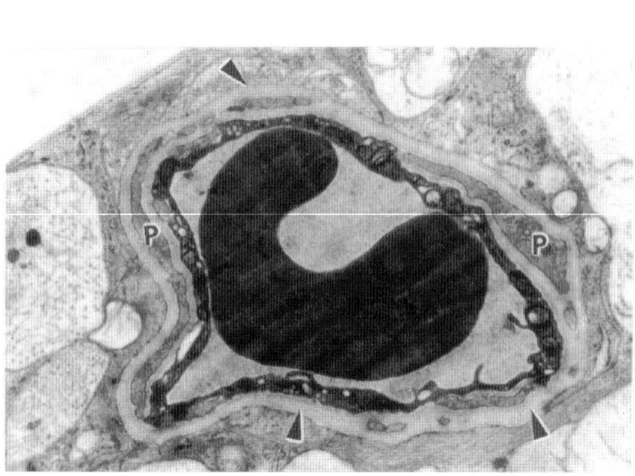
P
P

layers of the neurosensory retina — the photoreceptors, the outer nuclear and outer plexiform layers, the inner nuclear and inner plexiform layers, the ganglion cell layer and the nerve fibre layer (from choroid to vitreous). Müller (glial) cells extend vertically through the whole thickness of the retina. The high concentration of ganglion cells around the posterior pole leads to a layer four to six cells thick surrounding the fovea, but high resolution acuity at the fovea itself is facilitated by the displacement of all retinal elements aside allowing light energy to reach the photoceptors directly. This specialized area of the retina is known as the macula lutea because of the high concentration of visible yellow pigment and includes a central cone-rich area around the fovea which generates colour perception. The neurosensory retina is organized hierachically into networks of cells both vertically (first order cells connected to a smaller number of second order cells and second order cells connected to a smaller number of third order cells etc in an overall ratio of photoreceptor to ganglion cells of 130:1) and horizontally. Specific subsets of ganglion cells will depolarize strongly to specific stimuli applied in a specific retinal area — the receptive field. Parvocellular pathway ganglion cells tend to predominate in the fovea and magnocellular ganglion cells in the periphery. Ganglion cells of the magnocellular stream respond optimally to low spatial frequency, moving visual targets, whilst ganglion cells of the parvocellular stream respond optimally to high spatial frequency and fine static stereopsis (Horton, 1992).

Blood supply of the retina

The main branches of the central retinal artery and vein traverse the retina at the level of the inner plexiform layer: capillaries penetrate as deep as the inner nuclear layer only, and cells of the bipolar, outer plexiform, outer nuclear and photoreceptor layers are supplied from the choroid. The retinal blood vessels have autoregulatory properties capable of functioning without neural control. An increased pressure gradient across the vessel wall produced by a rise in intraluminal pressure and a fall in intraocular pressure results in vasconstriction both in arteries and veins.

OPTIC NERVE

Functionally, the optic nerve begins with the ganglion cells of the retina. Axons from ganglion cells in the macula area around the fovea form a spindle shaped papillo-macular bundle which enters the optic nerve head on the temporal side. Fibres from the remaining retina take an arcuate course to reach the optic nerve at the superior and inferior poles. Altogether, there are about 1 million axons in each optic nerve, conducting partially processed visual information from the retinal ganglion cells to the lateral geniculate ganglion.

The optic nerve can conveniently be described in terms of four parts: the optic nerve head, the intraorbital optic nerve, the intracanicular optic nerve, and the intracranial optic nerve.

The optic nerve head is further subdivided according to its relationship with the laminar cribrosa in the scleral canal into prelaminar, laminar and retrolaminar portions. Axons from the retinal ganglion cells exit the eye by turning 90 degrees to pass through the scleral canal and fibrous septa of the lamina cribrosa. At this point they become myelinated and the optic nerve head is formed. In some individuals the optic nerve exits the sclera at less than a 90 degree angle; as a result a halo shaped

Figure 1.2 Diagram of the retinal blood supply and electron micrograph of a retinal capillary containing an erythrocyte. Note the thickened basal lamina (arrowheads) surrounding the endothelial cell and the pericyte processes (P). Original magnification × 6000.

A

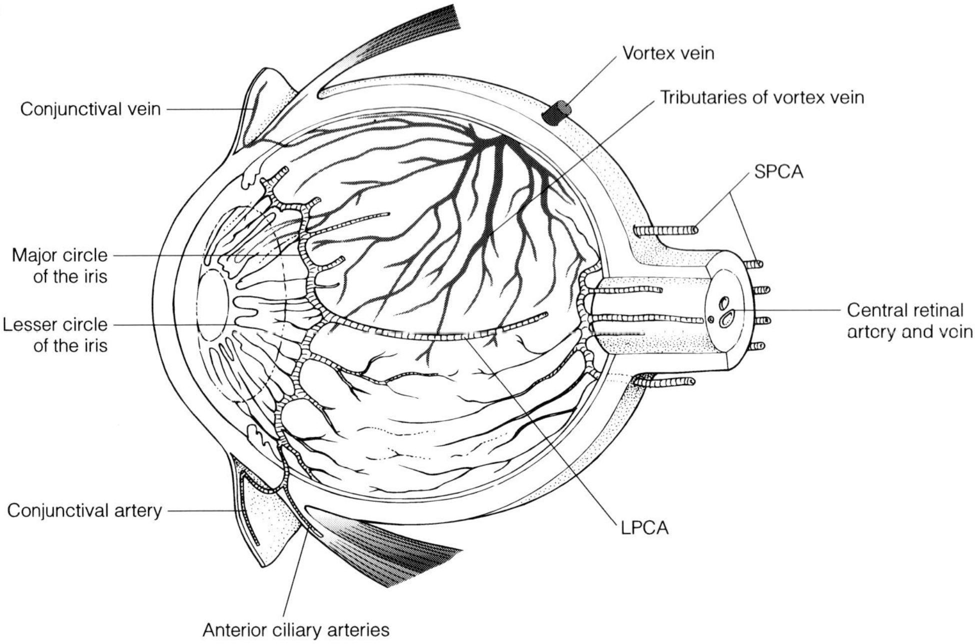
Vortex vein
Tributaries of vortex vein
Conjunctival vein
SPCA
Major circle
of the iris
Central retinal
artery and vein
Lesser circle
of the iris
Conjunctival artery
LPCA
Anterior ciliary arteries

D

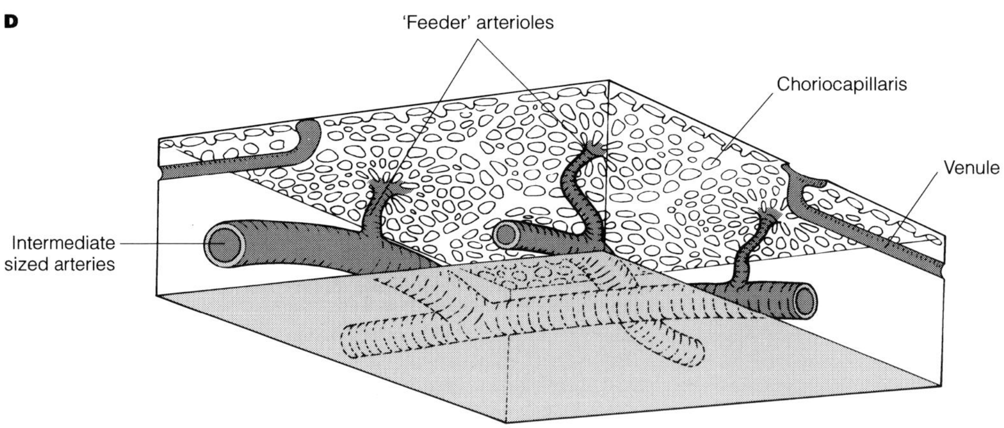
'Feeder' arterioles
Choriocapillaris
Venule
Intermediate
sized arteries

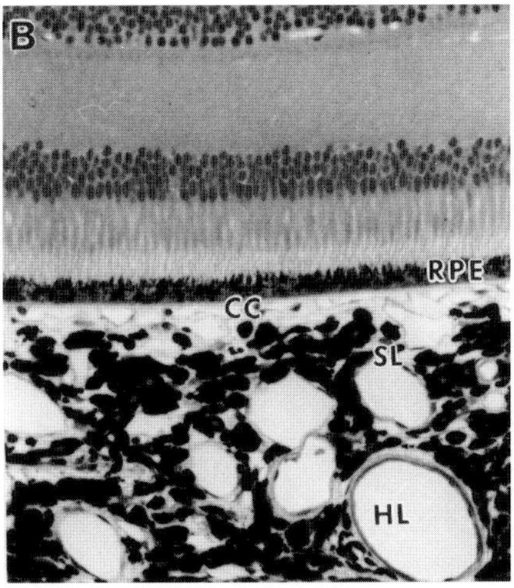

B

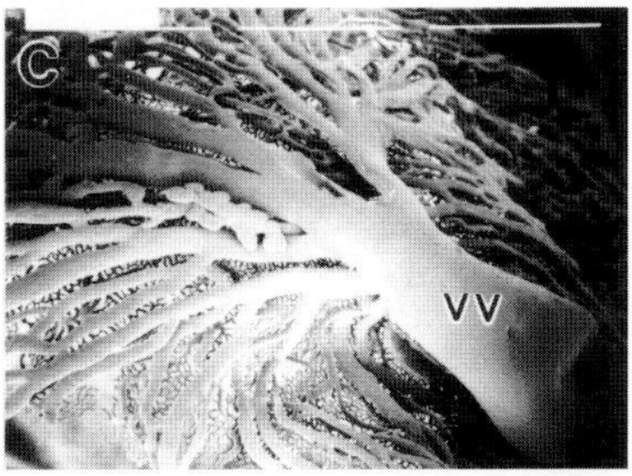

C

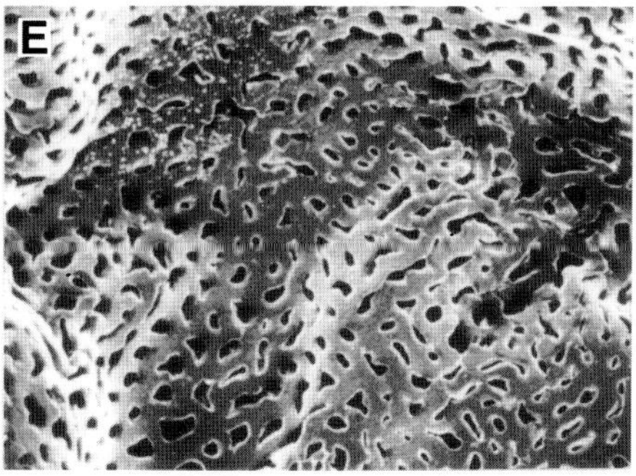

E

Figure 1.3 (**A**) Diagram of the choroidal blood supply. LPCA, long posterior ciliary artery; SPCA, short posterior ciliary artery. (**B**) Histologic section of the outer retina and choroid in a monkey eye. Note the heavy degree of pigmentation and the layers of the choroid. CC, choriocapillaris; HL, Haller's layer; SL, Sattler's layer. (**C**) Resin vascular cast of a quadrant of the choroid viewed from the external aspect; V V, vortex vein. (**D**) Resin vascular cast of the choriocapillaris viewed from the retinal aspect. (**E**) Schematic representation of the hexagonal units in the choriocapillaris fed by small arterioles. Original magnifications: **B** × 120; **C** × 35; **D** × 350.

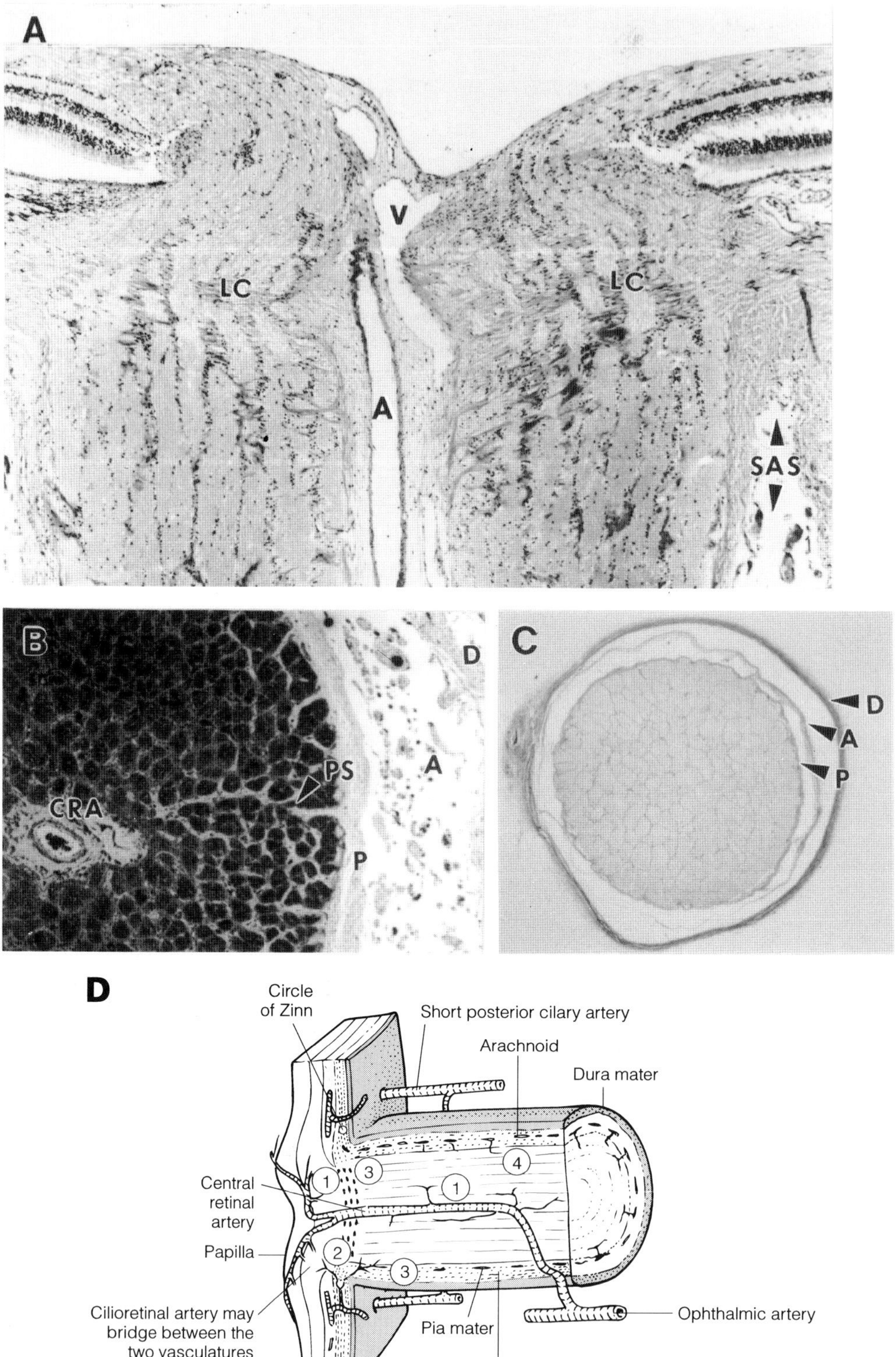
A
V
LC
LC
A
SAS
B
D
PS
A
CRA
P
C
D
A
P
D
Circle of Zinn
Short posterior cilary artery
Arachnoid
Dura mater
Central retinal artery
Papilla
Cilioretinal artery may bridge between the two vasculatures
Pia mater
Subarachnoid space
Ophthalmic artery
1
3
4
1
2
3

crescent of choroid and/or sclera is exposed at the nerve head margin on one side and an elevated sharply roled disc margin is seen opposite. This tilted disc is a common normal variant. In addition to axons, the nerve head is composed of supportive astrocytes, myelin forming oligodendrocytes and blood vessels. Blood vessels from the circle of Zinn supply the optic nerve head tissues while the central retinal artery and vein course through.

The orbital optic nerve is between 20 and 30 mm long and 3–4 mm in diameter, extending in an S shape from the globe to the optic foramen at the orbital apex. The nerve is surrounded by pia, arachnoid and dura — the latter layer forming in continuity with the sclera. At the apex of the orbit, elements of the dura fuse with periosteum and the origin of the extraocular muscles at the annulus of Zinn. Between 5 and 15 mm posterior to the globe the central retinal artery enters and the central retinal vein exits the nerve by the inferonasal margin. At the orbital apex the optic nerve is surrounded by the fibrous circle of Zinn — the origin of the four rectus muscles (see Fig. 1.4) The superior and medial recti also take origin from the nerve sheath itself. This has been offered as an explanation for the pain of eye movements which is a common symptom of inflammatory optic nerve disease, but the pain is probably due to dural movement in the central part of the nerve.

The intracanicular optic nerve passes thorough the optic canal, formed by the union of the two roots of the lesser wing of the sphenoid bone. Generally the canal is covered by bone and dura but the bony wall is often incomplete posterior to the foramen, particularly medially in relation to the sphenoid and posterior ethmoid sinuses. Each canal runs posteriorly and medially transmitting the optic nerve and ophthalmic artery tethered within a dural lining.

The intracranial optic nerve extends about 10 mm (3–16 mm) medially and posteriorly and superiorly to reach the chiasm. The frontal lobe of the brain lies superiorly, the anterior cerebral and anterior communicating arteries and olfactory nerve lie medially and the internal carotid and ophthalmic artery origin lie laterally. The sphenoid sinus lies inferiorly.

Vascular supply of the optic nerve head

At the most superficial level, the prelaminar portion of the optic nerve head derives its blood supply from direct branches of the central retinal artery. The laminar and retrolaminar portions are supplied by branches of the short posterior ciliary vessels via the anastomotic circle of Zinn-Haller. The circle of Zinn-Haller also derives potential input from the peripapillary choroid and the pial arterial network. Although autoregulation of blood flow is absent in the choroidal circulation (and present in the retinal), the healthy optic nerve head can maintain a steady blood flow in the face of fluctuations of intraocular and arterial perfusion pressure. These arrangements are of

Figure 1.4 (**A**) Histologic section of the optic nerve head. LC, lamina cribrosa; A & V, central retinal artery and vein; SAS, subarachnoid space. (**B**) Transverse section (Loyez stain) of the orbital portion of the optic nerve revealing the arrangement of the myelinated nerve fascicles (darkly stained) separated by pial septae (PS) which penetrate as far as the central retinal artery in the middle of the nerve. The three layers of meninges surrounding the nerve (dura mater (D). Arachnoid (A), and pia (P) are clearly visible in **B** and **C**. (**C**) Cross-section (trichrome stain) of an entire optic nerve and surrounding meninges posterior to the entry of the central retinal artery. (**D**) Blood supply of the optic nerve. The four sources of vessels supplying the optic nerve include: 1. branches from the central retinal artery or its branches: 2. branches from the circle of Zinn; 3. choroidal branches: 4. pial branches. Original magnifications: **A** × 60; **B** × 290: **C** × 40. (**D** Redrawn after Lee WR (1993) *Ophthalmic Histopathology*. Springer-Verlag, and reproduced courtesy of WR Lee and Springer-Verlag.)

great clinical importance because vascular insufficiency of the optic nerve head has been implicated in the commonest optic neuropathy of all — glaucoma — as well as in acute anterior ischaemic optic neuropathy (Anderson, 1970a; Hayreh, 1974).

OPTIC CHIASM

Because of its location at the floor of the third ventricle in the suprasellar cistern, diseases involving the optic chiasm result in specific combinations of abnormalities in afferent visual and eye movements, cerebrospinal fluid (CSF) flow and endocrine function, thereby drawing together the clinical specialities of ophthalmology,

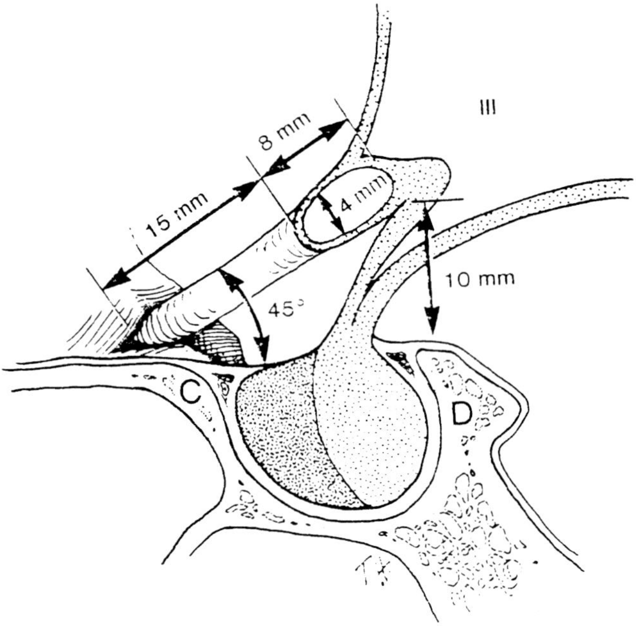

Figure 1.5 Relationship of the optic nerves and optic chiasm to the sellar structures and third ventricle (III). C: Anterior clinoid. D: Dorsum sellae. (From Glaser, 1990.)

neurology, endocrinology and neurosurgery. The inferior aspect of the chiasm lies about 10mm above the plane of the diaphragma sellae, and the plane of the visual pathways at this point is inclined some 45 degrees as nerve fibres sweep backwards and upwards into the optic tracts. Lateral to the chiasm lies the supraclinoid portion of the internal carotid artery: the anterior cerebral arteries pass over the dorsal aspect of the optic nerves as they converge. It is clear therefore that intrasellar tumours such as pituitary adenomas must expand some distance in the suprasellar cistern before impinging on the visual pathways (Fig. 1.5) For this reason, functioning adenomas are more likely to present to the endocrinologist and non-functioning tumours to the ophthalmologist (Horton, 1992; Hoyt, 1963).

THE ANTERIOR VISUAL PATHWAYS: NORMAL AND ABNORMAL DEVELOPMENT

The optic nerve develops from the neuroectoderm of the optic stalk which is first apparent in the 4 mm human embryo. By the 17 mm stage the stalk has elongated with a lumen communicating proximally with the forebrain cavity and with a distal segment invaginated by surface ectoderm. At this stage nerve fibres begin to grow from the ganglion cells of the retina and its embryonic cleft begins to close. Some retinal cells become isolated at the centre of the presumptive optic disc: these cells together with the hyaloid artery form the primitive epithelial papilla of Bergmeister. The lips of the distal embryonic cleft fuse to enclose the hyaloid artery, which eventually becomes the intraneural portion of the central retinal artery. After birth the intraocular hyaloid vessels disappear together with the papilla leaving the physiological optic disc cup. Entering the optic stalk, the nerve fibres invade the invaginating inner layer and proceed towards the brain. By the 25 mm stage the whole of the lumen has been filled with nerve fibres. The cavity of the optic vessicle no longer communicates with that of the forebrain where the site is marked by the optic recess in the floor of the third ventricle. Growing proximally to reach the optic recess, the fibres intermix to form the chiasmal decussation. The lateral geniculate body differentiates from the thalamus at the 30 mm stage and with the formation of the optic tract at 48 mm the anterior visual pathway is complete. Uncrossed fibres do not appear until the 59 mm (11th week) stage and by the 80 mm stage (13th week) the adult arrangement of partial decussation is complete. At 16 to 17 weeks of gestation a peak of 3.7 million axons can be identified in the optic nerve. This is followed by a very rapid decline to the normal adult number of 1.1 million by 31 weeks.

Primitive glial cells are formed from the same multipotential cells which at a very early stage and under both genetic and environmental regulation lose their bipotentiality and develop into cells which are committed to either neuronal or glial lineage. By the second half of the second month a dense network of neuroglial cells has formed in the distal part of the optic nerve which are orientated perpendicularly to the nerve fibres: these constitute the first elements of the lamina cribrosa. At this stage the network is entirely comprised of type 1 astrocytes, but during the fourth month type 2 astrocytes and oligodendrocytes differentiate under the regulation of various growth factors. Malfunctions of this differentiation underlie the pathogenesis of childhood optochiasmal glioma. Surrounding mesoderm also becomes incorporated into the optic nerve to form the system of septa. By the sixth and seventh months the arachnoid sheath has differentiated into pia and dura: the pia and the arachnoid being largely of the same neuroectodermal origin as the neurons and glial cells. During the eighth and ninth months mesodermal microglia appear and mesodermal elements also consolidate the structure of the lamina cribrosa. During this time the optic nerve increases in both diameter and length so that at birth it is approximately 2 mm in diameter and 24 mm long.

After the complete visual pathway has developed, myelination of nerve fibres occurs in the reverse direction to their growth. Myelination is wholly dependent on oligodendrocytes, and is first evident in the lateral geniculate bodies at about the fifth month. By the sixth month myelin reaches the optic tracts and chiasm and is apparent in the optic nerve by the eighth month. It slowly reaches the lamina cribrosa at or shortly after birth at which point the process normally ceases. In the phase of early postnatal visual development further myelination of the intraorbital optic nerve occurs in tandem with myelination of the posterior pathways.

Melanin is thought to play a role in axonal guidance during development of the

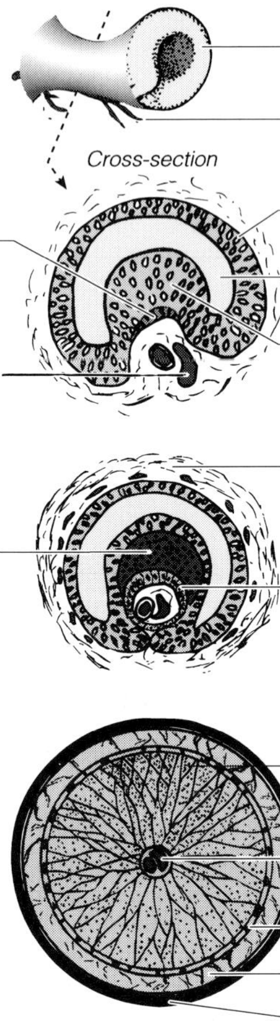

Figure 1.6 Embryology of the optic nerve.

anterior visual pathways, and major abnormalities of projection arise in human albinos (both oculocutaneous and ocular forms). The majority of fibres originating in the temporal retina are misdirected and decussate to the opposite lateral geniculate nucleus along with those from the nasal retina. As a result each hemisphere receives predominantly monocular input from the contralateral eye and failure to develop normal binocular function may explain in part the high frequency of strabismus and amblyopia in these patients (Silver and Sapiro, 1981).

Disruption of the process of controlled axonal loss in the second trimester of pregnancy may explain the dysplastic syndromes involving one or both optic nerves, the chiasm and other forebrain structures including the septum pellucidum and hypothalamus. For example, optic nerve hypoplasia may arise as a result of excess loss of axons during this period, although how this relates to specific teratogenic insults such as maternal alcohol and drug abuse is not clear. When the chiasm itself is dysplastic, there will be no decussation at all with retinofugal fibres projecting exclusively to the ipsilateral hemisphere. Such patients will not only have a bitemporal hemianopia but frequently have congenital see-saw nystagmus. The congenital nystagmus in these patients may reflect abnormalities in extrageniculostriate projections to subcortical structures. Because the nasal and temporal hemifields split the retina across the fovea and not across the optic nerve head, a very specific abnormality of the optic nerve head is seen when there is an absense or loss of crossing fibres. The optic nerve head will have deficient neuroretinal tissue at both nasal and temporal sides where nerve fibres serving the temporal hemifield enter, but not superiorly or inferiorly where fibres from the nasal hemifield enter. This is known as a 'bow-tie' disc or hemioptic hypoplasia when the cause is developmental. The appearance may be seen in some congenital retrogeniculate lesions reflecting the possibility of intrauterine transsynaptic degeneration (Provis *et al.*, 1985; Jacobson and Hirose, 1978; Silver and Sapiro, 1981; Beatty *et al.*, 1982).

THE POSTERIOR VISUAL PATHWAYS: OPTIC TRACTS, LATERAL GENICULATE NUCLEUS, VISUAL RADIATIONS AND VISUAL CORTEX

OPTIC TRACTS

The optic tracts form immediately posterior to the chiasm as retinofugal fibres pass posteriorly around the cerebral peduncles. The third ventricle lies superiorly, and the pituitary stalk medially. The uncal gyrus of the temporal lobe lies laterally; 90% of the fibres terminate in the ipsilateral lateral geniculate nucleus of the thalamus. The remainder are divided between those serving the afferent limb of the pupillomotor reflex which leave the tract to terminate in the pretectal nuclei of the rostral midbrain and others which synapse in the superior colliculus, the hypothalamus and the accessory optic system to serve foveational eye movements, neuroendocrine function (circadian rhthyms) and optokinetic eye movements respectively. These extrageniculate pathways are also of clinical importance in the residual vision of infants with major cortical abnormalities, and in the phenomena of 'blindsight' and statokinetic visual dissociation. Fibres from the superior retinas occupy the dorsomedial portion of the optic tract, while those from the inferior retinas occupy the ventrolateral tract (Sadun *et al.*, 1986 a,b).

LATERAL GENICULATE NUCLEUS

The lateral geniculate ganglion is a highly differentiated structure lying in the thalamus, the function of which is best considered as analagous to a relay station between retina and visual cortex. Crossed and uncrossed retinal fibres are organized into homonymous pairs. Six grey layers of cell bodies are discernable in humans. Crossing visual axons terminate in layers (also called laminae) 1, 4 and 6, while uncrossed ipsilateral axons end in layers 2, 3 and 5. Each layer contains a complete representation of the entire hemifield of vision.

Magnocellular retinal ganglion neurons project to layers 1 and 2; the smaller parvocellular neurons to layers 3, 4, 5 and 6. Central vision is thought to be mediated by the caudal portion of the lateral geniculate ganglion whilst peripheral vision is mediated ventrally where the six laminae fuse to become four. All six laminae are folded about a central hilum resulting in an exceedingly complex three-dimensional retinotopic pattern. Fibres from the superior retina pass to the medial aspect whilst those from the inferior retina pass to the lateral with the result that lesions of the lateral geniculate ganglion cause the most non-congruous hemianopias. It is intriguing to note that there are extensive projections of nerve fibres from the pre-striate cortex

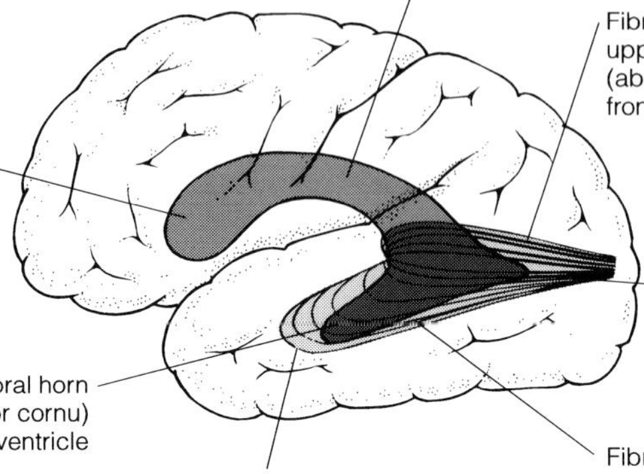

Figure 1.7 The optic radiation and its relation to the lateral ventricle, viewed from the left side.

back to the lateral geniculate ganglion, but there is little evidence as yet of functions other than the transmission of visual information from eye to cortex (Horton, 1992).

THE VISUAL (OPTIC) RADIATIONS

Myelinated fibres forming the geniculocalcarine tract exit from the dorsal aspect of the lateral geniculate ganglion to pass posteriorly and laterally to the ipsilateral occipital cortex. The most anterior and inferior fibres serving the upper visual quadrant form a loop reaching approximately 4 cm caudal to the anterior pole of the temporal lobe (Meyer's loop) by passing around the anterior tip of the temporal horn of the lateral ventricle whereas those serving the inferior quadrant pass on a more direct route through the parietal lobe. Lesions of the temporal lobe may therefore result in a superior quadrantic homonymous hemianopia.

OCCIPITAL CORTEX

The primary visual cortex (Brodmann area 17, or area VI) lies in the interhemispheric fissure in relation to the falx cerebri with a macular projection area extending laterally by about 1 cm onto the posterior cortical surface. Anteriorly the primary visual cortex lies superior and inferior to the calcarine fissure to reach the splenium of the corpus callosum. The term 'striate' cortex is also used: this denotes the fact that when viewed macroscopically, a section of the primary visual cortex shows a thin white band (stria of Gennari) of myelinated fibres within the cortical grey matter. At least 60% of the surface of the primary visual cortex is devoted to the representation of the central 10 degrees of vision, reflecting the superior acuity and colour vision capability of this part of the visual field. In spite of the hemidecussation of the visual pathways at the chiasm, the visual fields in the cortex do not completely overlap. In the deepest, most anterior part of each hemisphere there is a region serving the temporal peripheral field in which the outermost 30 degrees are seen monocularly. This means that occasionally lesions of the anterior occipital cortex result in a monocular field defect in spite of the fact that the lesion is post-chiasmal, and that more posterior lesions may spare this temporal crescent to produce a non-congruous hemianopia (Figs 1.8, 1.9).

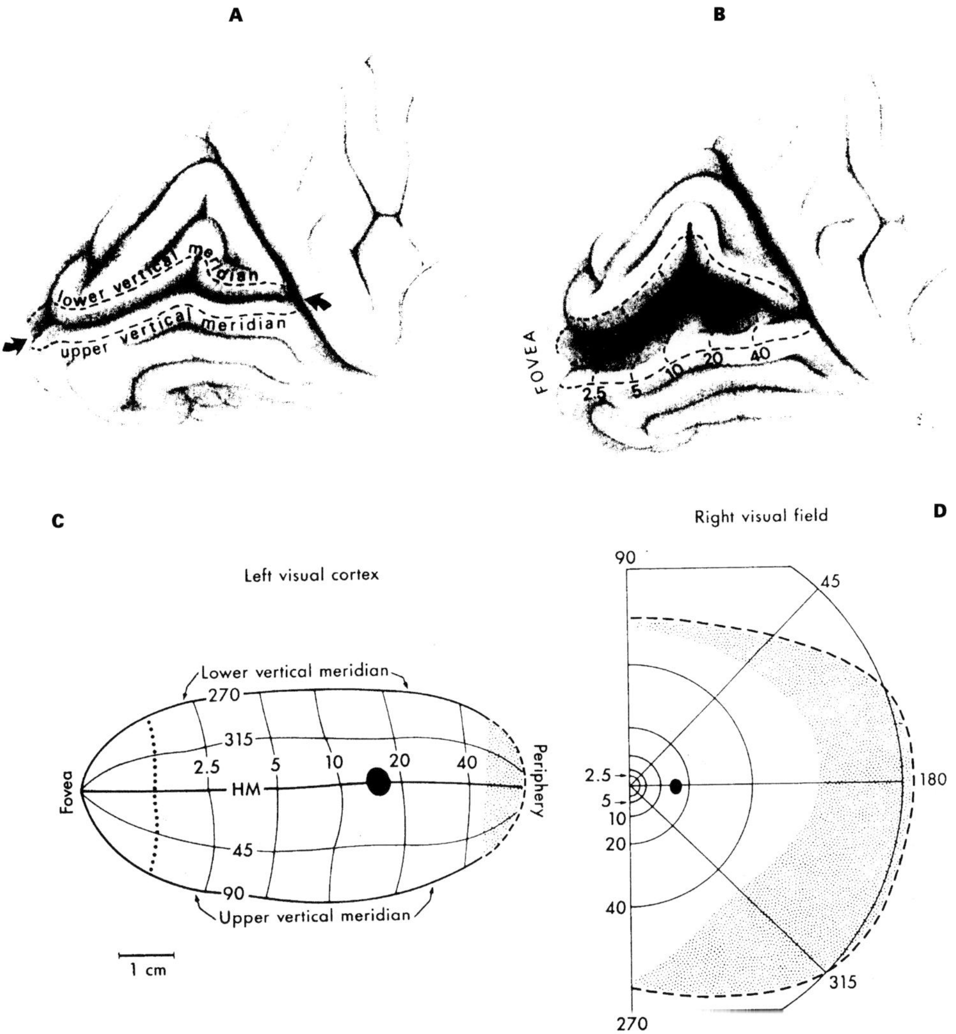

Figure 1.8 (**A**) Left occipital lobe showing location of striate cortex within the calcarine fissure. The boundary between striate cortex (V1) and extrastriate cortex (V2) contains the representation of the vertical meridian. (**B**) View of striate cortex after opening the lips of the calcarine fissue. The dashed lines indicate the co-ordinates of the visual field map. The representation of the horizontal meridian runs approximately along the base of the calcarine fissure. The vertical dashed lines mark the isoeccentricity contours from 2.5 degrees to 40 degrees. Striate cortex wraps around the occipital pole to extend about 1cm on to the lateral convexity where the fovea is represented. (**C**) Schematic map showing the projection of the right visual hemifield upon the left visual cortex by transposing the map illustrated in **B**) on to a flat surface. The row of dots indicates approximately where striate cortex folds around the occipital tip. The black oval marks the region of striate cortex corresponding to the contralateral eye's blind spot. (**D**) Right visual hemifield plotted with a Goldmann perimeter. The stippled region corresponds to the monocular temporal crescent which is mapped within the most anterior 8–10% of striate cortex. (From Horton, 1992.)

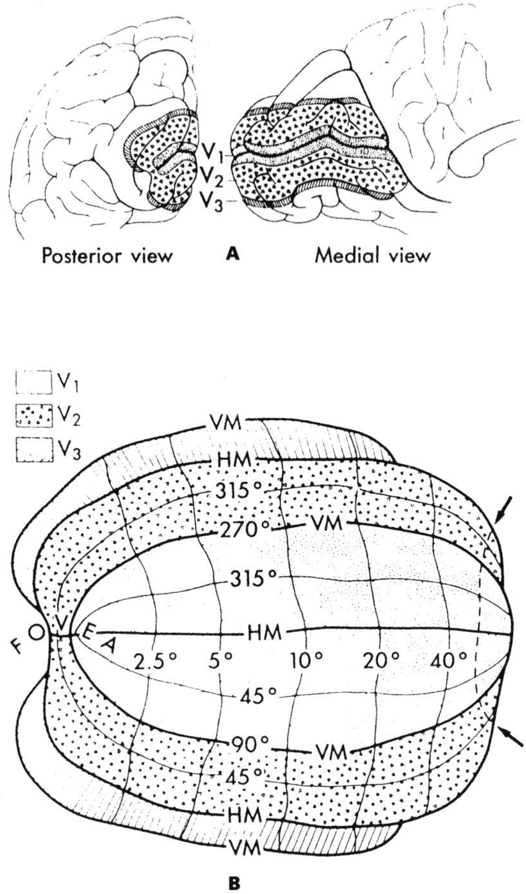

Figure 1.9 (**A**) Schematic diagram of the left occipital lobe of the human brain showing the arrangement of V1, V2 and V3 along the calcarine sulcus. (**B**) Flattened representation of the cortical areas shown in **A**) with co-ordinates of the right visual hemifield indicated directly onto the maps. Note that the horizontal meridian in V2 splits within a few degrees of fixation to wrap around the outside of V2 into dorsal and ventral halves representing the upper and lower quadrants of vision respectively. (From Horton, 1992.)

At a histological level, the six fundamental layers of the primate neocortex contain further subdivisions in the primary visual cortex reflecting functional anatomy. Magnocellular cells of the lateral geniculate ganglion project to layer IVC α and those of the parvocellular stream project to layer IVC β. Layer IVB includes the myelinated fibres referred to as the striae of Gennari. Axon terminals from the left and right eyes are not randomly distributed but are segregated into alternating parallel strips called ocular dominance columns which are only lacking at the monocular temporal crescent and at the cortical representation of the blind spot. Cells in the primary visual cortex are further arranged into those which respond maximally to stationary stimuli of specific orientation

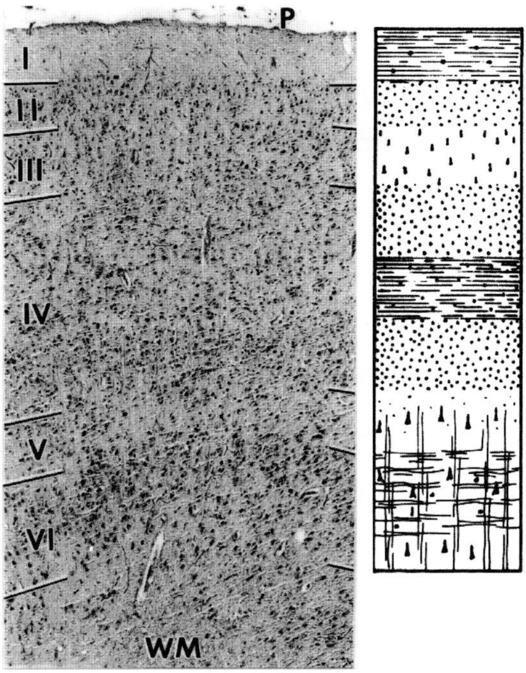

Figure 1.10 Histology and cytoarchitecture of the primary visual cortex. Layers I–VI are indicated on the micrograph and adjacent diagram. P, pia; WM, white matter. Original magnification × 35.

(simple cells), those which respond maximally to movement (complex cells) and those which are selective for both orientation and dimension (hypercomplex or end-stopped cells). In addition, cortical cells fall into the parvocellular and magnocellular subsets referred to above. Binocular integration occurs for the first time in the visual system in cells receiving inputs from monocular cells in layer IV (Livingstone and Hubel, 1988; Holmes, 1931, 1945).

Visual association areas

Further analysis, recognition and interpretation of afferent visual information takes place in the extrastriate (pre-striate) cortex. These higher visual association areas are referred to as Brodmann areas 18 and 19. Current understanding of the anatomy and physiology of these areas depends almost entirely on animal models of great complexity, where the terms areas V2, V3, V4 and V5 (or MT for middle temporal) are used. Areas 17, 18 and 19 in one hemisphere are extensively interconnected with equivalent areas in the other hemisphere principally via the splenium of the corpus callosum. Because the human cortex is a great deal larger and more complex than that of any animal model, the anatomical location of the human homologues of these areas remains to be elucidated fully. At a very simplistic level it is helpful to imagine that cortical area V1 projects via area V2 to two principal extrastriate territories: V4, served by the parvocellular system, and concerned with colour and form (the 'what?' area) and V5 (MT), served by the magnocellular system, and concerned with motion (the 'where?' area). Functional imaging of the human cortex has proved to be a valuable tool in efforts to extend the

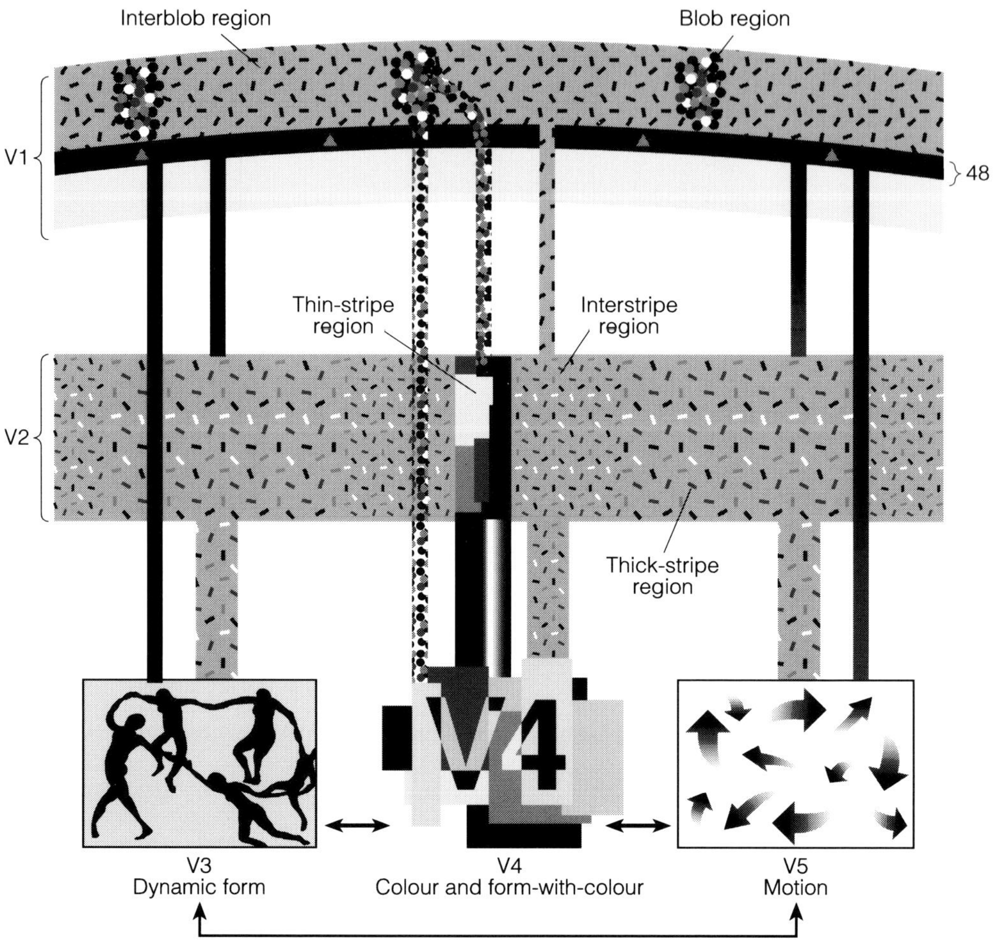

Figure 1.11 Visual perception at the cortical level. Mitochondrial cytochrome oxidase is present in high concentrations in highly metabolically active cells and this enzyme has been used to label 'hot' cells in the visual cortex. This has shown that cells in the visual cortex can be pigeon-holed into 'blob' and 'interblob' regions; blob cells exist as large columns particularly in layers 2 and 3 of the visual cortex, and receive information from the parvocellular neurons in the LGN. Magnocellular structures synapse in layer 4B of V1 and connect with areas V5 and V3. (From Zeki, 1993).

animal data to humans (Zeki, 1993; Corbetta *et al.* 1991; Felleman and van Essen, 1991; Goodale, 1993; Kosslyn *et al.*, 1993).

Vascular supply of the post-chiasmal pathways

The optic tract and lateral geniculate ganglion receive a dual blood supply from the anterior choroidal artery which is a direct branch of the internal carotid, and deep perforating thalamogeniculate branches of the posterior cerebral. The optic radiations

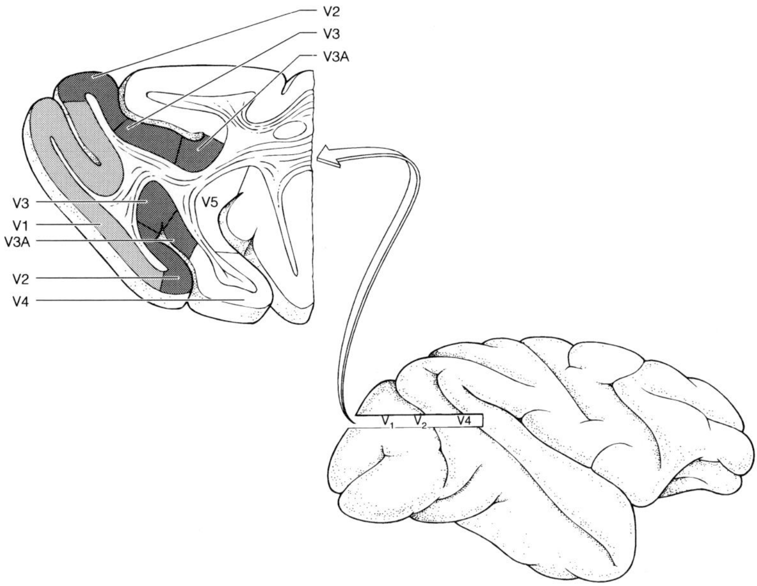

Figure 1.12 The extrastriate (visual association) cortex.

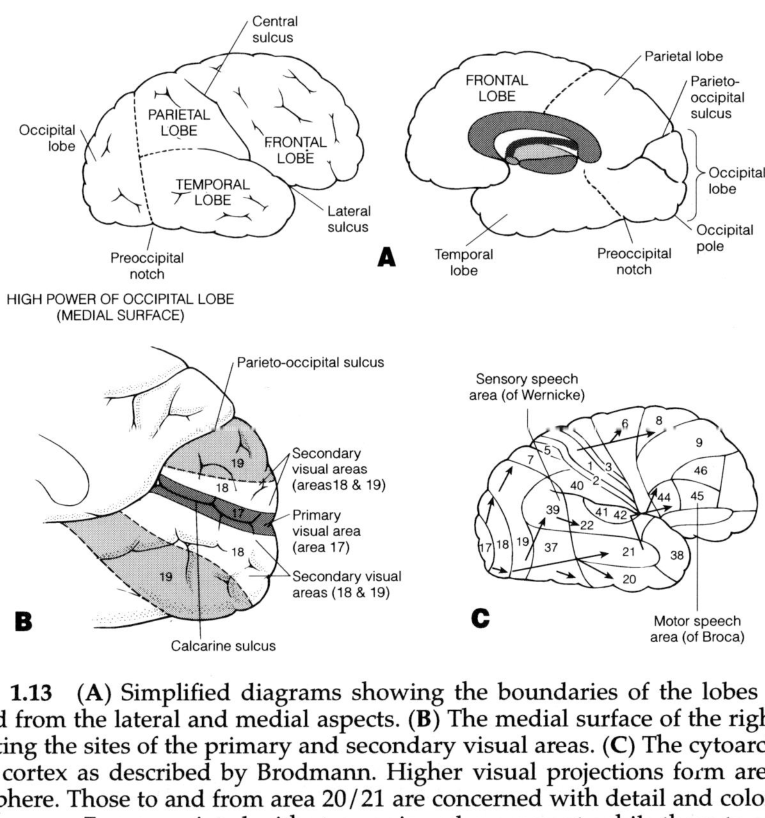

Figure 1.13 (**A**) Simplified diagrams showing the boundaries of the lobes of the brain as viewed from the lateral and medial aspects. (**B**) The medial surface of the right occipital lobe indicating the sites of the primary and secondary visual areas. (**C**) The cytoarchitectural areas of the cortex as described by Brodmann. Higher visual projections form area 17 of the left hemisphere. Those to and from area 20/21 are concerned with detail and color. Projections to and from area 7 are associated with stereopsis and movement, while those to and from area 39 are concerned with recognition of letters and numbers.

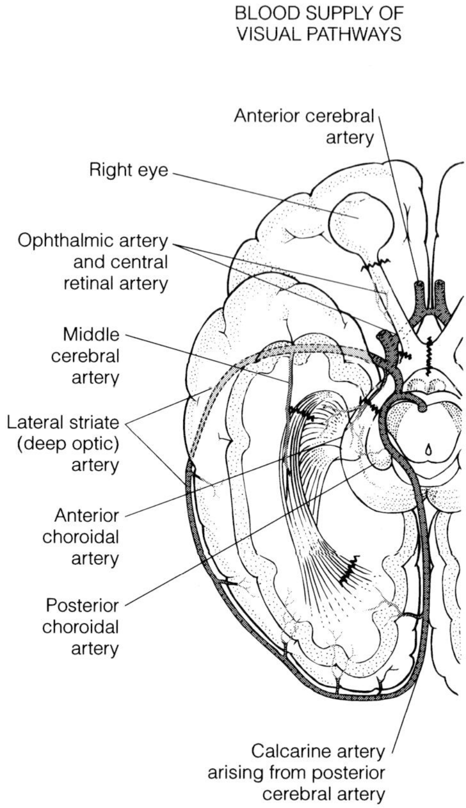

Figure 1.14 Diagram of the brain. The upper part summarizes the blood supply to the visual pathways.

- Intracranial optic nerve: ophthalmic artery (an important inferior relation) and pial branches of the hypophyseal artery.
- Optic chiasma: adjacent related vessels including the superior hypophysial, internal carotid, posterior communicating, anterior cerebral, and anterior communicating artery.
- Lateral root of the optic tract: anterior choroidal artery.
- Lateral geniculate body: anterior choroidal artery and branches of posterior cerebral artery.
- Commencement of the optic radiation (geniculocalcarine tract): anterior choroidal artery.
- Posteriorly directed fibres: lateral striate (deep optic) branch of the middle cerebral artery.
- Termination of geniculocalcarine tract and visual cortex: perforating branches of cortical arteries, principally the calcarine branch of the posterior cerebral although the middle cerebral may anastomose and aid in the supply of the cortex at the anterior end of the calcarine sulcus and at the posterior pole.

also receive a supply from both the posterior cerebral artery inferiorly and the middle cerebral superiorly. The occipital cortex principally derives its supply from parieto-occipital (superiorly), calcarine (centrally) and posterior temporal (inferiorly) branches of the posterior cerebral. However, at the occipital pole there is a rich anastomotic network incorporating terminal branches of the middle cerebral artery. This configuration may explain the apparent preservation of macular vision which is a characteristic finding of hemianopic field defects arising from vascular occlusion of posterior cerebral circulation to the occipital cortex (Smith and Richardson, 1966).

REFERENCES

Anderson DR (1970a). Ultrastructure of the optic nerve head. *Arch Ophthalmol* **83**:63–73.

Anderson DR (1970b). Vascular supply of the optic nerve of primates. *Am J Ophthalmol* **70**:341–351.

Beatty B, Sadun A, Smith L *et al.* (1982). Direct demonstration of transsynaptic degeneration in the human visual system: A comparison of retrograde and anterograde changes. *J Neurol Neurosurg Psychiat* **45**:143–146.

Belliveau JW, Kwong KK, Kennedy DN *et al.* (1991). Magnetic imaging mapping of brain function: human visual cortex. *Invest Radiol* **27**: S59–72.

Corbetta M, Miezin FM, Domeyer S *et al.* (1991). Selective and divided attention during visual discrimination of shape, colour and speed. *J Neurosci* **11**:2283–2402.

Felleman DJ and van Essen DC (1991). Distributed hierarchical processing in the primate cerebral cortex. *Cerbral Cortex* **1**: 1–47.

Glaser JS (1990). *Neuro-Ophthalmology* 2nd edn, p. 68. Philadelphia: Lippincott.

Goodale MA (1993). Visual pathways supporting perception and action in primate cerebral cortex. *Curr Opin Neurobiol* **3**: 578–585.

Hayreh SS (1974). Anatomy and physiology of the optic nerve head. *Trans Am Acad Ophthalmol Otolaryngol* **78**: 240–254.

Holmes G (1931). A contribution to the cortical representation of vision. *Brain* **54**: 470–479.

Holmes G (1945). The organisation of the visual cortex in man. *Proc R Soc Lond Biol* **132**: 348–361.

Horton JC (1992). The central visual pathways. *Physiology of the Eye* (ed. WM Adler), 9th edn, pp. 728–772. St Louis: Mosby Year Book.

Horton JC and Hoyt WF (1991). The representation of the visual field in the human striate cortex: a revision of the classic Holmes map. *Arch Ophthalmol* **109**: 816–824.

Hoyt WF and Luis O (1963). The primate chiasm: Details of visual fiber organization studied by silver impregnation techniques. *Arch Ophthalmol* **70**: 69.

Jacobson H and Hirose G (1978). Origin of the retina from both sides of the embryonic brain: A contribution to the problem of crossing at the optic chiasma. *Science* **202**: 637–639.

Kosslyn SM, Alpert NM, Thompson WL *et al.* (1993). Visual mental imagery activates topogroaphically organised visual cortex: PET investigations. *J Cogn Neurosci* 5, 263–287

Livingstone M and Hubel D (1988). Segregation of form, color, movement, and depth: Anatomy, physiology, and perception. *Science* **240**: 740–749.

Maunsell JHR (1992). Functional visual streams. *Curr Opin Neurobiol* **2**: 506–510.

Merigan WH and Maunsell JHR (1993). How parallel are the primate visual pathways? *Ann Rev Neurosci* **16**: 369–402.

Provis JM, Van Driel D, Billson FA *et al.* (1985). Human fetal optic nerve overproduction and elimination of retinal axons during development. *J Comp Neurol* **238**: 92–100.

Rademacher J, Galaburda AM, Kennedy DN *et al.* (1992). Human cerebral cortex: Localisation, parcellation and morphometry with magnetic resonance imaging. *J Cogn Neurosci* **4**, 352–374.

Sadun AA (1986). Parallel processing in the human visual system: A new perspective. *Neuro-Ophthalmology* **6**: 351–352.

Sadun AA, Johnson BM and Smith LEH (1986a). Neuroanatomy of the human visual system. Part II-Retinal projections to the superior colliculus and pulvinar. *Neuro-Ophthalmology* **6**: 363–370.

Sadun AA, Johnson BM and Schaechter JD (1986b). Neuro-anatomy of the human visual system. Part III: Three retinal projections to the hypothalamus. *Neuro-Ophthalmology* **6**:371–379.

Silver J and Sapiro J (1981). Axonal guidance during development of the optic nerve: The role of pigmented epithelia and other extrinsic factors. *J Comp Neurol* **202**:521–538.

Smith CG and Richardson WFG (1966). The course and distribution of the arteries supplying the visual (striate) cortex. *Am J Ophthalmol* **61**:1391–1396.

Zeki SM (1969). Representation of central visual fields in prestriate cortex of monkeys. *Brain Res* 14 : 271–291.

Zeki S (1993). *A Vision of the Brain*. Oxford: Blackwell Scientific Publications.

Zeki S, Watson JD, Lueck CJ *et al.* (1991). A direct demonstration of functional specialization in human visual cortex. *J Neurosci* **11**, 641–649.

2

Principles of clinical examination

THE VISUAL SENSORY SYSTEM

VISUAL ACUITY TESTING

Although acuity testing only measures the central 1–2 degrees of field at 100% contrast, this measurement of visual health is almost universally understood and changing levels of performance measured in this way sometimes assumes great medico-legal significance. The physiological basis and shortcomings in clinical practice may be less widely appreciated. The ability to discriminate small objects from their background may in fact mean different things: the 'minimal visible' is the criterion for the presence of a single feature, the 'minimal resolvable' is the criterion of the presence for identifiable features in a target, and the 'spatial minimal discriminable' is the criterion for the relative location of visible feature (hyperacuity or vernier acuity). The minimal resolvable or ordinary acuity is most applicable to everyday practice, involving the correct identification of a target characteristic. In health, there is a remarkable concordance between the observed minimal angle of resolution and the expected resolving capacity of the eye's optics. In disease, the observed minimal angle of resolution will drop not only as a result of defects in optical imagery, but also where abnormalities arise in foveal fixation, photoreceptor structure and function, photopic luminance levels, and full integrity of the neural pathways.

The purest visual acuity test uses a square wave grating comprising black and white stripes of equal width. Thus, 6/6 acuity equates to a grating made up of stripes each subtending 1 minute of arc at the testing distance, so that the separation between two black and two white stripes is 1 minute; pairs of stripes must therefore be repeated 30 times to subtend a visual angle of 1 degree. This is termed the spatial frequency and is measured in cycles/degree; the narrower the stripes the higher the spatial frequency. The highest frequency grating which elicits a response is the measure of the visual acuity. The correlation between Snellen values, stripe width and spatial frequency is shown in Table 2.1.

Grating acuities have been shown to be superior to visual acuity based on optotypes specially when there is foveal pathology or dense amblyopia. The stripes can be presented on a television screen and form the basis for the objective measurement of acuity using optokinetic nystagmus (rotating striped drum to elicit eye movements), visual evoked cortical potential and preferential looking techniques. Grating acuity techniques are in standard use in visual science and in the clinical assessement of visual function in infants.

For the remainder of clinical practice, acuity is measured by presenting a selection of

Table 2.1 Visual acuity and grating acuity equivalents

Acuity(m)	Acuity(ft)	Spatial fequency	Stripe width
6/6	20/20	30 cycles/degree	1
6/12	20/40	15	2
6/30	20/100	6	5
6/60	20/200	3	10

ordinary, recognizable targets or optotypes for the subject to choose between so that guessing is eliminated. A variety of optotype patterns can be used for the determination of the minimal resolvable acuity. The most familiar is the Snellen chart in which the standard pattern is enlarged so that resolution is achieved. For a normal observer in best focus the resolution limit is 30 to 60 seconds of arc. The E optotype for 6/6 vision (which uses a sans serif or gothic typeface) subtends 5 minutes of arc vertically and horizontally, and 1 minute between each stroke when viewed at 6 metres (or 20 feet). If the subject can only see at a distance of 6 metres an optotype which would subtend 1 minute of arc at 9 metres, then the acuity is said to be 6/9 and so on through to 6/60. Sometimes it is convenient to express acuity in terms of visual efficiency scores (for example in medico-legal work) or as Snellen acuities (for example when entering acuity data into automated perimetry equipment) (see Table 2.2).

Because some optotypes are easier to see than others, single letter charts have some advantages particularly when assessing patients with cognitive or reading difficulties. In the Landolt C test, the subject must identify the orientation of the C by finding the side of the gap in the curve and in the illiterate E test the direction of the bars must be recognized. If the minimal resolvable optotype size is 1 minute of arc then the acuity is said to be 6/6, but these tasks may be easier to perform than the task of reading a standard Snellen line

Table 2.2 Visual acuity equivalents in different notations

Minutes of arc (minimal angle of resolution – MAR)	Log MAR	Snellen acuity at 4 m	Snellen acuity at 20 ft	Snellen acuity at 6 m	Visual efficiency (%)	Snellen fraction
0.75			20/15	6/4.5	104	1.33
	–0.1	4/3.2	20/16	6/5		
1.0	0.0	4/4	20/20	6/6	100	1.0
1.25	+0.1	4/5	20/25	6/7.5	96	0.8
1.5			20/30	6/9	91	0.67
	+0.2	4/6.3	20/32	6/10		
2.0	+0.3	4/8	20/40	6/12	84	0.5
2.5	+0.4	4/10	20/50	6/15	76	0.4
3.0			20/60	6/18	70	0.33
	+0.5	4/12.6	20/63	6/20		
4.0	+0.6	4/16	20/80	6/24	58	0.25
5.0	+0.7	4/20	20/100	6/30	49	0.2
6.0			20/120	6/36	41	0.17
	+0.8	4/25	20/125	6/38		
7.5			20/150	6/45	31	0.133
	+0.9	4/32	20/160	6/48		
10.0	+1.0	4/40	20/200	6/60	20	0.10
20.0			20/400	6/120 (3/60)	3	0.05

and not strictly equivalent. Although the Snellen chart is well understood, the patient's performance may vary simply because of poor control of illumination and variable optotype complexity. As a general rule the smallest line that the individual can read is used to quantify visual acuity — one or two mistakes per line are often allowed. Changes in visual acuity over time are reported in units of 'number of lines lost or gained'. This method is subject to a number of limitatons: as each line becomes smaller the number of letters becomes greater and therefore harder to read; a two line loss from 6/20 to 6/60 is a tripling of the visual angle but a two line loss from 6/5 to 6/9 is less than double the visual angle and therefore is not comparable. In terms of visual pathophysiology, there may only be a weak correlation between the level of underperformance on a Snellen chart and the level of dysfunction of the visual apparatus and it is not correct to say that an eye with a Snellen fraction of 0.25 (6/24) has an disease process which is twice as severe as one with a fraction of 0.5 (6/12) (Frisen, 1980; Weatherill, 1993). For these reasons the 'Logmar' chart is preferable. The working distance is 4 metres. Each letter on a line has

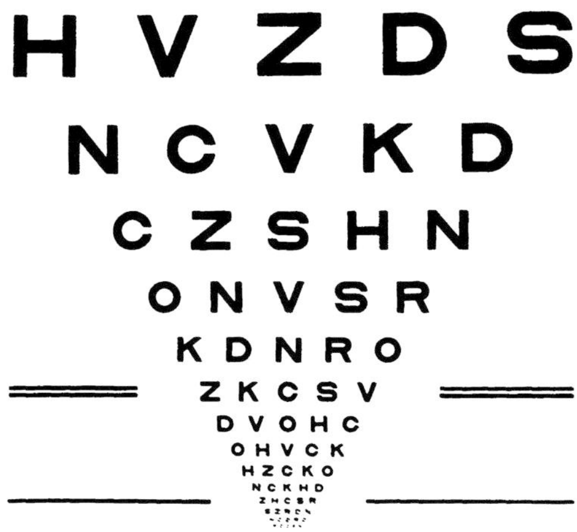

Figure 2.1 Logmar chart.

uniform difficulty, there are the same number of letters on each line, and the size increase from one line to the next is governed by a simple geometrical progression of the log of the minimal angle of resolution (Logmar). In conjunction with standardized illumination systems Logmar charts were first introduced into ophthalmology in 1982 for the early treatment of diabetic retinopathy and other multicentre prospective trials and are now widely used in clinical practice where accurate follow-up data is required (Ferris and Sperduto, 1982a; Ferris *et al.*, 1982).

NEAR VISION TESTING

Some patients experience difficulty in reading which is out of proportion to their Snellen acuity as a result of parafoveal scotomata or poor foveal fixation in certain eye movement disorders which prevent the whole word being seen at the same time. It is therefore extremely useful to determine acuity for near as well as for distance in all cases. In the UK, the current standard notation used is the N system where text printed in the Times Roman font is expressed in font sizes as points (multiples of 1/72nd of an inch) and the reading

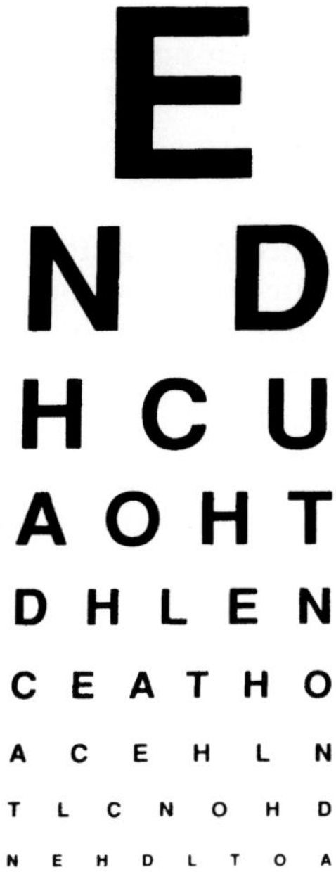

Figure 2.2 Standard Snellen chart.

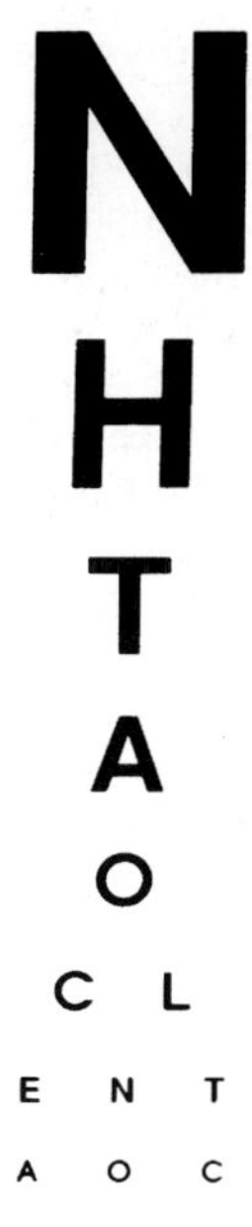

Figure 2.3 Reduced Snellen chart.

acuity is denoted as the minimum size comfortably seen at a normal reading distance (33 cm) with presbyopic correction when appropriate. This is likely to be replaced by reading versions of the Snellen and Logmar charts in the near future.

FACTORS INFLUENCING VISUAL ACUITY

In order to achieve peak performance referred to as normal visual acuity, all optical, anatomical and physiological elements must themselves perform normally. For example, acuity is readily degraded by refractive error so that 1 dioptre of defocus will reduce the Snellen fraction to about 0.3. Young hypermetropes (hyperopes) can accommodate to overcome their own refractive error, but myopes and presbyopes cannot. A pin-hole is a very helpful method of determining whether acuity is due to refractive error rather than ocular pathology or neurological disease. It is important to remember that a pin-hole, however, will only correct to 6/6 up to 4 dioptres of spherical and cylindrical error and that an up to date refraction is essential in all cases of unexplained visual loss. Optical quality also depends on pupil size: visual acuity remains approximately constant in the range of 2.5–6 mm after which the minimal angle of resolution falls off. In the elderly, as pupil size diminishes and lenticular opacities increase the spatial resolution of the eye may fall even in the absence of specific pathological conditions.

PHOTOSTRESS TESTING, AMSLER GRID AND ACUITY TESTING AT REDUCED ILLUMINATION

In all instances of deficient vision the clinician must ask whether the observed pathology matches the degree of visual loss. Normally this question lies within the province of the general ophthalmologist, but it is not unusual for a patient to have an apparently normal eye and yet still have poor vision. When this occurs in one eye only the problem probably will be localized to the optic nerve, especially when there is a marked colour vision deficit and a relative afferent pupil defect.

However, subtle retinal pathology involving the fovea and central vision may be overlooked and simple tests to distinguish macular from optic nerve lesions are sometimes helpful before recourse to more sophisticated electrodiagnostic methods. In the photostress test the subject fixates on a bright light for a defined period of time (about 30 seconds) and the time to recovery of acuity to the pre-test level after eventual disappearance of the induced positive scotoma is measured. In lesions of the choroid, retinal pigment epithelium or retinal photoreceptors, recovery from this bleaching is greatly prolonged, whereas in optic nerve disease photostressing does not produce the same effect as function does not depend on the rapid functioning of the visual cycle. The Amsler grid is a coarse high contrast grid against which small paracentral scotomas of macular disease can readily be seen.

An additional category of common difficulty arises in the discrimination between poor uniocular vision due to amblyopia ('lazy eye') dating from childhood strabismus or stimulus deprivation which the adult patient may only later become aware of, and an acquired cause of visual loss without evident intraocular pathology. When illumination is reduced (for example by using a standard neutral density filter), acuity is preserved in eyes with longstanding visual loss due to amblyopia, but is markedly degraded in an acquired optic neuropathy: this test is sometimes invaluable in distinguishing amblyopia from, for example, optic neuritis, but the results may be hard to interpret and usually when amblyopia is present the cause (microtropia, strabismus or anisometropia) is obvious. One other effect on simple testing of the amblyopic eye is that on single letter Snellen chart testing, acuity improves on the single letter per line format: this phenomenon is known as crowding (Han *et al.*, 1985; Greenwald and Fold, 1983).

FURTHER PSYCHOPHYSICAL TESTS OF VISION: CONTRAST SENSITIVITY, COLOUR VISION, VISUAL FIELDS

Contrast sensitivity

The patient who complains of 'faded' vision but who has a normal (high contrast) Snellen acuity can readily be shown to have defects in contrast sensitivity (Fredericksen *et al.*, 1991). The level of contrast at which a light and dark pattern is first discriminated is the contrast threshold. No consistent discrimination occurs for contrast below the subject's threshold for a particular spatial frequency. High spatial frequencies and very low spatial frequencies require higher contrast for resolution. Contrast sensitivity is the reciprocal of the contrast threshold. Contrast sensitivity is measured using sine wave (sinusoidal) gratings showing gradual change from light to dark. Measurement aims to record the patient's contrast threshold over a range of spatial frequencies using gratings of different contrast levels. Because two variables are involved (spatial frequency and contrast threshold) a graph must be constructed setting out the contrast threshold for each spatial frequency resulting in a contrast sensitivity curve. Pathological reduction in contrast sensitivity occurs in developmental and acquired visual defects when the contrast threshold can be raised for low, high or all spatial frequencies depending on the underlying cause (Travis and Thompson, 1989).

In formal systems, spatial vision is represented by sinusoidal or square wave gratings presented on a television monitor with frequencies ranging between 0.1 and 25 cycles / degree, with standardized visual angles of 5 degrees height and 32 degrees width and with additional counterphasing at a frequency of 0.6 / seconds to prevent afterimages. User-friendly book mounted charts introduced by Arden and Regan are commercially available. Wall-mounted charts are also useful; for example the VisTech and Pelli–Robson systems. In a VisTech chart photographs of sinusoidal gratings are presented and thresholds for different spatial frequencies are determined by the subject recognizing the correct orientation of the stripes, while in the simpler Pelli–Robson chart where standard sized optotypes of uniform spatial frequency are presented with decreasing contrast as the subject reads along a line allowing threshold detection (Pelli *et al.*, 1988). Computer generated presentations have the advantage of a capability to assess temporal effects (loss of contrast senstivity with time), and related functions including motion detection thresholds and flicker modulation sensitivity (Arden and Jacobsen, 1978; Pardhan, 1993; Arden, 1988; Regan and Neiman, 1983).

In visual science, contrast sensitivity forms the basis of one of the most important psychophysical methods for measuring visual function: for example allowing the demonstration that neurons of the visual system are sensitive to limited ranges of spatial frequency and orientation. In clinical practice these methods allow the detection of otherwise subclinical pathology and offer a sensitive way of following patients with chronic disease such as optic nerve function after an episode of optic neuritis.

Colour vision

It is a characteristic of certain disorders of the anterior visual pathways that sensitivity to hue discrimination (colour vision) may be impaired while luminance and contrast-based functions (acuity) are preserved. At the level of retinal photoreceptors, colour vision is a function of three classes of cones of overlapping spectral sensitivities for red, green and blue so that colours are represented by differential matching of the output of each group. At a neural level, colour vision is processed according to a colour-opponent code whereby certain colour pairs appear as mutually exclusive opposites such as red-green and blue-yellow. The physiological substrate for colour opponent encoding lies within the neural elements of the retina. In clinical terms, these concepts are reflected in the classification of congenital defects of colour vision according to whether one or more classes of

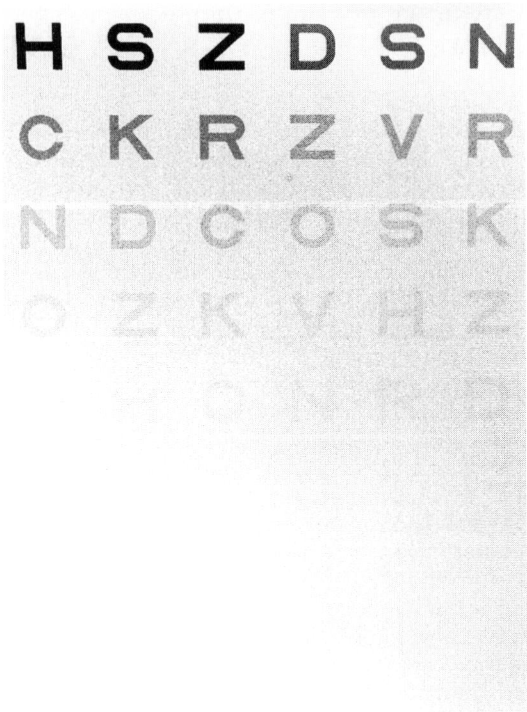

Figure 2.4 The Pelli-Robson contrast charts for vision.

photoreceptor are missing (dichromats and monochromats) or have anomolous sensitivity (anomalous trichromats) (Table 2.3).

The inherited dyschromatopsias are binocular, symmetrical and and do not change over time. Monochromats have major cone defects and have poor acuity as well, but dichromats and anomalous trichromats have normal acuity.

Acquired dyschromatopsias are different to congenital defects in several respects. First, they are noticeable to the patient. Second they may be monocular or even restricted to one part of the visual field. Third, although colour defects may be much more marked than acuity defects, acuity is generally reduced to some degree (Hart, 1987) (Table 2.4).

According to Kollner's rule, patients with neural disorders have a preponderance of damage to red-green discrimination with preservation of blue-yellow discrimination (type I and II defects), while those with retinal and choroidal disease may show selective loss of blue-yellow discrimination (type III defects). However, some optic neuropathies — especially those associated with preserved acuity — may show type III defects. Because blue cones are not found in the central 0.5 degrees of field, disease processes which selectively damage the extrafoveal visual field will leave the patient with normal acuity and normal red-green discrimination. Examples of this include glaucoma, dominant optic atrophy, chronic papilloedema and early chloroquine retinal toxicity. More typically, optic neuropathies which involve the fibres of the maculopapillar bundle such as retrobulbar neuritis, Leber's disease and extrinsic compression will damage neural elements serving foveal function and green-red discrimination will be damaged, often out of proportion to acuity loss.

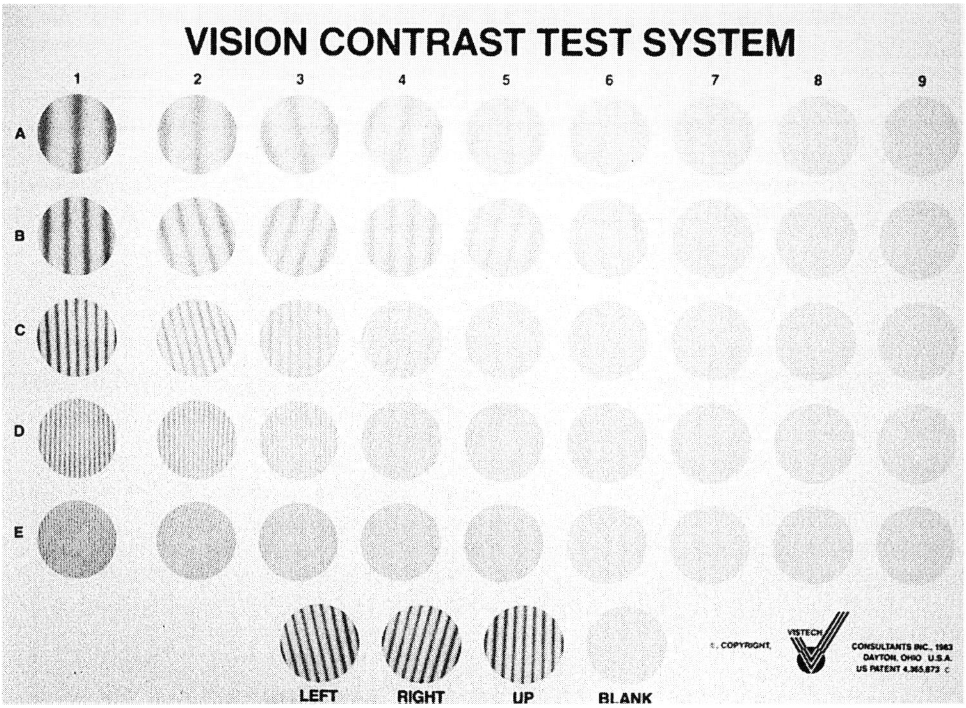

Figure 2.5 The VisTech contrast charts for vision.

Table 2.3 Classification of congenital colour deficiency

	Red deficient	Green deficient	Blue deficient
Anomalous trichromats	Protanomal	Deuteranomal	Tritanomal
Dichromats	Protanope	Deuteranope	Tritanope
Monochromats	Blue-cone monchromats / Rod monochromats		

Table 2.4 Classification of acquired colour deficiency

Name	Alternative name	Hue discrimination defect	Visual acuity loss
Type I	Red / green 'protan-like'	Red / green discrimination loss: Preserved blue / yellow discrimination	Moderate to severe
Type II	Red / green 'deutan-like'	Red / green discrimination loss plus mild blue / yellow impairment	Moderate to severe
Type III	Blue / yellow 'tritan-like'	Blue / yellow confusion	Mild to moderate

Formal colour vision testing using spectral light sources graded for luminance changes is very demanding and time-consuming, and not very practicable in the clinical setting. Pseudo-isochromatic plates are very widely used because of their portability, low cost and ease of use. The plates consist of a series of dots of various colours and sizes that are clustered together into carefully arranged patterns of various hues. These hues can readily be distinguished by a normal trichromat but not by those with defective colour vision. The patterns form highly legible figures which are visible even to those with relatively poor acuity. An initial test plate excludes subjects whose acuity or reading skills do not allow them to perform the test. Commercially available pseudo-isochromatic plates (Ishihara and Hardy, Ritter, Read (HRR)) are designed to detect individuals with congenital dyschromatopsias, but do not allow protan-deutran distinctions or the separation of anomalous trichromats from dichromats. They are also of practical use in the qualitative assessment of acquired colour defects.

A greater quantitative element is supplied by the Farnsworth-Munsell 100-hue test in which the subject is required to arrange a series of coloured discs in sequence between pairs of reference discs (MacFadyen, 1988). The order of discs is then plotted in a circular diagram so that the degree of error is represented by points far away from the centre of the diagram. Characteristic patterns for errors along the red-green and blue-yellow axis will emerge allowing full characterization of the dyschromatopsia. Even with automated, computer-assisted versions, this test is rather inconvenient and time consuming and is not greatly used for this reason. The Farnsworth D-15 (dichotomous) panel test simplifies matters by recording confusions in the allocation of non-adjacent hues into their correct colour grouping.

Other techniques include the Pickford-Nicholson anomaloscope in which the subject views a translucent panel through a monocular objective and has to match pairs of coloured lights. A more modern alternative is provided by computer-assisted colour contrast sensitivity systems in which standard optotypes are presented in colour against a coloured background and the contrast thresholds measured in each of the colour confusion axes. It is likely that in many clinics a psychophysical central vision assessment package can be used where thresholds for acuity tasks, contrast sensitivity and colour contrast sensitivity can all be presented in a sequence of quick user-friendly formats with a microprocessor and standard computer monitor (Arden, 1988).

Visual field testing

The analysis of the visual fields retains central importance in the localization of defects in the visual system, and for monitoring the natural history of a condition and responses to therapy. Simple confrontation testing (qualitative) remains useful in clinic-based and bedside topical diagnosis, but semi-quantitative and quantitative methods are essential for accurate documentation, detection of more subtle defects and for assessing progress. The diagnostic value of field testing rests on the principle of the retinotopic organization of the afferent visual system whereby nerve fibres from retinal ganglion cells serving defined parts of the visual field project in an anatomically consistent arrangement. Fibres from the inferior retina will pass inferiorly in the optic nerve and chiasm. Fibres serving central vision (the papillomacular bundle) tend to move from the temporal or lateral side of the optic nerve anteriorly to occupy the central core posteriorly. As these fibres make up the majority of all fibres in the optic nerve, the hallmark of optic nerve lesions is a central scotoma, together with acuity loss and colour vision defects. However, other patterns are possible, and the precise characterization of the nature of the field defect in acquired optic nerve diseases may carry important diagnostic implications (Table 2.5).

At the chiasm, inferonasal fibres serving the upper temporal field loop anteriorly into the distal contralateral optic nerve (von Wilbrand's knee) before passing into the contralateral optic tract. Crossing fibres at the chiasm appear to be more sensitive to

Table 2.5 Specific types of field loss in optic nerve disease

Field defect	Pathophysiology	Common causes
Arcuate scotoma	Retinal nerve fibre bundle damage selectively involving fibres entering disc at 12 o'clock and 6 o'clock	Glaucoma, Optic disc drusen, optic neuritis, ischaemic lesions
Centrocaecal scotoma	Selective damage to fibres of papillomascular bundle serving central vision and lying in the temporal side of the anterior optic nerve	Leber's hereditary optic neuropathy, Toxic optic neuropathies — ethambutol, ethanol, methanol, tobacco, rarely optic neuritis
Altudinal scotoma	Selective damage to upper or lower poles of the optic nerve: reflecting susceptibility at these points to reduced vascular perfusion pressure in the anastomotic circle of Zinn-Haller deriving from branches of the short posterior ciliary vessels and lying at the level of the lamina cribrosa	Anterior ischaemic optic neuropathy, rarely optic neuritis and compressive lesions

pathological processes than non-crossing fibres and the hallmark of chiasmal disease is the bitemporal hemianopia or one of its variants. The pathophysiological reason for this differential sensitivity remains unclear. It is at the chiasm that the visual system becomes functionally divided about the vertical through the fixation point (represented in the fundus by the fovea, NOT the optic nerve head). At the chiasm and posteriorly in projections throughout the optic radiations to the cortex, the lateral separation of blended hemifields from each side is inviolate. In any technique of assessing the visual field in suspected abnormalities of the visual pathways it is therefore essential to pay close attention to the vertical meridian.

In testing the visual field it is helpful to employ Traquair's analogy of the hill of vision. The field is represented as a three dimensional hill with the base plane representing the horizontal and vertical dimensions of visual space and the hill representing the sensitivity of the retina to stimulation by a focal light at different places. At the pinnacle of the hill is the fovea where even the dimmest and smallest target can be detected. This concept allows for the representation of relative field loss as alteration in the slope of the hill, as well as constriction ('coast erosion') and absolute loss (the blind spot for example). Lines joining points of equal sensitivity are isopters, and using the standard manual perimeter (Goldmann), the isopters are determined either by moving a spot of light from periphery to centre until it hits the hill and is perceived (kinetic testing), or by increasing the intensity of stimulus at one spot until threshold is reached (static testing). The concept of the hill of vision is also useful in confrontation testing, where relative defects can be detected by eliciting differential brightness of say a hand, or a red bottle top in opposite hemifields. In other individuals, however, it is not practicable to depend on the subjects's conscious response, and an involuntary saccadic eye movement to fixate on a peripherally placed stimulus may serve as a sensitive test for obtunded or pre-verbal patients (Table 2.6, Fig. 2.6A).

Table 2.6 Confrontation techniques in visual field testing

Confrontation with neurological pins
Visually elicited eye movements
Infants
Obtunded adults
Finger mimicking
Pre-verbal children
Dysphasic adults
Hand and colour comparison
Children and adults
Blinking to menace and flashing lights
Children and obtunded adults

Techniques which allow the depiction of the hill of vision in the form of isopters on a chart include the semiquantitative tangent screen and quantitative Goldmann kinetic perimetry (Fig. 2.6B). The task is always hampered by the need for highly trained and experienced perimetrists who can reliably distinguish between pathology and artifact (Wellings, 1989). Now automated perimetry machines are widely available (Keltner and Johnson, 1986; Yabuki *et al.*, 1989).

These can now generate numerical indices of point-by-point deviations in retinal thresholds supported by reliability scores and statistical analysis to help determine the significance of any departure from age matched controls. Ease of data storage and standardization of presentation are advantages. With increasing sensitivity however,

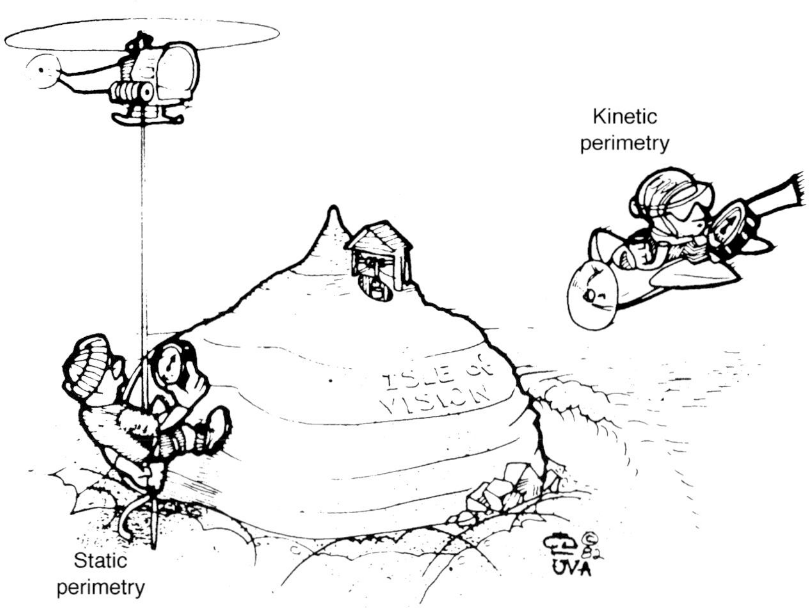

A

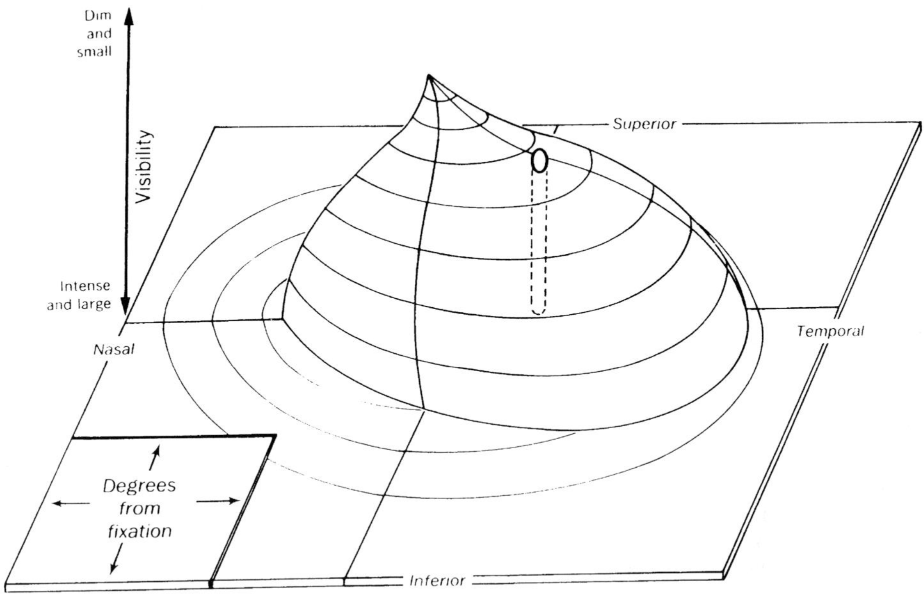

B

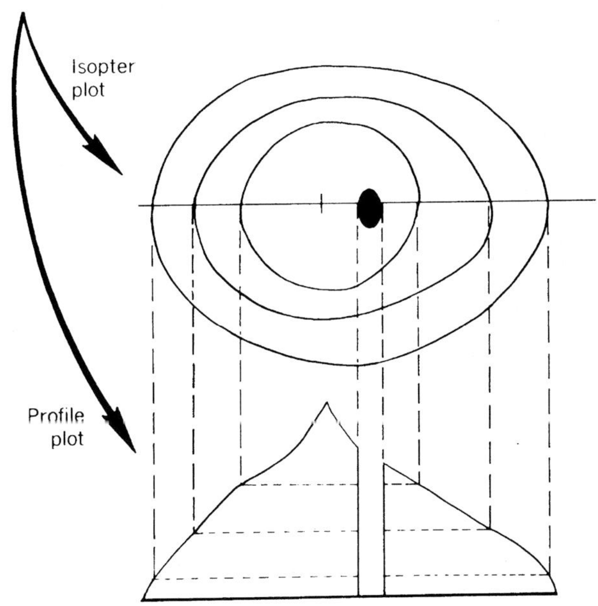

Figure 2.6 The 'island' or 'hill' of vision proposed by Traquair is surrounded by a 'sea of blindness'. The height of the island represents increasing sensitivity. Using kinetic perimetry, the island is intercepted by a moving target of fixed size. Using static perimetry, a target's visibility is increased in size or luminosity until it descends on to the island. The blindspot located 15 degrees temporal to fixation is absolute, creating a small 'well' in the sensitivity contour. (**A** Cartoon by Dr Steven Newman, redrawn from Feldon, 1989; **B** from Anderson 1982.)

specificity is lost and although it is now possible to explore the visual field at the limits of complex physiological measurement even to the extent of measuring differential function in ganglion cell subpopulations according to their motion detection and luminance functions, it is important to deploy strategies which support practical management decisions (Safran and Glaser, 1980; Zappia *et al.*, 1971). Automated systems measuring static and/or motion detection thresholds are primarily designed for the detection of subclinical disease states which will not be detectable by confrontation, in particular early glaucomatous optic neuropathy, and are not necessarily suitable for characterizing patterns of field defect which is so important in topical neuro-ophthalmic diagnosis (Beck *et al.*, 1985; McCary and Feigon, 1979). Other problems include patient learning effects, physiological variation in field performance over time, and fatigue (Wildberger and Robert, 1988; Searle *et al.*, 1991).

In addition, test strategies emphasize threshold changes across the horizontal meridian, but in neuro-ophthlamic assessment, the vertical meridian is of crucial diagnostic importance, and fixation testing strategies rely on repeated blind spot checking which is of course lost in bitemporal defects of chiasmal disease. One ingenious way of making automated devices more user-friendly is to move the subject's eye and not the stimulus. In oculokinetic perimetry, this is achieved by requiring the subject to follow a moving target on a computer screen and count numbers presented peripherally (Damato, *et al.*, 1989). Arcuate, quadrantic, hemianopic, altitudinal and nasal step defects can all be readily detected in this way. Other user-friendly techniques which may shortly enter general clinical use are high-pass resolution perimetry and white noise perimetry. A further alternative, which also dispenses with the entire psychophysical paradigm is pupil perimetry whereby the timing and amplitude of pupilary contractions to focal light stimuli are recorded using a computerized infrared pupillometer linked to an automated Humphrey perimeter. The results correlate well with those of standard static threshold perimetry, and the consistent finding of pupillary defects in patients with homonymous field loss is of great interest as this supports observations suggesting the suprageniculate influence on the pupillary light reflexes (Kardon *et al.*, 1991, 1993).

COLOUR PERIMETRY

As described in the section on colour vision testing, acquired lesions of the optic nerve characteristically show chromatic defects which may precede luminance defects. It follows that in some circumstances colour visual field testing is more sensitive than using white test targets of differing sizes and light intensities. Following Kollner's rule, optic neuropathies frequently manifest red-green discrimination defects which are readily picked up using a red target on confrontation methods ('in which hemifield is the colour brighter?') especially with the tangent screen. In other instances where blue-yellow defects are conspicuous, short wavelength automated perimetry (SWAP) may be useful.

FUNDOSCOPY — DIRECT AND INDIRECT OPHTHALMOSCOPY, SPECIAL TECHNIQUES

The direct ophthalmoscope incorporates a light source focused directly onto the retina through a small angled mirror which fills either half or the whole of the aperture. The mirror centre is unsilvered so that the illuminated fundus can be seen through it. Between the returning light rays and the examiner's eye there is a revolving magazine of lenses which usually range from –30 to +30 dioptres to correct any inherent refractive error in either the patient or the examiner. In practice, it may be easier to view the fundus of a patient with a larger refractive error by leaving the glasses on and turning the ophthalmoscope lens to zero. Changing the ophthalmoscope lens power will also change

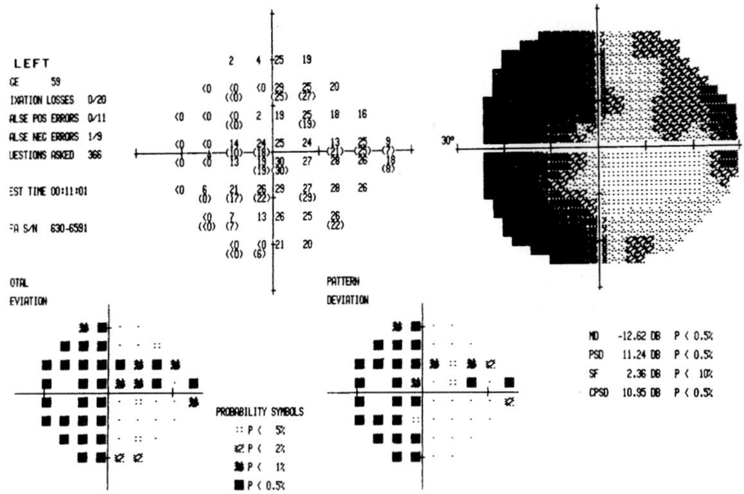

A

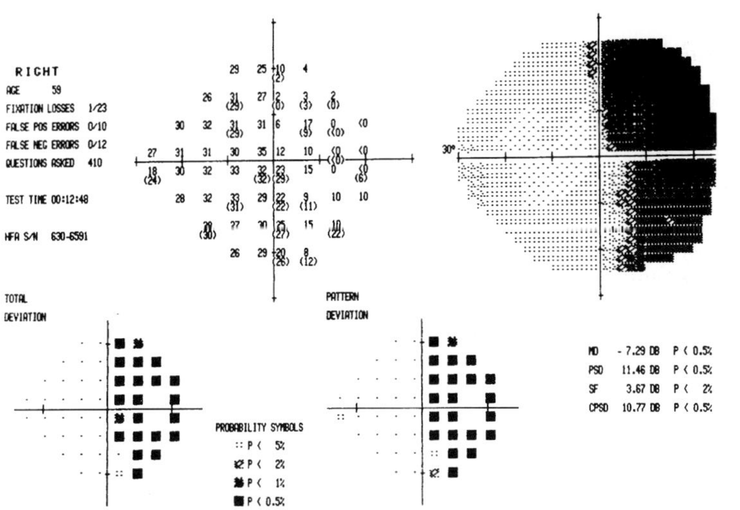

B

Figure 2.7 Humphrey central 24 degrees threshold field illustrating bitemporal hemianopia.

the depth of focus within the eye and allow examination of media opacities, especially in the lens. The field of view with the direct ophthalmoscope is small, approximately 6 degrees with a magnification of ×15; the image is erect and real. A green or 'red-free' filter is useful for examining nerve fibre detail, retinal vessels, haemorrhages and microaneurysms. The examiner views the patients' right eye with his right eye and reverses eyes to view the left. Pupillary dilatation with tropicamide, cyclopentolate or phenylephrine drops is essential for the best retinal view. The risk of precipitating an attack of acute angle closure glaucoma by using dilating drops is very low and is usually outweighed by the benefits of achieving an adequate view.

The direct ophthalmoscope, by virtue of its small field and high magnification, is particularly suitable for viewing the optic nerve head. However, when a wider field and an appreciation of stereoscopic depth detail is required, indirect ophthalmoscopy is used. In this technique a light source is directed into the eye and the reflected light is gathered by a hand-held condensing lens to form a virtual inverted image of the retina. The size of the image varies according to the power of the condensing lens: the greater the power the smaller the image. A +13D lens magnifies the retina approximately four times and a +30D lens by two. Indirect ophthalmoscopy has the advantage of providing high intensity illumination, stereopsis and a wide field of view as well as allowing dynamic assessment of vitreoretinal pathology. Disadvantages include the inverted image, the requirement for wide pupillary dilation and the considerable practice needed to master the technique.

Other methods for viewing the fundus require a slit lamp and are especially helpful in the assessment of stereo detail in macular pathology. These include fundus contact lenses and the non-contact Hruby and Volk lenses.

PUPILS — PRINCIPLES OF CLINICAL EXAMINATION AND DIAGNOSIS

SYNOPSIS OF ANATOMY AND PHYSIOLOGY

The pupillary light reflex pathway is a three-neuron reflex arc:

1) afferent neurons from retinal ganglion cells to the pretectal area,
2) interneuron from the pretectal complex to the parasympathetic motor pool (Edinger–Westphal nucleus) of the oculomotor complex,
3) parasympathetic efferent fibres with the oculomotor nerve to the ciliary ganglion and then to the pupil sphincter muscle.

The integrity of pupil function therefore depends on normal function in the retinal photoreceptors, the retinal ganglion cells, the axons within the optic nerve, chiasm and optic tract, the brachium of the superior colliculus, the pretectal area of the midbrain, interneurons in the midbrain, the oculomotor nuclear complex, the parasympathetic pathway via the ciliary ganglion and the efferent sympathetic pathways from hypothalamus to the pupillary dilator. The afferent limb of the pupillary light reflex is therefore a retinomesencephalic projection. At the optic chiasm, a slightly higher proportion of afferent axons cross to the contralateral tract than remain uncrossed (ratio 53:47). This may explain the presence of an afferent pupil defect in patients with isolated retrochiasmal lesions. Within the oculomotor complex, a midline dorsal cell mass contains the oculomotor neural pool: a rostral portion which is associated with accommodation and a caudal portion which is associated with pupil constriction. In the peripheral oculomotor nerve, pupillomotor fibres are superficially located, lying just internal to the epineurium leaving them especially vulnerable to compression. In the more anterior portion this separation is less distinct and compressive lesions within the cavernous sinus may result in a complete external ophthalmoplegia with preserved pupil function.

The ocular sympathetic pathways begin in the posterolateral hypothalamus and descend uncrossed through the brain stem to terminate in the spinal cord between C8 and T2. Second order neurons exit the spinal cord primarily with the ventral root of T1 to enter the cervical sympathetic chain via white rami communicantes. The fibres ascend through the inferior and middle cervical ganglia without synapsing to terminate in the superior cervial ganglion at the skull base. Third order post-ganglionic fibres destined for the eye ascend the internal carotid to enter the skull, whilst those serving facial sweat and piloerection follow the external carotid and its branches. Oculosympathetic fibres to the eye pass through the ciliary ganglion without synapsing and include orbital vasomotor fibres, pupillary dilators, smooth muscles of the upper and lower lids (Müller), lacrimal gland, and trophic fibres to uveal melanophores.

The pupillary near response

Accommodative effort, caused either by retinal image blur or conscious near fixation, results in the activation of the 'near triad' of lens accommodation, convergence of the visual axes and pupillary constriction (see Chapter 8 — vergence eye movements). Loss of the pupillary light reaction with preservation of the near response (light-near dissociation) is a feature of range of neural lesions, but loss of the near response with preservation of the light response does not occur.

COMMON ABNORMALITIES OF THE PUPILS AND EXAMINATION TECHNIQUES

In clinical records in the UK it is very common to find the acronym PERLA entered to describe the bedside examination of the pupils. This stands for Pupils Equal and Reacting to Light and to Accommodation and does not indicate whether the examiner has taken the step of studying the consensual reflexes.

Afferent and relative afferent pupil defects

The pupil of an eye that is blind from retinal or optic nerve disease will fail to react directly to light but will contrict consensually when the other healthy eye is stimulated. The blind eye shows an afferent pupil defect. Much more commonly, however, a disease process will leave one eye with a degree of visual impairment and direct stimulation will still result in pupillary constriction. In these circumstances it is important to perform a swinging light test to look for relative afferent pupillary defects. Relative afferent pupillary defects are best seen by moving a hand-held light from one eye to the other holding the light to each eye for about one second. As the light shifts from the eye with normal vision to the eye with reduced vision, the direct light stimulus is no longer sufficient to keep both pupils small; thus they both dilate. The test is very quick and easy to perform and is sufficiently sensitive to detect residual optic nerve dysfunction after an episode of retrobular neuritis and recovery of acuity to 6/6. Only one working iris sphincter is necessary to perform this test. For example, a third nerve palsy or anterior ocular segment disruption as a result of trauma, inflammation or surgery will not stop the examiner from observing the direct and consensual responses of the intact pupil as each is alternately stimulated. A dim side light is invaluable especially in patients with dark irides to observe the pupillary movements. The afferent pupil defect may also be quantified by using a series of neutral density filters over the good eye to reduce the stimulus to the point at which a balance point is reached. The magnitude of the defect is then given by the density of the filter required for neutralization in log units (Thompson, *et al.* 1981).

Afferent pupil defects are absent in functional visual loss and are very small when visual loss is due to a macular lesion of the retina or to amblyopia (Greenwald and Fold, 1983). More extensive retinal lesions such as a complete retinal detachment will show marked afferent pupil defects. Optic nerve lesions typically produce marked defects and hence the test of great value in cases of otherwise unexplained visual loss. When optic neuritis has been diagnosed and there is no relative afferent pupillary defect, the diagnosis is either wrong or else there is bilateral disease. Rarely, afferent pupil defects arise in post-chiasmal lesions either of the optic tract or, conceivably, of the pretectal mesencephalon in which case there will be no field loss (Kardon *et al.*, 1993).

Efferent pupil defects

A dilated pupil which does not respond to direct or consensual light stimulation must always suggest the possibility of a partial oculomotor nerve palsy with the implication of significant intracranial pathology such as an unruptured posterior communicating artery aneurysm. Normally however a degree of ptosis and ophthalmoplegia will also be present on careful examination and although exceptions to this rule have been reported another explanation is much more likely if the lid positions and eye movements are completely normal.

Abnormally large pupils

A dilated pupil which does not respond to light or to the near reflex raises the possibility of accidental or deliberate instillation of a pharmacologically active agent such as atropine, scopolamine or some plant juices containing belladonna alkaloids. In distinction to mydriasis resulting from parasympathetic paralysis, oculomotor nerve palsy or a tonic pupil, the dilated pupil is not reversed by instilling pilocarpine 1%. In clinical practice, only a limited range of problems present with unequal pupils. A history of previous intraocular surgery or trauma should be excluded as this is a frequent source of confusion. The combination of pupillary inequality with reduced visual acuity or pain mandates immediate ophthalmological referral because of the possibility of acute angle closure glaucoma.

Tonic pupil (Holmes–Adie syndrome)

Probably the commonest cause of abnormal pupillary light reactions and a large pupil in one eye is the tonic pupil. A tonic pupil is the result of damage to the ciliary ganglion or short ciliary nerves producing in addition to a poor pupillary light reaction, accommodative paresis, cholinergic supersensitivity and a response to near vision which is strong and tonic. A tonic pupil may result from local infection or injury of the ciliary body or form part of a widespread peripheral neuropathy such as alcohol toxicity, diabetes and amyloidosis (Smith and Smith, 1983). When there is no local cause and the deep tendon reflexes are absent, the patient has Adie's syndrome (Holmes–Adie pupil plus tendon areflexia). The term tonic describes the fact that the near pupil response is slow and steady and on looking back into the distance the pupil holds its contraction for a few seconds. As a result of denervation hypersensitivity, the tonic pupil constricts with a low concentration of pilocarpine 0.125% but a normal pupil will not. The onset of symptoms in Adie's syndrome is often abrupt, with a dilated pupil, but early symptomatic accommodation paresis soon recovers: later the dilated pupil constricts and the anisocoria may disappear. The abnormal light reaction will not recover. There is a strong tendency towards eventual bilaterality and females are much more often affected than males (Loewenfeld and Thomson, 1981).

Light-near dissociation

Light-near dissociation will arise in major anterior visual pathway disease if both eyes are blind from an optic nerve or retinal cause and the patient can generate a near response by converging. Lesions of the midbrain can selectively interrupt the pretectal pupillomotor fibres as they pass from the optic tract to the Edinger-Westphal nucleus. Supranuclear inhibitory fibres may also be implicated. Commonly this is seen in Parinaud's syndrome, pinealoma, demyelination and in neurosyphilis (Argyll Robertson pupils) when the resting pupil size is usually very small (Thompson *et al.*, 1981, Loewenfeld, 1969).

Horner's syndrome

Unequal pupils may also be due to failure of the sympathetic supply to the dilator pupillae resulting in poor dilation in the dark. Horner's syndrome of ptosis, miosis and facial anhidrosis may arise from interuption of the sympathetic pathways at any point along the course of the central, the pre-ganglionic (second order), or the post-ganglionic (third order) neurons. Localization is often achieved by the association of other physical signs. Horner's syndrome due to central or second order neuron damage is therefore likely to be associated with abnormalities referable to the brain stem (e.g. lateral medullary syndrome), cervical spine or thoracic outlet (Pancoast's syndrome), while Horner's due to third order neuron impairment will often be associated with ipsilateral vascular headache syndromes implicating the carotid artery or a history of basal skull trauma. Sometimes there are no clinical clues to help localize the lesion, but the task is important because of the association between pre-ganglionic disruption and neoplastic disease, especially in children. Only if the sympathetic pathway is intact will 4% cocaine dilate the pupil and help to confirm the existence of a deficit but not localize the lesion. Hydroxyamphetamine 1% has traditionally been used to localize by only causing mydriasis when post-ganglionic fibres are intact and are able to relase noradrenaline. In a post-ganglionic lesion there will be no mydriasis but amphetamine will dilate a pupil when there is a pre-ganglionic lesion. Nowadays amphetamine is no longer available to most clinicians but the synthetic sympathomimetic pholedrine serves the same purpose. When iris heterochromia accompanies Horner's syndrome, the cause is usually either congenital or the result of perinatal injury reflecting the common derivation from neural crest tissue of both iris stromal pigment and the oculosympathetic pathways (Grimson and Thompson, 1975).

Physiological anisocoria

Up to one-fifth of the normal population is said to have unequal pupils (anisocoria) in a dim light of 0.4 mm or more. However, careful examination shows that there is no evidence of abnormal peripheral innervation to the iris and no further investigation is required (Lam *et al.*, 1987).

REFERENCES

Arden GB (1988). Testing contrast sensitivity in clinical practice. *Clin Vis Sci* **2**: 213–224.

Arden GB and Jacobsen JJ (1978). A simple grating test for contrast sensitivity: Preliminary results indicate value in screening for glaucoma. *Invest Ophthalmol Vis Sci* **17**: 23–32.

Arden GB, Grundez K and Perry S (1988). Colour vision testing with a computer graphics system. *Clin Vis Sci* **2**: 303–320.

Beck RW, Bergstrom TJ and Lichter PR (1985). A clinical comparison of visual field testing with a new automated perimeter, the Humphrey Field Analyser, and the Goldmann perimeter. *Ophthalmology* **92**: 77–82.

Dagi LR, Chrousos GA and Cogan DC (1987). Spasm of the near reflex associated with organic disease. *Am J Ophthalmol* **103**: 582.

Damato BE, Ahmed J, Allen D *et al.* (1989). The detection of glaucomatous visual field defects by oculo-kinetic perimetry. *Eye* **3**: 727–731.

Ferris FL III and Sperduto RD (1982). Standardised illumination for visual acuity testing in clinical research. *Am J Ophthalmol* **94**: 97–98.

Ferris FL III, Kassof KA, Brenick GH and Bailey I (1982). New visual acuity charts for clinical research. *Am J Ophthalmol* **94**: 91–96.

Frederiksen JL, Larsson HB, Ottovay E and Stigsby B (1991). Acute optic neuritis with normal visual acuity: comparison of symptoms and signs with psychophysiological, electrophysiological and magnetic resonance imaging data. *Acta Ophthalmol* **69**: 357–366.

Frisen L (1980). The neurology of visual acuity. *Brain* **103**: 639–670.

Greenwald MJ and Folk ER (1983). Afferent pupillary defects in amblyopia. *J Ped Ophthalmol Strab* **20**: 63–67.

Grimson BS and Thompson HS (1975). Drug testing in Horner's syndrome. In *Neuro-Ophthalmology Symposium* (eds JS Glaser and JL Smith), Vol VIII, pp. 265–270, St Louis: CV Mosby.

Han DP, Thompson HS and Folk JC (1985). Differentiation between recently resolved optic neuritis and central serous retinopathy. *Arch Ophthalmol* **103**: 394–396.

Hart WM (1987). Acquired dyschromatopsias. *Surv Ophthalmol* **32**: 10.

Hitchings RA, Migdal CS, Wormald R *et al.* (1994). The (Glaucoma) Primary Treatment Trial: Changes in visual field analysis by computer assisted perimetry. *Eye* **8**: 117–120.

Kardon RH, Aydin-Kirhali P and Thompson HS (1991). Automated pupil perimetry I. Pupil field mapping in patients and normal subjects. *Ophthalmology* **98**: 485–496.

Kardon RH, Haupert CL and Thompson HS (1993). The relationship between static perimetry and the relative afferent pupil defect. *Am J Ophthalmol* **115**, 351–356.

Keltner JL and Johnson CA (1986). Current status of automated perimetry. Is the ideal automated perimeter available? *Arch Ophthalmol* **104**: 347–349.

Lam BL, Thompson HS and Corbett JJ (1987). The prevalence of simple anisocoria. *Am J Ophthalmol* **104**: 69–73.

Loewenfeld IE (1969). The Argyll Robertson pupil, 1869–1969: A cricial survey of the literature. *Surv Ophthalmol* **14**: 199–299.

Loewenfed IE and Thompson HS (1985). Mechanism of tonic pupil. *Ann Neurol* **10**: 275–276.

MacFadyen DJ, Drance SM, Chisholm IA *et al.* (1988). The Farnsworth-Munsel 100-Hue color vision score and visual evoked potentials in multiple sclerosis. *Neuro-Ophthalmology* **8**: 289–298.

McCary JA and Feigon J (1979). Computerized perimetry in neuro-ophthalmology. *Ophthalmology* **86**: 1287–1301.

Pardhan S (1993). Binocular performance in patients with unilateral cataract using the Regan test. *Eye* **7**: 59–62.

Pardhan S and Gilchrist J (1993). The importance of measuring binocular contrast sensitivity in unilateral cataract. *Eye* **5**: 31–35.

Pelli DG, Robson JG and Wilkins AJ (1988). The design of a new letter chart for measuring contrast sensitivity. *Clin Vis Sci* **2**: 187–189.

Regan D and Neiman D (1983). Low-contrast letter charts as a test of visual function. *Ophthalmology* **90**: 1192–1200.

Safran AB and Glaser JS (1980). Statokinetic dissociation in lesions of the anterior visual pathways. *Arch Ophthalmol* **98**: 291–295.

Searle AET, Wild JM, Shaw DE and O'Neill EC (1991). Time-related variation in normal automated static perimetry. *Ophthalmology* **98**: 701–707.

Smith SA and Smith SE (1983). Evidence for a neuropathic aetiology in the small pupil of diabetes mellitus. *Br J Ophthalmol* **67**: 89–93.

Thompson HS, (1991). Asymmetry of pupillomotor input. *Eye* **5**: 36–39.

Thompson HS and Kardon RH (1991). Pretectal pupillary defects: editorial comment. *Ophthalmology* **11**: 173–174.

Thompson JS, Corbett JJ and Cox TA, (1981). How to measure the relative afferent pupillary defect. *Surv Ophthalmol* **26**: 39–42.

Travis D and Thompson P, (1989). Spatiotemporal contrast sensitivity and colour vision in multiple sclerosis. *Brain* **112**: 283–303.

Weatherill JR (1993). Visual acuity assessment. *Eye* **7**: 26–29 [Published erratum appears in *Eye* 1993; **7**: 604].

Wellings PC (1989). Detection and recognition of visual field defects resulting from lesions involving the visual pathways. *Austral N Z J Ophthalmol* **17**: 331–335.

Wildberger H and Robert Y (1988). Visual fatigue during prolonged visual field testing in optic neuropathies. *Neuro-Ophthalmology* **8**: 167–174.

Yabuki K, Sakai M, Suzumara H *et al.* (1989). A comparison of kinetic and static perimetry for lesions in the visual pathway. In *Perimetry Update 1988/89* (ed A Heijl). Amsterdam: Kugler and Ghedini.

Zappia RJ, Enoch JM, Stamper R *et al.* (1971). The Riddoch phenomenon revealed in non-occipital lobe lesions. *Br J Ophthalmol* **55**: 416–420.

3

Specialized investigations in neuro-ophthalmology

FLUORESCEIN ANGIOGRAPHY

Fluorescein angiography provides an important adjunct to the ophthalmoscopy of diseases of the retina and the optic nerve head by demonstrating evidence of disease activity and by providing a permanent record (Sanders, 1970). Following an intravenous injection, a dilute solution of fluorescein in the blood will absorb blue light at a peak of 480nm and emit it as green-yellow at a peak frequency of 530nm. By using appropriate filters on flash fundus photography the exciting blue light can be separated from the emitted light and the retinal and choroidal circulations studied. Dynamic studies of the passage of dye from the arterial to venous sides of the circulation in the two vascular beds are obtained. In the evaluation of optic disc swelling, true disc oedema can be distinguished from the pseudopapilloedema of buried optic disc drusen or elevated discs in hypermetropic eyes by demonstrating the presence of dilated capillaries on the disc surface during the arterial phase of the angiogram, and hyperfluorescence in the late

Table 3.1 Common indications for fluorescein angiography in neuro-ophthalmology

Clinical problem	Comment
Optic disc swelling	Distinction between true acquired pathological disc swelling of raised intracranial pressure or local disease and pseudopapilloedema of hypermetropic eyes, buried disc drusen and other anomalies
Unexplained optic neuropathy	Subtle or subclinical retinal vasculitis indicates an inflammatory cause (multiple sclerosis, sarcoidosis or Behcet's)
Unexplained visual acuity loss with a central scotoma	Subtle macular pathology (age related macular degeneration, branch retinal vein occlusion, retinal dystrophies) well demonstrated
Unexplained neuromuscular disease	Mild or severe forms of retinal pigment epithelial degeneration well shown in the mitochondrial myopathies (Kearns–Sayre syndrome)
Unexplained (aseptic) meningitis	Demonstration of choroidal abnormalities in the uveomeningeal syndromes (Vogt–Koyanagi–Harada syndrome)

venous phase. In addition, buried disc drusen may fluoresce without any injection of dye – a phenomenom known as autofluorescence; thus avoiding unnecessary imaging and cerebrospinal fluid (CSF) studies and sometimes shunting procedures as well. Further examples are given in Table 3.1 (see also Fig. 3.1).

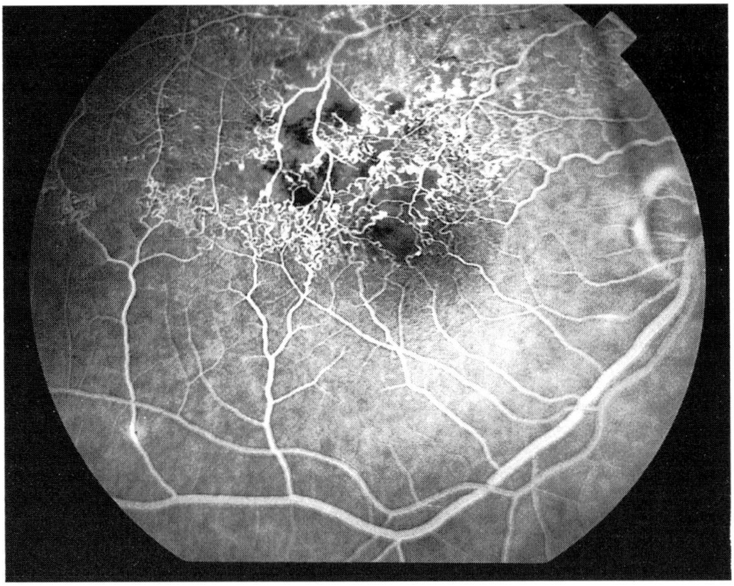

Figure 3.1 Microvascular changes in the paramacular circulation following a branch retinal vein occlusion.

It is important to remember that fluorescein angiography is an invasive study. Patients frequently experience nausea and occasionally vomit shortly after injection. They should be warned that the skin (but not the sclera) appears icteric for a few hours and that urine passed during this time will be fluorescent. Rarely, hypersensitivity reactions occur – probably due to the presence of macromolecular impurities because fluorescein itself has a low molecular weight and does not provoke an antigen–antibody reaction. This usually takes the form of urticaria and transient bronchospasm but may occasionally give rise to anaphylactic shock. Full resuscitation equipment is mandatory and the investigation is contraindicated in patients with a history of adverse reactions to radiological contrast media or asthma.

CLINICAL ELECTROPHYSIOLOGY

Psychophysical methods of acuity measurement, contrast function, motion detection, perimetry and colour vision all depend on a stimulus-response paradigm which is mediated by the subject's conscious understanding of the test, and certain assumptions must be made about the correlation of these stimulus-response properties to physiological events. The clinical electrophysiology of vision bypasses this area of theoretical and practical complexity and allows closer correlation with physiological functions (Plant, 1995). There is the added advantage of being suitable for the assessment of vision in preverbal children, and in neurologically impaired subjects. The chief disadvantage is the high degree of technical expertise required to give consistent results, and for this reason tests are used selectively (Fig. 3.2).

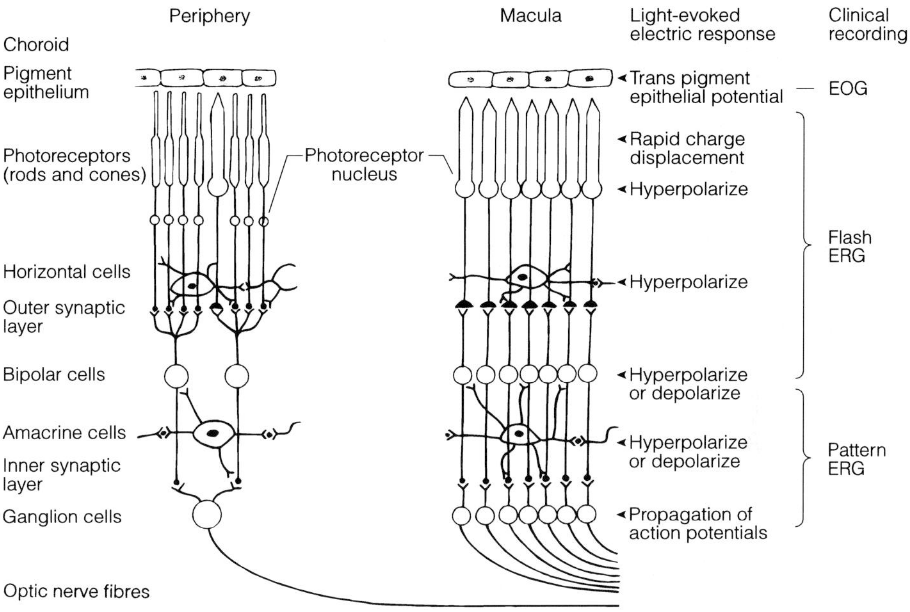

Figure 3.2 Electrophysiological recording of visual function.

VISUAL EVOKED POTENTIALS

Following repetitive visual stimulation using flashes of light or sudden changes in a grid pattern, a cortical potential is detectable which may be summated and averaged using microprocessors after repeated testing to yield the visual evoked cortical potential (VECR) or visual evoked response (VER). The VER reflects the integrity of the central visual field throughout the entire afferent visual system but is non-specific in localizing a lesion to the retina, optic nerve or cortex. The VER primarily represents the central visual field for the reason that most of the occipital cortex is concerned with the central 10 degrees, and also because the central field has the most posterior location in the cortex and is therefore the most detectable. A flash-generated VER is stimulated by luminance change while a pattern VER is stimulated by contrast change. The complex wave form is described in terms of amplitude and latency according to characteristics of the P_1 wave which is a large positive deflection occuring at around 100ms. Amplitude varies widely amongst normal subjects but latency is constant.

Pathological conditions of the anterior visual pathways yield relatively non-specific abnormalities of the VER, but the test is nonetheless useful especially when carried out in conjunction with flash and pattern generated electroretinograms (see below). Latency delay with relative amplitude preservation is found in demyelination, even long after the acute episode and following visual recovery and also in optic nerve compression. Amplitude reduction is a feature of ischaemic optic neuropathy and other conditions where axonal loss is prominent compared with conduction block (Halliday, 1976). By careful choice of stimulus parameters (check size and reversal speed in the pattern-generated VEP), the effects of optical blurring can be minimized and the test made sufficiently sensitive to be useful in those patients with moderate or minimal acuity loss. For example, the persistent latency changes of optic neuritis are best demonstrated and the effects of optical defocus minimized by using high contrast squares, each subtending 50 minutes of arc.

Additional specificity can be achieved by half field testing whereby differences in amplitude and latency recorded from each hemisphere after uniocular stimulation can be used to assess abnormalities of the optic chiasm. Further refinements in VER techniques, which are currently undergoing clinical evaluation, include differential testing of the parvo and magnocellular systems by use of test targets which selectively stimulate chromatic, temporal and spatial functions, and also the discrimination between striate, extrastriate and subcortical responses (Berninger, 1989). These are likely to be of value in the early detection of subclinical abnormalities such as glaucomatous optic neuropathy and in the assessment of residual vision in those with cortical visual impairment, especially children (Kriss, 1992).

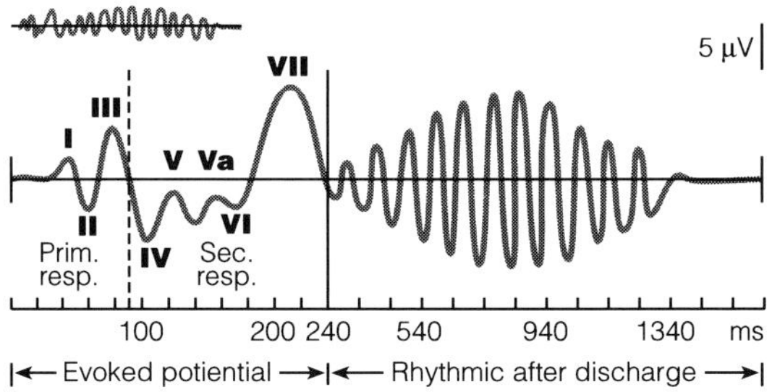

Figure 3.3 The flash visual evoked response.

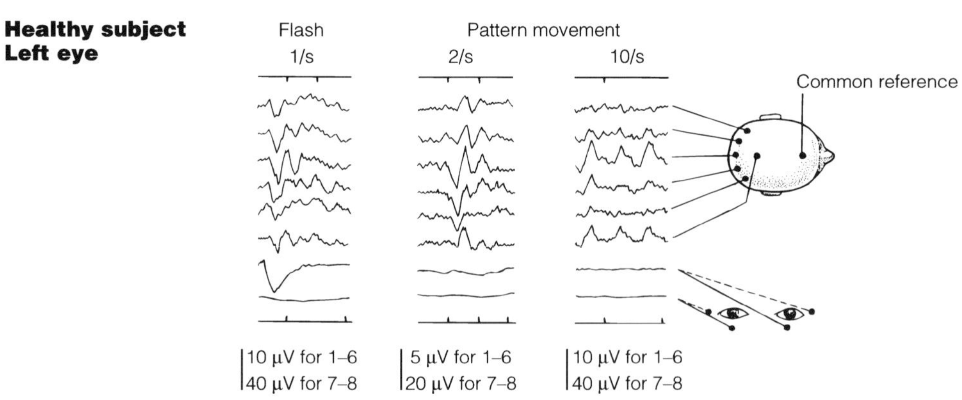

Figure 3.4 Flash and pattern visual evoked responses.

ELECTRORETINOGRAPHY

Stimulation of the eye with either a flash or a pattern reversal system results in a recordable potential from the retina which has two principle components: the a-wave which reflects the activity of the photoreceptors, and the b-wave which arises from the inner nuclear layer and the Müller cells (International Standardization Committee, 1989).

Disorders predominantly involving cones can be distinguished from those involving rods by performing the test in light (photopic) and dark (scotopic) conditions. In primary retinal diseases, such as diabetic retinopathy, pigmentary retinopathies and dystrophies, and in toxic degenerations, both the a-wave and the b-wave are abnormal. Exceptions to this are seen in central retinal artery occlusion where in the acute phase the photoreceptors which derive their blood supply from the choriocapillaries are preserved and therefore the a-wave persists while the b-wave is extinguished. Superimposed on the b-wave in a normal retina are a series of rhythmic oscillations referred to as oscillatory potentials which may be of diagnostic importance when lost in the early stages of both diabetic retinopathy and in pigmentary retinopathies. Recently it has been possible to demonstrate properties of the b-wave which may reflect abnormalities of post-photoreceptor processing (Sieving, 1994). When visual loss results from diseases which involve the ganglion cells or optic nerve such as Tay Sachs disease, glaucoma or optic neuritis, the electroretinograph (ERG) in response to flashes of light is usually normal. Only in advanced cases of retinal ganglion cell loss does the flash ERG become abnormal, as a result of secondary transsynaptic degeneration of outer retinal elements (bipolar cells and photoreceptors) (Fig. 3.5).

In practice, the clinician must distinguish between visual acuity loss of retinal and optic nerve origin. Sometimes, a pattern ERG (PERG) is useful. Just as the use of pattern reversal stimuli instead of flash offers greater sensitivity in the VEP, so it does with the ERG. Although the origins of the PERG are not entirely clear, it is accepted that the response does arise from retinal structures proximal to the photoreceptors, and it is this anatomical localization which, together with the fact that pattern reversal stimuli test the central retina only, gives the test its potential power (Plant, 1986). Unlike the flash ERG, the late components of the PERG are abnormal in optic nerve and retinal ganglion cell

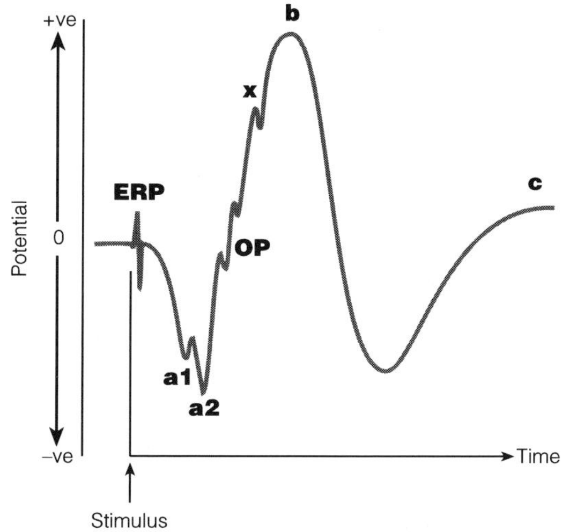

Figure 3.5 The flash electroretinograph.

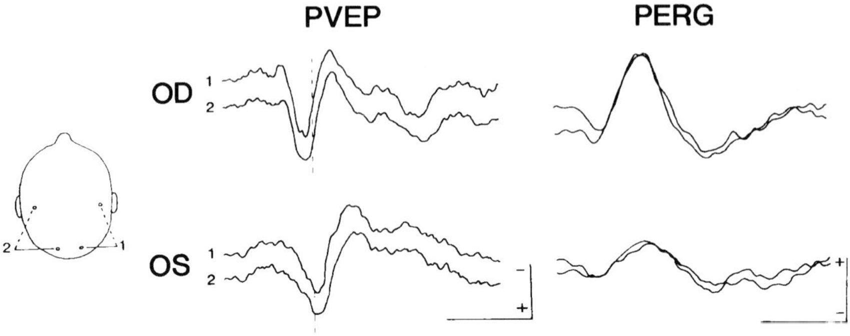

Figure 3.6(A) PERG and PVEP recordings in a 39-year-old male with moderate left visual impairment (acuity reduced to 6/12). The left eye PVEP shows a 20ms delay but the PERG shows a moderate P50 component abnormality in keeping with dysfunction distal to the optic nerve: the diagnosis was central serous retinopathy. (Courtesy of Dr G Holder.) (From Holder, 1989.)

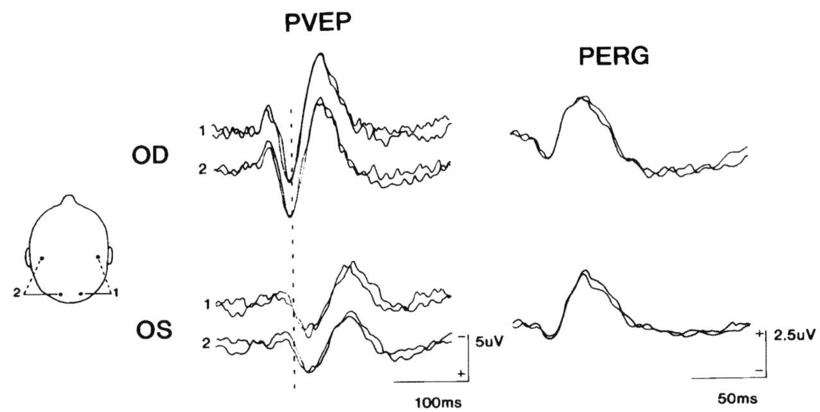

Figure 3.6(B) PERG and PVEP recordings in a 35-year-old male with asymptomatic optic disc pallor (normal acuities). Left eye PVEP markedly delayed; left eye PERG shows reduced N95 component consistent with retinal ganglion cell or nerve fibre loss. (Courtesy of Dr G Holder.) (From Holder, 1991.)

layer disorders. Therefore, the PERG may be of value in discriminating subtle cases of central visual loss of central retinal origin, when early and late components will be abnormal from visual loss of optic nerve origin when the late component alone is abnormal (Lorenz *et al.*, 1989; Holder, 1987; Ryan and Arden, 1988). Recent refinements in recording techniques may allow separation of chromatic and achromatic responses (Morrone *et al.*, 1994). Unfortunately, the technical difficulties associated with obtaining reproducible PERG results are considerable, and this useful investigation is not as yet widely available. By using specialized light projection systems it is possible to test cone function by projecting a spot stimulus to the fovea rather than across the entire field (ganzfeld) and foveal ERGs may develop as an alternative to the PERG. With the increasing recognition that subclinical abnormalities of retinal function may be of diagnostic importance in for example tapetoretinal degenerations and mitochondrial cytopathies, the use of electroretinography is likely to gain in importance in clinical neuro-ophthalmology (Figs 3.6 A,B).

ULTRASOUND, DOPPLER AND COLOUR DOPPLER FLOW MAPPING (COLOUR DOPPLER IMAGING)

Real-time B-mode ultrasound is an important alternative to computed tomography (CT) scanning in the examination of orbital structures, and in particular the anterior optic nerve where calcified buried drusen causing pseudopapilloedema (Fig. 3.7), and optic nerve sheath distension in chronic papilloedema can readily be demonstrated. Disc swelling due to local scleral or optic nerve sheath swelling can also be shown (scleritis and perineuritis), and also optic nerve calcification in cases where the distinction between meningioma and glioma is difficult (Attah, 1988).

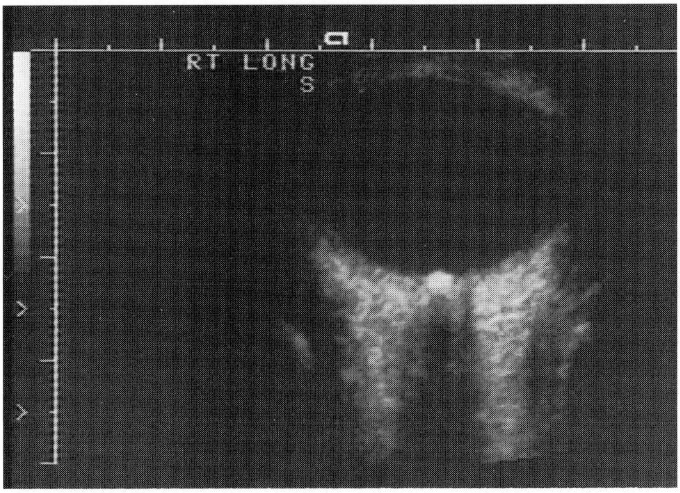

Figure 3.7 B-Mode ultrasound of optic nerve head showing calcific drusen.

However, it is in investigation of patients with vascular disease that sonographic methods have the most to offer. Although selective intra-arterial angiography may remain the definitive examination technique for extracranial carotid disease, these techniques have reached the point where non-invasive assessment is sufficiently accurate to be useful in screening for atherosclerotic disease, allowing the use of angiography, either by intravenous digital subtraction or by arterial cannulation, to be restricted to selected cases (Davies and Humphrey, 1993). Indirect tests of vascular patency such as simple Doppler imaging of directional blood flow have been superceded by direct B-mode ultrasonographic scanning of the vascular lumen and athersclerotic plaque. The duplex scanner combines simultaneous real-time B-mode arterial images and pulsed Doppler so that both lumen patency and flow velocity can be estimated. Interpretative caution is required however, as these methods do not allow the distinction to be made between a severe stenosis and complete occlusion, and there may be difficulties in distinguishing between internal and external carotid lesions in patients with a high bifurcation, and in obtaining adequate studies in the obese patient (Steinke *et al.*, 1990; Sellar, 1995) (Fig. 3.8). Other non-invasive tests of extracranial carotid function may also be useful, ranging from simple observation of central retinal artery patency as the intraocular pressure is raised in ophthalmodynanometry, to ocular suction cup devices in ophthalmo-pneumoplethysmography (Gee, 1985).

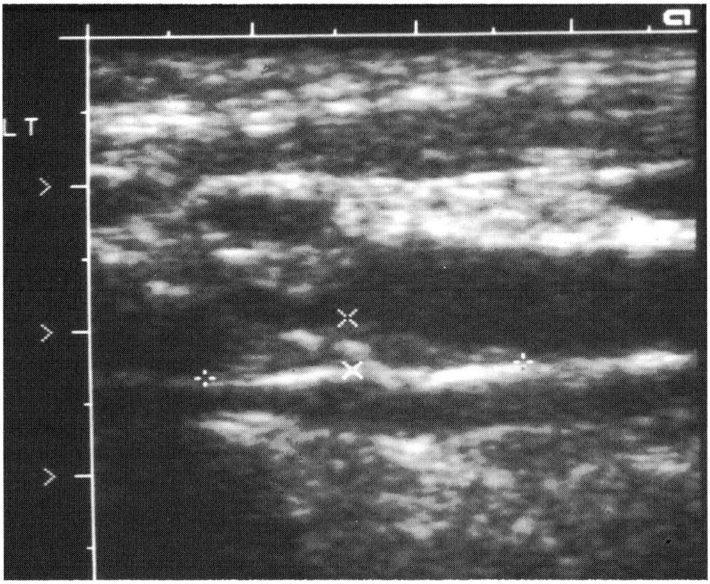

Figure 3.8 Duplex Doppler study of atherosclerotic carotid stenosis.

Colour Doppler flow mapping is a further refinement where the spatial and temporal distribution of the colour-coded Doppler signal can be visualized in real time and superimposed on a high resolution grey scale image of the tissue and vessel morphology. This has been applied to the study of extracranial carotid disease, but may be of greater clinical value in the assessment of vascular lesions of the cavernous sinus and orbit (Lieb *et al.*, 1991; Aburn and Sergott, 1993). The demonstration of reversed blood flow with an arterial wave form in the superior opthalmic vein is of diagnostic importance in patients with carotid-cavernous and dural fistulas, and is a parameter which can be used to monitor clinical progress (Flaherty *et al.*, 1991; Spector, 1991). In addition, reduced ophthalmic artery blood flow may be shown in cases where chronic ocular ischaemia complicates occlusive carotid disease. These developments have led investigators to study smaller and smaller vessels in the orbit and in particular the central retinal artery and the short posterior ciliary arteries which supply the choroid and retrolaminar optic nerve. However, reproducible results have been difficult to obtain as these vessels are multiple and there is considerable inter-individual variation in their disposition. In addition, the normal vascular lumen of a short posterior ciliary artery is too small to be measured by sonographic methods, so total blood flow measurements cannot reliably be obtained (Williamson *et al.*, 1993).

NEUROIMAGING

The use of imaging in the assessment of visual failure requires an appreciation of the complementary roles of magnetic resonance imaging (MRI) and CT, and in particular, an understanding of the contribution specific MRI strategies and sequences can make to the solution of specific clinical problems (Anderson, 1992; Kwan, 1990; Slamovits and Gardner, 1989). In general terms, MRI is preferrable to CT, with the following exceptions:

1) demonstation of bone lesions (fractures, neoplastic erosion) and dystrophic calcification
2) acute haemorrhage (blood invisible on MRI initially)
3) MRI contraindicated by cardiac pacemaker, transcutaneous neural stimulators, metallic intraocular foreign bodies and magnetic aneurysm clips
4) definition of orbital structures (unless surface coils and fat suppression techniques available).

Intravenous injection of contrast enhancing agents (iodinated compounds for CT and paramagnetic gadolinium for MRI) help the resolution of lesions associated with blood–brain barrier abnormalities or increased vasculature.

GLOBE

Magnetic resonance imaging is contraindicated by the possibility of a ferromagnetic foreign body, where torque created by the high magnetic field may dislodge the fragment and cause further intraocular damage. Titanium or cobalt-nickel retinal tacks, or intraocular lens loops made of platinum or titanium are not contraindications; CT is superior to MRI in retinoblastoma and astrocytic hamartoma because of the clinical importance of detecting intraocular calcification, but MR may be useful in the assessment of solid retinal detachment as the paramagnetic properties of melanin in choroidal melanoma lead to a bright signal T1-weighted images (Bloom *et al.*, 1992) (Fig. 3.9). B-mode ultrasound remains the investigation of choice in most other posterior ocular segment diseases where there is media opacity.

ORBIT

Routine brain CT scans do not give good orbital images, and in order to obtain these special head postioning is required. Coronal imaging is preferable, but on CT this requires the patient to lie prone with the neck extended, which may not be well tolerated. With this method, the bony orbital walls, rectus muscles and their relationship to the optic nerves may all be studied. Computer facilitated three-dimensional image reconstruction is valuable in the assessment of facial and orbital trauma. A CT scan will demonstrate the hyperostosis and calcification associated with a meningioma, and is suitable for the detection of both ferrous and non-ferrous foreign bodies with and without an acute haematoma. Also, CT effectively demonstrates orbital calcification, masses, the extraocular muscles, optic nerves and paranasal sinuses.

However, in a number of specific instances, MRI offers certain advantages especially when high resolution is facilitated by the use of fat signal suppression techniques and headcoils (Tien *et al.*, 1991). In cavernous haemangioma, the bright signal on T2 and hypo-intense signal of T1 sequences may allow radiographic distinction from a glioma or meningioma, which may be valuable where the lesion is at a site inaccessible to biopsy,

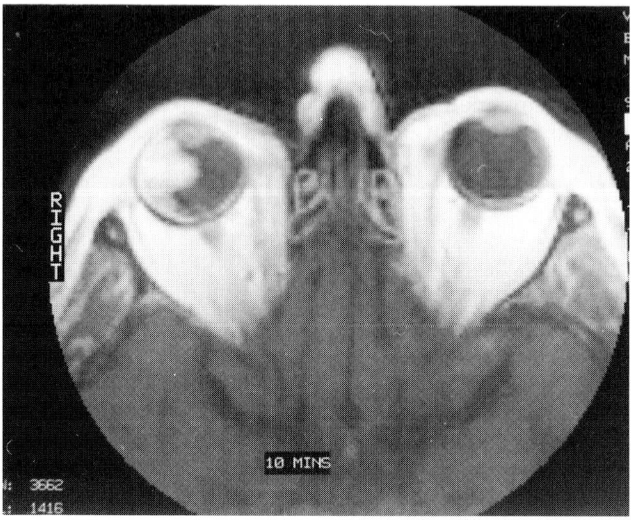

Figure 3.9 MRI of intraocular choroidal melanoma.

such as the orbital apex. It is known that MRI can identify feeder vessels in a lymphangioma prior to surgery and also distinguish fluid levels, septa and lobulated structures, reflecting the non-encapsulated structure of this lesion. The superior ophthalmic vein is well seen on contrast-enhanced CT and on MRI: sudden worsening in patients with carotid-cavernous fistula due to thrombosis of the superior ophthalmic vein may be indicated by a high signal on T1-weighted images.

In primary optic nerve sheath meningiomas, Gadolinium-enhanced MRI is superior to CT in evaluating intracanalicular and intracranial extension, and also in distinguishing perioptic tumour growth from distal cystic change. Fat-suppression T1-weighted imaging gives superior delineation of tumour surface adjacent to orbital fat, and demonstrates the tram-tracking sign characteristic of meningiomas by enhancing the contrast between tumour and the perineural subarachnoid space (Lindblom, 1992a, b; Zimmerman *et al.*, 1990a) (Fig. 3.10). In optic glioma, MRI can distinguish between perineural growth giving rise to arachnoid gliomatosis and a dilated patulous optic nerve sheath (Imes and Hoyt, 1991).

Inflammatory and neurodegenerative diseases of the optic nerve are also suitable for study with MRI (Table 3.2). Long areas of abnormal signal on fat-suppression short tau inversion (STIR) sequences in acute optic neuritis may correlate with poorer prognosis for visual recovery (Miller *et al.*, 1988; Blackwell and Beck, 1989). The absence of abnormal signals arising from the cortex and brain stem in Leber's hereditary optic neuropathy may help in the distinction from optic neuritis (Kermode *et al.*, 1989). Periventricular high signal lesions on T2-weighted sequences are also seen in ischaemic gliosis, and therefore may lose clinical significance in subjects over the age of 40 years. Transient gadolinium leakage reflecting breakdown of the blood–brain barrier is seen in sarcoid optic neuropathy and in the early stages of an episode of acute idiopathic optic neuritis (Guy *et al.*, 1992; Engelken *et al.*, 1992). Gadolium enhancement of a lesion which does not give rise to abnormal signal without the use of contrast is seen months after the onset of visual loss in radionecrosis of the anterior visual pathways (Zimmerman *et al.*, 1990b; Hudgins *et al.*, 1992).

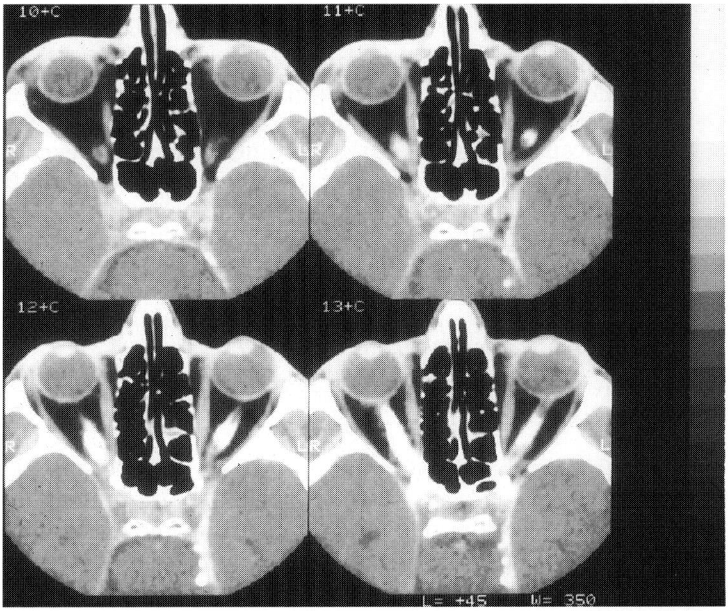

Figure 3.10 Optic nerve sheath calcification in bilateral meningioma on CT scan.

Table 3.2 Some MRI features of optic nerve disease

Intrinsic lesions	
Optic neuritis	Increased signal on fat-supression STIR sequences
Radionecrosis	Late gadolinium enhancement
Neurosarcoid	Meningeal enhancement associated with optic nerve signal
Optic glioma	Demonstration of perineural arachnoid gliomatosis
Extrinsic lesions	
Perioptic meningioma	Gadolinium enhancement and demonstration of intracranial extension in primary optic nerve sheath meningioma

SELLAR AND PARASELLAR REGION

Generally, MRI is preferable to CT in the assessment of lesions in the sellar and parasellar regions for the following reasons: direct coronal images may be more readily obtained, interruption or invasion of the flow voids in the cavernous sinus and carotid artery by disease processes allow detailed imaging, neurovascular-CSF interfaces are clearly shown, subacute haemorrhage in pituitary apoplexy is easier to demonstrate, and finally meningeal enhancement distinct from bone signal is readily seen. However, CT may supply additional information, for example detecting calcium in craniopharyngioma, hyperostosis in meningioma and bone distraction in nasopharyngeal carcinoma or metastases. Both MRI and CT may fail to detect pituitary microadenomas or to allow the distinction from other intrasellar lesions such as pars intermedia cysts (Hamed *et al.*, 1993).

POSTERIOR FOSSA

In studying the brain stem and cerebellum MRI offers advantages over CT because of the absence of beam hardening artifacts arising from the petrous ridge. However, MRI artifacts may arise from pulsatile blood flow in the carotids, jugular and torcula. Sagittal imaging from the mesencephalic junction to the foramen magnum is especially useful in patients with gaze palsies, internuclear ophthalmoplegia or nystagmus. Cryptic infratentorial arteriovenous malformations are well seen because of high signal arising from haemosiderin associated with previous overt or clinically silent haemorrhage. Also MRI may show aberrant vessels at the pontomedullary junction in hemifacial spasm and in some cases of trigeminal neuralgia: such patients may benefit from decompression surgery. Magnetic resonance angiography and three-dimensional MRI imaging are further refinements which are rapidly becoming available.

MAGNETIC RESONANCE ANGIOGRAPHY (MRA)

Selective intra-arterial angiography continues to set the gold standard for vascular imaging in the head and neck because of its excellent spatial resolution. However, the infrequent but real risks of vascular damage, adverse systemic reactions, transient and permanent neurological defects and even death have stimulated the development of alternative techniques. Intravenous contrast-enhanced digital subtraction angiography (DSA) is limited by the need to insert central venous catheters, by poor image quality, and by systemic reactions. Ultrasonographic methods are non-invasive but are highly operator dependent and limited in anatomical coverage because of the signal attenuating effects of bone and the inability to distinguish between tight stenosis and complete extracranial carotid occlusion (Sellar, 1995).

Magnetic resonance angiography is a non-invasive technique whereby it is possible to generate high contrast between stationary tissue and flowing blood by suitable manipulation of imaging parameters. Interpretation depends on a computerized depiction of data based on the haemodynamic properties of flowing blood rather than on actual vessel anatomy. Because of the physiology of blood flow, the diameter of vessels may sometimes appear smaller on MRA techniques than with conventional arteriography, primarily because of the slower laminar flow near the vessel wall. As a result, aneurysms and ulceration of atheromatous plaques may not be well seen. There are extracranial applications for MRA as an adjunctive method for the study of carotid occlusive disease and disections. Intracranial application include the study of dural and carotid-cavernous fistula (although conventional angiography is required to distinguish a direct carotid origin from one arising from a dural vessel, and to allow endovascular therapy), screening for intracranial aneurysms in high risk patients with positive family history, polycystic renal disease (Huston *et al.*, 1994; Litt, 1994), fibromuscular dysplasia and aortic coarctation, and in the detection of supratentorial arteriovenous malformations, and perhaps most importantly in the diagnosis of dural venous sinus obstruction by thrombus infiltration or compression (Fig. 3.11).

INTERVENTIONAL NEURORADIOLOGY

The endovascular therapy of central nervous system (CNS) vascular lesions has developed as the logical extension of refined diagnostic neuroangiography, employing advances in real-time imaging, new coaxial catheter systems, new embolic agents and balloon techniques. The principle conditions in neuro-ophthalmology in which these

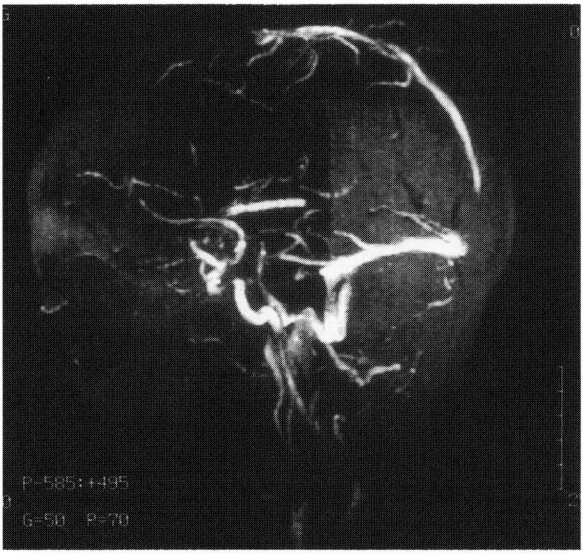

Figure 3.11 Venous study on MRA showing superior sagittal sinus occlusion.

methods are now important are direct carotid-cavernous fistula, dural arteriovenous fistulae involving the cavernous sinus, and intracranial aneurysms (Kupersmith *et al.*, 1984; Kwan, 1989; Higashida *et al.*, 1990; Vargas *et al.*, 1994). In addition, patients with supratentorial and infratentorial arteriovenous malformations may present to the ophthalmologist, or require ophthalmic follow-up. The majority of these procedures on adults are performed with sedation only, using a transfemoral approach for catheterization, and following anticoagulation with heparin. Transvenous approaches are reserved for patients with prior carotid ligation or other significant carotid pathology (Teng *et al.*, 1995).

There is now abundant evidence that in carotid cavernous fistulae of both traumatic and non traumatic origin the prognosis for vision is much improved by treatment with these methods when compared with direct carotid ligation procedures. Simple reduction of the arterial pressure on its own will exacerbate ocular ischaemia, and it is only by closing a fistula directly that the venous pressure in the eye and orbit can be reduced and normal perfusion gradients restored. Indirect dural arteriovenous fistula results in a less severe initial clinical picture with insidious onset, but there may still be considerable ocular morbidity. Selective and superselective catheterization of internal and external carotids bilaterally is required to assess the possibility of multiple feeder vessels and transarterial or transvenous embolization routes employed (Kupersmith *et al.*, 1986, 1988; Brosnahan *et al.*, 1992). The treatment of intracranial aneurysms by interventional methods is reserved for those unsuitable for surgical clipping. This applies in particular to giant intracavernous and carotid-ophthalmic aneurysms. A detachable balloon is used to either embolize an aneurysm or feeder vessels directly, or sometimes to occlude the internal carotid artery proximal to the neck of an aneurysm. Neuro-ophthalmic symptoms due to local cranial nerve compression resolve as the balloon induces intraluminal thrombosis and shrinkage.

REFERENCES

Aburn NS and Sergott RC (1993). Orbital colour Doppler imaging. *Eye* **7**: 639–647.

Anderson ML (1992). Imaging advances in neuro-ophthalmology. *Curr Opin Ophthalmol* **3**: 615–619.

Atta HR (1988). Imaging of the optic nerve with standard echography. *Eye* **2**: 358–366.

Berninger TA, Arden GB, Hogg CR and Franto T (1989). Separable evoked retinal and cortical potentials from each major visual pathway: preliminary results. *Br J Ophthalmol* **73**: 502–511.

Blackwell CL and Beck RW (1989). MRI in optic neuritis. (Letter) *Arch Ophthalmol* **107**: 789.

Bloom PA, Ferris JD, Laidlaw DA and Goddard PR (1992). Magnetic resonance imaging – diverse appearances of uveal malignant melanomas. *Arch Ophthalmol* **11**: 1105–1111.

Brosnahan D, McFadzean RM and Teasdale E (1992). Neuro-ophthalmic features of carotid cavernous fistulas and their treatment by endoarterial balloon embolisation. *J Neurol Neurosurg Psychiat* **55**: 553–556.

Davies KN and Humphry PR, (1993). Complications of cerebral angiography in patients with symptomatic carotid territory ischaemia screened by carotid ultrasound. *J Neurol Neurosurg Psychiat* **56**: 967–972.

Engelken JD, Yuh WTC, Carter KD and Nerad JA (1992). Optic nerve sarcoidosis: MR findings. *Am J Neuroradiol Res* **13**: 228–230.

Flaharty PM, Lieb W, Sergott RC *et al.* (1991). Color Doppler imaging: A new noninvasive technique to diagnose and monitor carotid cavernous sinus fisutulas. *Arch Ophthlamol* **109**: 522–526.

Gee W (1985). Ocular pneumoplethysmography. *Surv Ophthalmol* **29**: 276–292.

Guy J, Moa J, Bidgood D, Mancuso A and Quisling RG (1992). Enhancement and demyelination of the intraorbital optic nerve on fat suppression magnetic resonance imaging. *Ophthalmology* **99**: 713–719.

Halliday AM, Halliday E, Kriss A *et al.* (1976). The pattern evoked potential in compression of the anterior visual pathways. *Brain* **99**: 357–374.

Hamed LM, Silberger J, Silberger M *et al.* (1993). Magnetic resonance angiography of vascular lesions causing neuro-ophthalmic defects. *Surv Ophthalmol* **37**: 425–434.

Higashida RT, Halbach VV and Dowd C (1990). Endovascular detachable balloon embolisation therapy of cavernous carotid artery aneuysms: results in 87 cases. *J Neurosurg* **72**: 857–863.

Ho AC, Lieb WE, Flaharty PM *et al.* (1992). Color Doppler imaging of ocular ischaemic syndrome. *Ophthalmology* **99**: 1453–1462.

Holder GE (1987). Significance of abnormal pattern electroretinography in anterior visual pathway dysfunction. *Br J Ophthalmol* **71**: 166–171.

Holder GE (1989). Pattern electroretinography in patients with delayed pattern visual evoked potentials due to distal anterior visual pathway dysfunction. *J Neurol Neurosurg Psychiat* **52**: 1364–1368.

Holder GE (1991). The incidence of abnormal pattern electroretinography in optic nerve demyelination. *Electroenceph Clin Neurophysiol* **78**: 18–26.

Hudgins PA, Newman NJ, Dillon WP and Hoffman JC (1992). Radiation induced optic neuropathy: characteristic appearances on gadolinium enhanced MR. *Am J Neuroradiol* **13**: 235–238.

Huston J III, Nichols DA, Luetmer PH *et al.* (1994). Blinded prospective evaluation of sensitivity of MR angiography to known intracranial aneurysms: Importance of aneurysm size. *Am J Neuroradiol* **15**: 1607–1614.

Imes RK, Hoyt WF (1991). Magnetic resonance imaging of optic gliomas in neurofibromatosis I. *Am J Ophthalmol* **111**: 729–734.

International Standardization Committee of the International Society for the Clinical Electrophysiology of Vision (1989). Standard for clinical electroretinography. *Arch Ophthalmol* **107**: 816–819.

Kermode AG, Moseley IF and Kendall BE (1989). Magnetic resonance imaging in Leber's optic neuropathy. *J Neurol Neurosurg Psychiat* **52**: 1671–1674.

Kriss A and Russell-Eggitt I (1992). Electrophysiological assessment of visual pathway function in infants. *Eye* **6**: 145–153.

Kupersmith MJ, Berenstein A, Choi IS *et al.* (1984). Percutaneous transvascular treatment of giant carotid aneurysms: neuro-ophthalmologic findings. *Neurology* **34**: 328–335.

Kuppersmith MJ, Berenstein A, Flamm E and Ransohoff J (1986). Neuro-ophthalmic abnormalities and intravascular therapy of traumatic carotid cavernous fistulas. *Ophthalmology* **93**: 906–912.

Kuppersmith MJ, Berenstein A. Choi IS *et al.* (1988). Management of nontraumatic vascular shunts involving the cavernous sinus. *Ophthalmology* **85**: 121–130.

Kwan ES (1990). Radiologic evaluation of neuro-ophthalmic disease. *Curr Opin Ophthalmol* **1**: 484–498.

Kwan E, Hieshima GB, Higashida RT *et al.* (1989). Interventional neuroradiology in neuro-ophthalmology. *J Clin Neuro-Ophthalmol* **9**: 83–97.

Lieb WE, Flaharty PM, Sergott RC *et al.* (1991). Color Doppler imaging provides accurate assessment of orbital blood flow in occlusive carotid artery disease. *Ophthalmology* **98**: 548–552.

Lindblom B, Truwit CL and Hoyt WF (1992a). Optic nerve sheath meningioma. Definition of intraorbital, intracanalicular and intracranial components with magnetic resonance imaging. *Ophthalmology* **99**: 560–566.

Lindblom B, Norman D and Hoyt WF (1992b). Perioptic cyst distal to optic nerve meningioma: MR demonstration. *Am J Neuroradiol* **13**: 1622–1624.

Litt AW (1994). MR angiography of intracranial aneurysms: Proceed, but with caution. *Am J Neuroradiol* **15**: 1615–1616.

Lorenz R, Dodt E and Heider W (1989). Pattern electroretinogram peak times as a clinical means of discriminating retinal from optic nerve disease. *Doc Ophthalmol* **71**; 307–320.
Miller DH, Newton MR, van der Poel JC *et al.* (1988). Magnetic resonance imaging of the optic nerve in optic neuritis. *Neurology* **38**: 175–179.
Morrone C, Poriatti V, Fiorentini A and Burr DC (1994). Pattern reversal electroretinogram in response to chomatic stimuli: I. Humans. *Vis Neurosci* **11**: 861–871.
Plant GT (1995). Recent advances in the electrophysiology of visual disorders. *Curr Opin Ophthalmol* **6**: 54–59.
Plant G, Hess R and Thomas S (1986). The pattern evoked electroretinogram in optic neuritis. A combined psychophysical and electrophysiological study. *Brain* **109**: 469–490.
Ryan S and Arden GB (1988). Electrophysiological discrimination between retinal and optic nerve disorders. *Doc Ophthalmol* **68**: 247–255.
Sanders MD (1970). A classification of papilloedema based on a fluorescein angiographic study of 69 cases. *Trans Ophthalmol Soc UK* **89**: 177.
Sellar RJ (1995). Imaging blood vessels in the head and neck. *J Neurol Neurosurg Psychiat* **59**: 225–237.
Sieving PA, Murayama K and Naarndorp F (1994). Push-pull model of the primate optic electroretinogram: A role for hyperpolarising neurons in shaping the b-wave. *Vis Neurosci* **11**: 519–532.
Slamovits TL and Gardner TA (1989). Neuro-imaging in neuro-ophthalmology. *Ophthalmology* **96**: 555–568.
Spector RH (1991). Echographic diagnosis of dural carotid-cavernous sinus fistulas. *Am J Ophthalmol* **111**: 77–83.
Steinke W, Kloetzsch C and Hennerici M (1990). Carotid artery disease assessed by color Doppler imaging: correlation with standard Doppler sonography and angiography *Am J Neuroradiol* **11**: 259–266.
Teng MWH, Lirng J-F, Chang T *et al.* (1995). Embolisation of carotid-cavernous fistula by means of direct puncture through the superior orbital fissure. *Radiology* **194**: 705–711.
Tien RD, Chu PK, Hesselink JR and Szumowski J (1991). Intra and paraorbital lesions: value of fat suppression MR imaging with paramagnetic contrast. *Am J Neuroradiol* **12**: 245–253.
Vargas ME, Kupersmith MJ, Setton A *et al.* (1994). Endovascular treatment of giant aneurysms which cause visual loss. *Ophthalmology* **101**: 1091–1098.
Williamson, Baxter GM and Dutton GN (1993). Colour Doppler velocimetry of the arterial vasculature of the optic nerve head and orbit. *Eye* **7**: 74–80.
Zimmerman CF, Schatz NJ and Glaser JS (1990a). Magnetic resonance imaging of optic nerve meningiomas. *Ophthalmology* **97**: 585–591.
Zimmerman CF, Schatz NJ and Glaser JS (1990b). Magnetic resonance imaging of radiation optic neuropathy. *Am J Ophthalmol* **110**: 389–394.

4

Retinal disorders in neuro-ophthalmology

RETINAL DYSTROPHIES AND DEGENERATIONS

The terms retinitis pigmentosa, pigmentary retinopathy tapeto-retinal degeneration and retinal dystrophy are often used interchangeably to describe degenerative disease of the outer retina (photoreceptors and/or retinal pigment epithelium). The process may be confined to the retina or may be a manifestation of a systemic process with neurological consequences in addition to visual loss. Secondary degeneration (pseudoretinitis pigmentosa) arises as a consequence of inflammation, toxic agents, ischaemia and trauma. The clinical picture is of bilateral symmetrical chronic progressive visual failure with constricted fields, waxy disc pallor (often with hyaline bodies or disc drusen), attenuated retinal arteries and 'bone spicules' of abnormal pigment deposits in the peripheral fundus (Fig. 4.1). In typical cases the visual fields may be reduced to a 5 degree arc tunnel with preserved central acuity as rod photoreceptors are destroyed while the cones at the fovea are relatively preserved. Such patients will be especially incapacitated

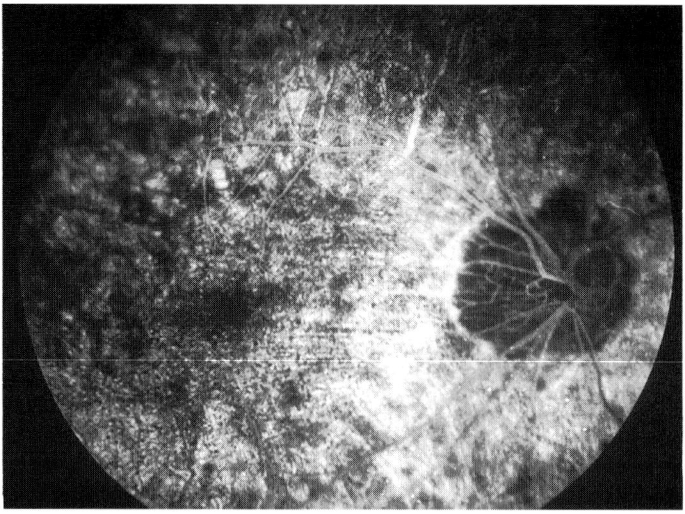

Figure 4.1 Fundus fluorescein angiogram showing advanced retinal pigment epithelial degeneration in Kearns-Sayre syndrome.

in scotopic conditions (night-blindness). Other variants include cone-rod dystrophies in which central macular, colour and high acuity vision are destroyed first giving rise to central scotomata, nystagmus and a bull's eye macular appearance. In other instances, pigmented spicules are absent and there is diffuse mottling of the retinal pigment epithelium ('salt and pepper retinopathy'). In some cases, white spots appear across the fundus, limited sectors of the retina appear to be involved, or the retina may appear to be clinically normal in spite of severe loss of function. The aetiology is usually genetic with autosomal dominant, autosomal recessive, X-linked and mitochondrial patterns of inheritance all occurring. The diagnosis of retinal photoreceptor degeneration can often be made clinically, but fundus fluorescein angiography and electrodiagnostic testing (visual evoked potential: VEP; and electroretinograph; ERG) are essential for a full characterization of the phenotype (Pagon, 1988; Newsome, 1988). The ERG is especially helpful in elucidating those cases where the clinical appearances do not necessarily match the degree of visual loss.

With the advent of modern molecular genetics, numerous gene defects have been reported to be associated with retinal photoreceptor dysfunction — principally within the genes for rhodopsin and peripherin (Rosenfeld *et al.*, 1994). Much of the classification of the retinal dystrophies and degenerations given here appears in standard texts but certain topics require special attention.

VOLUNTARY MUSCLE DISEASE AND RETINAL PHOTORECEPTOR DEGENERATION (see Table 4.2)

Kearns-Sayre syndrome

The Kearns-Sayre-syndrome is a subset of chronic progressive ophthalmoplegia (CPEO) with onset before the age of 20 years, progressive ophthalmoplegia, retinal degeneration and at least one of the following: cardiac conduction abnormalities, elevated cerebrospinal fluid (CSF) protein, or cerebellar dysfunction. Deletion of segments of mitochondrial DNA have been implicated in the pathogenesis of this condition. Over 90% of patients with Kearns-Sayre syndrome will have mitochondrial DNA deletions on

Table 4.1 Classifications of retinitis pigmentosa

By electrophysiology
Typical retinitis pigmentosa
Cone-rod dystrophy
By mode of inheritance
Autosomal dominant
Autosomal recessive
X-linked recessive
Mitochondrial transmission
By clinical appearance (Ripps, *et al.*, 1987)
Typical retinitis pigmentosa
Aytpical retinitis pigmentosa
• sine pigmenta
• puncta albescens
• inversus
• pericentral and central
• sectoral
By age of onset (Schroeder *et al.*, 1987)
Congenital (Leber's hereditary amaurosis)
Childhood onset
Juvenile onset
Adult onset

Table 4.2 Typical patterns of retinal involvement in selected neurodegenerative syndromes

Retinal involvement	Neurodegenerative syndrome
1.Typical retinitis pigmentosa	Abetalipoproteinaemia (Bassen-Kornsweig disease) Refsum's disease, Charcot-Marie-Tooth disease
2. 'Salt-and-pepper' retinopathy without typical bone spicules	Kearns-Sayre syndrome Usher's syndrome
3. Cone-rod dystrophy with predominantly central acuity loss	Olivocerebellopontine degeneration type III Harding type 2 autosomal dominant spinocerebellar
4. Isolated optic atrophy or disc swelling	Krabbe's disease Mucopolysaccharidosis II – Hunter's disease

skeletal muscle biopsy but the proportion falls to 50% in those with mitochondrial disease and CPEO only. There is a poor correlation between the size or site of deletion and the clinical profile. In the majority of cases, family members are not affected and deletions are not found in muscle biopsies of the proband's parents. In such sporadic cases the deletion is likely to occur during embryogenesis (Fig. 4.1).

A 'salt-and pepper' retinopathy reflecting retinal pigment epithelial degeneration is most frequently encountered with fine pigment dusting throughout the fundus rather than the the appearance of classical bone spicules. Fluorescein angiography is helpful to confirm subtle changes. The ERG is a sensitive indicator of subclinical retinal involvement. Rarely, pigmentary retinopathy may be a manifestation of mitochondrial diseases such as MELAS (mitochondrial myopathy, encephalopathy, lactic acidosis and stroke-like episodes) in which CPEO does not occur (Mullie *et al.*, 1985; Holt *et al.*, 1990; Harding, 1993). In both Becker and Duchenne-type muscular dystrophy, scotopic ERG abnormalities are characteristic, and overt macular degeneration has also been reported (Sigismund *et al.*, 1994).

SPINOCEREBELLAR DEGENERATIONS

In Harding type 2 spinocerebellar degeneration, visual symptoms consist of bilateral blurring and reduced central visual acuity, without poor night vision, and the ERG initially shows abnormalities of the photopic response. This reflects the predominant cone involvement of this disease process (Enevoldsen *et al.*, 1994; Grouw *et al.*, 1994).

TOXIC RETINAL DEGENERATIONS

Retinal degeneration is seen in association with long-term medication with phenothiazines (thioridazine, chlorpromazine), amiodarone, tamoxifen and chloroquine. Large daily doses of tamoxifen (> 80 mg) are strongly associated with retinal degenerative changes but this effect is only rarely seen in patients receiving the current standard dose of 20 mg daily. With regard to chloroquine, there are significant differences in safe doses between the base and its salts.

Ocular toxicity is very unlikely with doses of less than 4 mg per kg lean body weight per day of chloroquine phosphate and the equivalent doses for sulphate and base forms are 3.2 mg/kg/day and 2.4 mg/kg/day respectively. Very few cases of toxicity have been reported when the total dose of phosphate has been less than 300 g (Moorsman *et al.*, 1990).

Hydroxychloroquine is a much less likely cause of retinal toxicity: retinal damage is highly unlikely if the daily dose is less than 6.5 mg/kg/day of sulphate, or if the cumulative dose does not exceed 200 g. Unfortunately there are no clinical features of diagnostic tests which can reliably detect the retinopathy at a reversible stage although field loss to a red target at 4 to 9 degrees from fixation may be the most sensitive index of early problems.

PARANEOPLASTIC RETINAL DEGENERATIONS; CANCER ASSOCIATED RETINOPATHY AND MELANOMA ASSOCIATED RETINOPATHY

The chief symptomatic complaint in cancer associated retinopathy (CAR) is of bizarre entoptic phenomena — intermittent spontaneous shimmering lights, floaters or flashing lights, together with declining vision and field defects. Typically a ring scotoma develops from arcuate defects and fundoscopy shows conspicuous retinal arterial narrowing. The ERG is often helpful, and an autoimmune pathogenesis based on the presence of anti-photoreceptor antibodies has been implicated. The search for infective and toxic aetiologies is negative and within a few months remote cancer is discovered (Berson and Lessell, 1988; Chung and Selhorst, 1992; Jacobson *et al.*, 1990; Thirkill *et al.*, 1987; Alexander *et al.*, 1992).

RECENTLY DESCRIBED SPECIFIC IDIOPATHIC RETINAL DEGENERATIONS; ACUTE ZONAL OCCULT OUTER RETINOPATHY (AZOOR); BIG BLINDSPOT SYNDROME; MULTIPLE EVANESCENT WHITE DOT SYNDROME

AZOOR and related conditions are idiopathic syndromes of rapid visual loss of one or more large zones of outer retinal function, photopsia, minimal fundoscopic abnormalities together with electroretinographic abnormalities affecting one or both eyes predominantly in young women. Fluorescein angiography in the acute stages is normal. One variant of AZOOR is the acute idiopathic blindspot enlargement syndrome (AIBSES) in which the dense scotomas are concentrated around the normal blindspot. In another variant there are fundal abnormalities in the acute phase: the multiple evanescent white dot syndrome (MEWDS) is associated with the appearance of rapidly fading white outer retinal lesions and vitreous haze at the time of visual loss. On follow-up the field defects and photopsia persist and areas of retinal pigment epithelial atrophy develop. The

Table 4.3 Differential diagnosis of retinitis pigmentosa (pseudoretinitis pigmentosa)

Inflammatory conditions
Intrauterine infection with rubella, cytomegalovirus, syphilis
Toxic
Thioridazine
Chlorpromazine
Chloroquine
Tamoxifen
Uniocular
Trauma
Diffuse unilateral subacute neuroretinitis (DUSN)
Paraneoplastic retinopathies
Cancer associated retinopathy
Melanoma associated retinopathy
Specific idiopathic retinal degenerations
Acute zonal occult outer retinopathy (AZOOR)
Big blindspot syndrome
Multiple evanescent white dot syndrome (MEWDS)

differential diagnosis includes retrobulbar neuritis, retrochiasmal visual disturbance, CAR and diffuse unilateral subacute neuroretinitis (Fletcher *et al.*, 1988; Gass, 1993; Hamed *et al.*, 1989; Miller, 1977; Singh *et al.*, 1991).

UVEOMENINGEAL SYNDROMES

INFLAMMATORY INTRAOCULAR AND INTRACRANIAL DISEASE

The uveomeningeal syndromes are a mixture of diseases with shared involvement of retina, uveal tract (choroid, ciliary body and iris) and brain. In some cases the presentation may be with neurological abnormalities and the ocular features may be asymptomatic and only discovered on careful examination after pupillary dilation; in others the presentation may be with visual loss but there is a relatively asymptomatic CSF pleocytosis. Idiopathic inflammatory disease is the most common cause of this group in current UK hospital practice, amongst which neurosarcoidosis, Behçet's disease, multiple sclerosis and the Vogt–Koyanagi–Harada syndrome are the most noteworthy (Mann and Katz, 1992; Rosenbaum, 1989).

SARCOIDOSIS

Sarcoidosis is a systemic disease of unknown aetiology characterized by the presence of non-caseating granulomata together with an increased number of T-helper/inducer cells in peripheral blood. The eye is involved in 25% of cases while thoracic disease (hilar adenopathy, lung parenchymal involvement) is present in over 75%. Extrathoracic disease of skin and joints is frequent but sarcoidosis of the nervous system (neurosarcoid) is relatively uncommon occurring in only 5% of cases. Neurosarcoidosis can involve cranial and peripheral nerves, the meninges and brain and spinal cord parenchyma resulting in mixed combinations of peripheral and cranial neuropathies, encephalopathy, meningitis and seizures. Involvement of the visual pathways can cause visual acuity loss and field defects. Anterior pituitary insufficiency, hypothalamic syndromes and diabetes insipidus can also occur; 20% of cases of posterior uveitis due to sarcoidosis are associated with central nervous system (CNS) disease (Stern, 1985).

Active ocular disease in the presence of undiagnosed systemic involvement is common and is the presenting mode in 20% of all cases. Anterior uveitis (typically acute granulomatous iritis) arises most commonly but 30% of ocular sarcoid is confined to the posterior ocular segment. The vitreous body, choroid and optic nerve can all be involved by granulomatous infiltration and the retina shows characteristic periphlebitis (vasculitis). Keratoconjunctivitis sicca mimicking Sjörgren's syndrome is the consequence of lacrimal gland damage, often with associated enlargement.

The diagnosis of neurosarcoidosis often rests with the ophthalmological findings supported by evidence of systemic disease (abnormal chest X-ray, gallium scan, elevated serum angiotensin converting enzyme (ACE) levels, cutaneous anergy, positive Kveim test and pulmonary function tests). Histological confirmation of non-caseating granulomas is invaluable, and conjunctival biopsy may have a yield of 40–50% when suspicious nodular lesions are present; this may avoid the requirement for either a Kveim test which takes 6 weeks to perform and more invasive biopsy (liver, endobronchial, mediastinal). Management is based on immunosuppression titrated against clinical indices of disease activity (Gass, 1976; Jabs and Johns, 1986; Delaney, 1977; Brod, 1990).

BEHÇET'S DISEASE

In Behçet's disease the protean manifestations include ocular, neurological and systemic features. Ocular involvement occurs in 70–85% of patients, including iridocyclitis with hypopyon, focal retinitis, retinal vein occlusions with vasculitis and ischaemic optic neuropathy. Neurological features include meningoencephalitis with CSF pleocytosis, dural sinus thrombosis and focal lesions of cortex, cerebellum and brain stem. Systemic Behçet's classically consists of orogenital ulceration, arthritis and dermatoses together with superficial and deep venous thrombosis. Recently purely neuro-ophthalamic Behçet's ('Behçet's MINUS' — *M*ultiple *I*ntermittent *N*eurological episodes with *U*veitis *S*yndromes) has been described (Lueck *et al.*, 1993). The natural history is of relapse and remission with a gradual downhill course which may be ameliorated by immunosuppression (Barnes, 1984; International Study Group, 1990).

VOGT–KOYANAGI–HARADA SYNDROME

The Vogt–Koyanagi–Harada syndrome comprises a pan-uveitis with neurological and dermatological abnormalities. The ocular abnormalities typically include serous retinal detachment and small creamy white peripheral fundal lesions together with inflammatory cells in anterior chamber and vitreous. Neurological changes include symptoms of meningeal inflammation, CSF pleocytosis, cranial neuropathies and specific features of VIIIth nerve involvement (dysacusis and tinnitus). Changes in the skin include poliosis, viteligo and alopecia. It is interesting to note that the focal fundal lesions bear resemblances to the Dalen Fuchs nodules of sympathetic ophthalmia, and that the cochlea shares certain melanosomal structures with the retinal pigment epithelium, suggesting that the pathogenesis may be an organ-specific autoimmune process Current therapy is based on steroid-sparing immunosuppression titrated against clinical features of disease activity (Chan, 1988; Johnson, 1990; Wright *et al.*, 1978; Moorthy *et al.* 1995).

ACUTE MULTIFOCAL PLACOID PIGMENT EPITHELIOPATHY

Acute multifocal placoid pigment epitheliopathy (AMPPE) is a related ocular disease in which multiple pale yellow-white placoid subretinal lesions are seen across the posterior fundus. The disease may be unilateral or bilateral and an overlap with the Vogt–Koyanagi–Harada syndrome may be seen with associated serous retinal detachment and meningism. The differential diagnosis includes sarcoidosis, syphilis, Lyme disease and tuberculosis (Frohman *et al.* 1987; Kirkham *et al.*, 1972).

Table 4.4 The uveomeningeal syndromes

Infectious causes
Syphilis, TB, Fungi
CMV, Varicella, HSV
Idiopathic inflammatory
Behçet's,
Sarcoid,
Vogt-Koyanagi-Harada syndrome
Multiple sclerosis
Acute multifocal posterior pigment epitheliopathy (AMPPE or placoid)
B-Cell lymphoma and paraneoplastic syndromes

THE PHAKOMATOSES IN NEURO-OPHTHALMOLOGY

The phakomatoses have generated intense interest in this modern era of molecular genetics because as familial cancer syndromes they serve as models for the genetic regulation of tumour growth. The following account emphasizes the ocular and neuro-ophthalmic features, the presence of which may be of great clinical significance. Genetic counselling has assumed greater importance as a part of management and screening for ophthalmic involvement as a standard element in the management of individuals who are first degree relatives of affected patients.

NEUROFIBROMATOSIS (NF) TYPES 1 AND 2

It is now recognized that although they have overlapping features, including a propensity to neurofibromas and tumours of the CNS, NF1 and NF2 are separate diseases which map to separate chromosomes — 17 for NF1 and 22 for NF2. Developmental hamartomas arise in both types (Narod *et al.*, 1992; Ragge, 1993; Gutman and Collins, 1992).

NF1 is the most common with a frequency of about 1 in 3000. The gene has 100% penetrance but variable expression; NF1 is inherited as an autosomal dominant trait but about 50% of new cases are considered to be new mutations. The diagnostic criteria for NF1 are met if a person has two or more of the following:

1) six or more café-au-lait spots over 5 mm in greatest diameter in prepubertal individuals and 15 mm in postpubertal individuals.
2) two or more neurofibromas or one plexiform neuroma.
3) axillary or inguinal freckles
4) optic glioma
5) two or more Lisch nodules
6) distinctive osseous lesions (e.g. sphenoid dysplasia)
7) a first degree relative with NF1.

Ocular features of NF1 include iris hamartomas — Lisch nodules or melanocytic naevi which are detectable in about 50% of 5-year-olds, 75% of 15-year-olds and 95–100% of adults over 25 years. Individuals with NF1 may also have congenital glaucoma, anterior subcapsular cataract, posterior segment hamartomas, retinal vascular occlusions (Moadel *et al.*, 1994) and pulsating exophthalmos due to sphenoid dysplasia. Retinal and choroidal hamartomas are occasionally seen (Savino *et al.*, 1977), but these are a more typical feature of NF2. Controversy continues as to whether the optic gliomas of NF1 are benign hamartomas or true neoplasms (see Chapter 4) and the results of long-term follow-up and analysis are awaited. Spinal cord tumours including intramedullary astrocytomas and neurofibromas may cause significant CNS morbidity. The gene for NF1 is located in the long arm of chromosome 17 — band q11.2. Within this gene is an area coding for a GAP-like protein which may act as a growth regulator interacting with an oncogene to produce benign and occasionally malignant tumours. The unpredictability of disease severity even in the same NF1 gene mutation makes genetic counselling exceedingly difficult.

Neurofibromatosis 2 is a much rarer disease than NF1 with a population incidence of 1 in 33 000 to 1 in 40 000. At least 50% of new cases appear to be new mutations. Like NF1, NF2 has an extremely high penetrance. The hallmark of NF2 is the presence of bilateral vestibular nerve schwannomas (Fig. 4.2): diagnostic criteria are met if a person has either of the following:

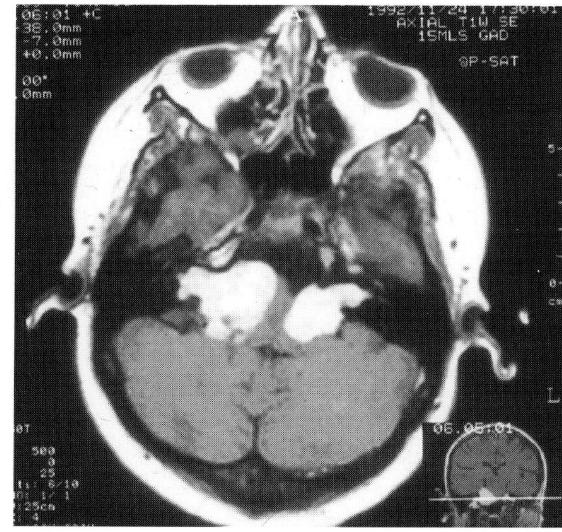

Figure 4.2 MRI scan of posterior cranial fossa showing bilateral vestibular schwannomas in NF2.

1) bilateral VIIIth nerve masses seen with appropriate imaging
2) a first degree relative with NF2 and either unilateral VIIIth nerve mass or one of the following:

- neurofibromas
- meningioma
- glioma
- schwannoma
- juvenile posterior subcapsular lenticular opacity

Patients with NF2 tend to develop tumours of neural converings and sheaths — meningiomas including optic nerve sheath meningiomas, schwannomas, ependymomas whereas those with NF1 tend to develop neural or astrocytic tumours — astrocytomas and gliomas. Although presentation is typically the result of hearing loss, more than 75% of patients with NF2 have premature visual loss as a result of cataract, and occasionally optic nerve sheath meningioma. Other ocular findings include combined retinal pigment epithelial and retinal hamartomas, epiretinal membranes, optic disc gliomas, retinal haemangiomas, medullated nerve fibres, choroidal naevi, uveal melanoma, and choroidal hamartoma. Lisch nodules are occasionally seen.

The NF2 gene is located on chromosome 22q band 11.2. The same genetic locus may be responsible for the sporadic tumours of the type seen in NF2. In sporadic forms of the disease the vestibular schwannomas develop at a later age and may occur unilaterally.

VON HIPPEL-LINDAU DISEASE

Von Hippel-Lindau (VHL) disease is a pleiotrophic autosomal dominant inherited familial cancer syndrome characterized by a predisposition to develop haemangioblastomas of CNS and retina, renal cell carcinoma, phaeochromcytoma and renal, pancreatic and epididymal cysts. The minimum birth incidence in the UK is 1 in 36 000. The gene for VHL disease has been mapped to chromosome 3p25-p26, and the clinical importance lies in the fact that long-term morbidity and mortality can be reduced by presymptomatic diagnosis of ocular, CNS and renal involvement.

Although clinical heterogeneity is common, retinal angiomatosis is the most frequent initial manifestation and develops in more than 70% of patients by the age of 60 years. Retinal haemangiomas (or more correctly, haemangioblastomas) are most commonly seen in the peripheral retina but may also occur on the optic disc and at the ora serrata (Figs 4.3, 4.4). Ophthalmological screening requires dilated direct and indirect fundoscopy together with fluorescein angioscopy for the detection of nascent, preclinical lesions (Maher *et al.*, 1990, 1991; Moore *et al.*, 1991; Richards *et al.*, 1993).

Current criteria for diagnosis are: no family history and two of the following features:

1) retinal or CNS haemangioblastoma
2) phaeochromocytoma
3) renal cell carcinoma
4) renal / pancreatic / epididymal cysts;

or a positive family history and one of the above features.

Current screening recommendations in an affected individual are:

1) annual physical examination and urinalysis including VMAs
2) annual ophthalmological examinations
3) brain imaging 3-yearly to age 50, then 5-yearly
4) annual renal ultrasound and 3-yearly abdominal CT scanning.

When screening of an at-risk relative is required, this protocol is modified so that the eyes are examined from the age of 5 years (with fluorescein angioscopy from age 10), brain imaging is undertaken 3-yearly from the age of 15 to 40 and then 5-yearly, and abdominal imaging is commenced from age 20.

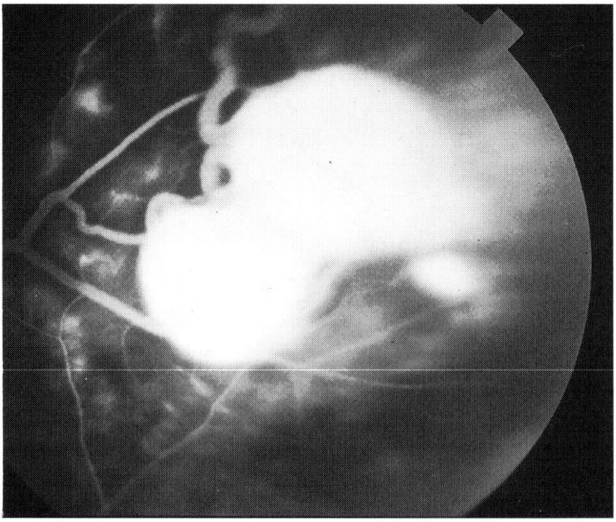

Figure 4.3 Fundus fluorescein angiogram appearances of a large retinal angioma in von Hippel–Lindau disease.

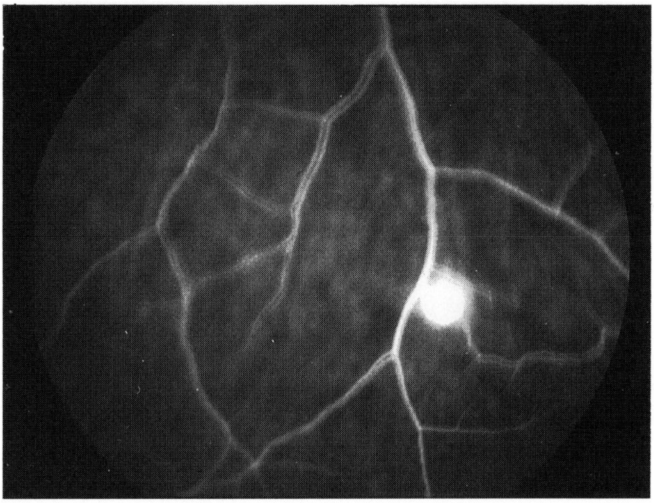

Figure 4.4 Subclinical von Hippel–Lindau retinal angiomas.

TUBEROSE SCLEROSIS

The triad of epilepsy, retinal tumours and adenoma sebaceum referred to as tuberose sclerosis or Bourneville's disease has now been widened and the term tuberose scelerosis complex (TSC) is applied. All tissues are involved, most typically brain and retina but also skin, heart, kidneys and lungs. Inherited as an autosomal dominant trait, TSC shows marked genetic heterogeneity. It appears that different families may have different mutations; in some pedigrees the mutation location is at chromosome 9q34.1-q34.2 and in others it is at 11q14-q23. Diagnosis is based on the presence of (Johnson and Gomez, 1991):

1) cortical tubers, or
2) multiple hamartomas associated with cortical tubers:

- subependymal nodules
- facial angiofibromas
- renal angiomyofibroma
- cortical tubers
- giant cell astrocytomas
- retinal hamartoma
- ungual fibroma
- fibrous forehead plaque

Retinal or optic nerve hamartomas are found in 50% of patients: other ocular abnormalities include adenoma sebaceum on the eyelids and colobomas. A wide range of neuro-ophthalmic features including retrochiasmal field defects, ocular motility abnormalities and papilloedema reflect intracranial involvement (Fig. 4.5). The retinal hamartomas may be calcified or non-calcified lesions of both glioblastic and angioblastic origin — patches of focal congenital retinal pigment epithelial hypertrophy may also be seen. In contrast to von Hippel Lindau disease, retinal hamartomas in TSC are only rarely associated with visual loss. The differential diagnosis of non-calcified hamartomas includes retinoblastoma in infants, and calcified hamartomas on the optic nerve may

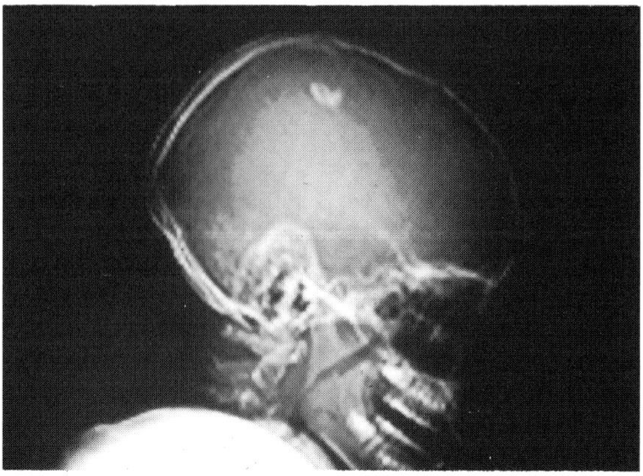

Figure 4.5 Scout CT scan showing intracranial calcification in tuberose sclerosis.

resemble florid calcified peripapillary disc drusen seen in retinitis pigmentosa (Altman *et al.*, 1988; Zimmer Galler and Robertson, 1993).

ENCEPHALO-TRIGEMINAL ANGIOMATOSIS (STURGE–WEBER SYNDROME)

Sturge–Weber is a further vascular neurocutaneous syndrome classed with the phakomatoses, but which unlike von Hippel–Lindau disease, does not appear to have a familal basis. Facial cavernous angiomas are commonly found in the distribution of the ophthalmic division of the trigeminal nerve. Intracranial calcifying occipitoparietal leptomeningeal angiomata on the same side as the facial lesion result in underlying cortical abnormalities with epilepsy, homonymous hemianopia and, in some cases, mental retardation. Ipsilateral ocular involvement is characteristic with glaucoma and haemangiomas of choroid, conjunctiva and episclera arising in over half of all cases. In other patients, asymptomatic retinal vascular tortuosisty and iris heterochromia have been noted (Sullivan *et al.*, 1992). Some patients have isolated facial or intracranial lesions.

RETINAL VASCULAR DISEASE

RETINAL TIAs AND STROKES

Transient monocular blindness (amaurosis fugax) and acute monocular visual failure are usually the result of temporary or permanent occlusion of the central or branch retinal arteries or of the blood supply to the optic nerve head.

Transient monocular blindness

This term is used to cover a variety of symptoms, including typical amaurosis fugax in which the patient reports the drawing of a black veil across the visual field vertically, horizontally or obliquely to extinguish vision either completely or in a hemifield and lasting for a period of 1 to 10 minutes. Complete recovery follows in about 15 to 20 minutes with gradual clearing in a reverse direction. The precise local anatomical and pathophysiological mechanisms underlying this evolution of events are not well understood. This history is strongly suggestive of the passage of an embolism across the retinal circulation resulting in an initial proximal occlusion of either the central retinal artery or one of its main branches before breaking up and dispersing into the periphery. The differential diagnosis of transient visual loss becomes much narrower if these details can be elicited — in particular the monocular nature and the time course. By contrast, transient visual loss due to raised intracranial pressure with papilloedema is typically very fleeting, with momentary monocular or binocular fading of vision on coughing, Valsalva manoeuvre or sudden postural change. Sometimes benign orbital tumours present with gaze evoked amaurosis in which vision is lost only when the eye turns in a particular direction as a result of intraorbital ophthalmic artery compression. Stuttering visual loss in which field or acuity fade, partially recover and then fade again suggests the onset of ischaemic optic neuropathy, whilst a more sustained gradual fading of vision particularly after exposure to bright light with positive visual phenomena is indicative of retinal ischaemia arising from chronic hypoperfusion (Furlan *et al.*, 1979).

Table 4.5 Conditions associated with transient monocular blindness

Intraocular
Glaucoma (intermittent angle closure causing corneal oedema)
Anterior ischaemic optic neuropathy
Intraorbital (mass effect causing gaze evoked amaurosis)
Haemangioma
Meningioma
Intracranial
Raised intracranial pressure (visual obscurations)
Carotid artery
Thromboembolism
Stenosis and occlusion
• arteritis
• fibromuscular dysplasia
• dissecting aneurysm
• radiation angiopathy
Cardiac
Valvular emboli
• calcific aortic stenosis
• endocarditis
• mitral valve prolapse
Mural thrombosis
• cardiac dysrhythmias
• postinfarction
Atrial myxoma
Miscellaneous
Migraine
Paradoxical embolism

Central retinal artery (CRA) occlusion

Sudden painless blindness is the presenting symptom of a CRA occlusion unless a cilioretinal artery is present to supply blood to the macula. Examination of the pupils confirms a relative afferent pupil defect, and the ophthalmoscopic appearances depend upon how soon after the onset of symptoms the examination is performed. In the first few minutes 'cattle-truck' segmentation of the venous blood column is seen with arterial attenuation. Mild digital pressure on the globe will induce segmentation of the arterial blood column confirming slow circulation. In ophthalmic artery occlusion the intraocular pressure is reduced. After an hour or so the ischaemic retina developes a white appearance with a cherry-red spot at the fovea due to the normal red colour of the choroid showing through the small area with a deficiency of the neurosensory retina. Within a few days the cherry-red spot and retinal opacification disappears leaving optic atrophy and retinal artery attenuation.

Five causes of central retinal artery occlusion are described:

1) embolic obstruction
2) occlusion *in situ* in association with atheroma with superimposed thrombosis or haemorrhage
3) inflammatory arteritis e.g. temporal arteritis
4) vasospasm e.g. migraine
5) arterial occlusion secondary to low perfusion pressure in carotid stenosis, aortic arch syndrome or iatrogenic globe compression.

Amaurosis fugax as a premonitory symptom of CRA suggests an embolic cause. In patients under 40 years of age, the heart is the most common source, due to rheumatic valve disease, mitral valve prolapse, endocarditis, or atrial myxoma and careful cardiological assessment is essential. When standard echocardiography is negative, a transoesophageal study may be helpful. In older patients the source may be cardiac or arterial from atheromatous ulceration of the aorta or ipsilateral internal carotid artery.

Although irreversible damage to the retina occurs after 2–4 hours, prompt initial treatment may help to restore at least some degree of vision. This should include ocular massage to lower the intraocular pressure and help dislodge an embolus into the peripheral retinal circulation, CO_2 rebreathing and intravenous Diamox. Paracentesis may be of value if the patient presents immediately. Heparin anticoagulation may be helpful in impending CRA occlusion and high dose corticosteroids are indicated if giant cell arteritis is suspected. As a general rule, when a CRA is due to giant cell arteritis, co-existing features of ischaemic optic neuropathy (pallid disc swelling with flame haemorrhages are likely to be present (Wilkinson and Russell, 1972). This applies even if visible emboli are not present. In giant cell arteritis the elastic lamina of the ophthalmic artery is involved in 90% of cases and as 90% of the ocular blood supply flows into the posterior ciliary vessels to supply the disc and choroid it is unusual for a patient with this condition to develop a central retinal artery occlusion without also having a disc infarction.

Branch retinal artery (BRA) occlusion

The lodging of an embolus at a first or second order bifurcation of the CRA results in a branch retinal artery occlusion, producing an area of pallid retinal oedema and sudden and permanent loss of the corresponding visual field. Emboli can often be seen in the fundus: the most common form is a fibrinplatelet Hollenhorst plaque derived from an ulcerated atheromatous cartotid artery plaque. Other materials include calcific deposits from a cardiac valve or atheromatous plaque, amniotic fluid, fat in pancreatitis and long bone fractures, and foreign bodies such as talcum powder in intravenous drug abusers. Sometimes asymptomatic emboli are discovered: these patients should be treated as though they were at the same risk of stroke as those with visual loss.

Reducing the risk of cerebral hemisphere stroke in CRA and BRA

To reduce the risk of stroke (Savino *et al.*, 1977; Howard and Russell, 1987; Hankey *et al.*, 1991; Poole and Russell, 1985), all patients are evaluated for associated hypertension, cardiac disease, arterial vascular disease and the presence of antiphospholipid antibodies. The fact that there are abundant data to suggest that the annual risk of cerebral hemisphere stroke is less (about 3%) after amaurosis fugax than after a cerebral hemisphere transient ischaemic attack (TIA) (about 6%) does not alter the need to investigate all patients with amaurosis thoroughly. The most likely explanation for the discrepancy in figures is not that amaurosis is somehow a more benign condition, but simply that in the retinal circulation relatively small embolic events are much more likely to be symptomatic than in the cerebral circulation. A carotid bruit may be heard, but its absence does not necessarily mean normal vessels.

Doppler ultrasonography of the carotid bifurcation is widely used and together with duplex imaging of the lumen and plaque dimensions provides useful non-invasive data on the degree of stenosis, the presence of calcification and ulceration, and haemodynamic abnormalities across the stenotic lesion. There are, however, a number of limitations to this technique which mean that many patients require angiography as well (see Chapter 3). First, the technique is very operator-dependent and distinguishing external and internal carotids in patients with fat necks may be difficult. Second, there are difficulties in distinguishing a very tight stenosis from a complete occlusion, and third, the clinically significant lesion may not always be at the bifurcation but may lie distally in the region of the foramen lacerum. However, a normal, technically satisfactory study does seem to exclude a significant lesion at the bifurcation.

With respect to angiography, intravenous digital subtraction angiography and magnetic resonance angiography provide alternatives to direct arterial puncture techniques with less morbidity but less resolution. Selective arterial angiography remains the gold standard investigation, and it was on this technique that the important collaborative studies on carotid endarterectomy were based. It is evident that only those patients with a stenosis occluding between 70 and 99% of the vascular lumen are significantly less likely to develop a cerebral hemisphere stroke if they undergo endarterectomy as opposed to optimal medical management with antiplatelet agents. Patients with symptomatic carotid stenosis of less than 30% do not appear to benefit from surgery and do just as well with optimal medical therapy (careful management of hypertension and use of anti-platelet agents) (Hass *et al.*, 1989). The selection of patients for endarterectomy must also depend on the assessment of risk of death from coronary artery disease which usually is also present, and on the morbidity and mortality of angiography and surgery at the centre offering treatment. The important consequence of these studies is that in practice only a minority of patients who present with retinal TIA (amaurosis fugax), retinal strokes (artery occlusions) or cerebral hemisphere TIAs will definitely be helped by endarterectomy. The results of trials determining the benefits for endarterectomy in patients with moderate (30–70%) stenosis are awaited with interest (Trobe, 1987; Warlow, 1984; North American Symptomatic Carotid Endarterectomy Trial Collaborators, 1991; European Carotid Surgery Trial Collaborative Group, 1991; Easton and Wilterdink, 1994; Streifler *et al.*, 1995).

The diagnostic approach to patients with amaurosis fugax or retinal artery occlusion who do not appear to have carotid disease leads to other possiblities, although it is important to emphasize that the absence of visible emboli in the retinal circulation does not rule out an embolic source. The ophthalmic artery may serve as a local origin of embolus and local vasospasm or retinal migraine may accompany a migraine attack or may occur in a person with a strong history of migraine. There are isolated documented accounts of reversible spasm of the retinal arteries in these cases. The diagnosis is always one of exclusion in otherwise well young adults or children. Usually recovery is full after each attack, but permanent visual loss may follow either from retinal artery occlusion and retinal infarction, or from ischaemic optic neuropathy.

There are also reports of retinal artery occlusion in patients who are normotensive and have the lupus anticoagulant or anti-cardiolipin antibodies. These procoagulant defects usually arise in association with systemic lupus erythematosis (SLE) but are occasionally found in isolation and should always be considered in the differential diagnosis of retinal artery occlusion and stroke in younger patients (Acheson *et al.*, 1991; Greaves, 1993). Sterile (Libmann-Sacks) endocarditis may also be a source of embolic disease in SLE. All patients with carotid disease should have an electrocardiogram to assess the possibility of additional ischaemic heart disease and patients who do not have carotid lesions will normally have standard two-dimensional echocardiography to study the possibility of occult valvular heart disease.

Recently, the technique of transoesophageal echocardiography has been introduced and is said to offer increased visualization of the mitral valve and facilitate diagnosis of mitral valve prolapse and of persistent patency of the foramen ovale which may dispose towards paradoxical embolus (Klötzsch, 1994). However, it should be noted that asymptomatic mitral valve prolapse and minor ostium secundum defects of the foramen ovale are common and that transoesphageal echocardiography is an invasive technique with associated morbidity. Therefore the use of this technique and the evaluation of the clinical significance of these minor cardiac lesions in the pathogenesis of retinal or cerebral TIAs must be governed by the clinical assessment of the patient by a cardiologist.

In addition to the antiphospholipid antibody syndromes, retinal arterial occlusion without detectable embolization or hypertension has also been reported to occur in Wegener's granulomatosis, Goodpasture's syndrome, and in Loeffler's eosinophilic syndrome (Sanders, 1987). In primary idiopathic retinal arteritis, otherwise well young patients suffer recurrent branch artery occlusions without associated systemic disease (Gass *et al.*, 1986; Johnson *et al.*, 1994). In other patients there is associated encephalopathy, white and grey matter infarcts on MRI, CSF pleocytosis and elevated protein with bilateral hearing loss — a constellation known as Susac's syndrome (Susac, 1994).

VENOUS STASIS RETINOPATHY AND CHRONIC OCULAR ISCHAEMIA

Chronic severe ocular ischaemia may produce a constellation of symptoms, beginning initially with venous stasis retinopathy in the posterior pole and progressing to anterior segment abnormalities (Riordan-Eva *et al.*, 1994) (Table 5.6).

The retinal changes are not specific to carotid disease and may also be seen in patients with other disease processes which interfere with the oxygen carrying capacity of blood in the retinal circulation, such as blood dyscrasias, hyperviscosity syndromes and severe anaemia. The patient may complain of mild to severe blurring of vision and of dazzling in bright light which may relect photoreceptor hypoxia. Diabetic retinopathy and

Table 4.6 Ocular findings with venous stasis retinopathy and ischaemic oculopathy

Venous stasis retinopathy
Dot and blot retinal haemorrhages
Microaneurysms
Venous congestion
Irregular calibre of retinal veins
Neovascularization
Macular oedema
Mid disc swelling
Diffuse oculopathy
Iris/angle neovascularization
Intraocular pressure change
Corneal oedema
Uveitis
Sluggish pupillary light reactions
Episcleral vascular congestion

central retinal vein occlusion may share overlapping features reflecting the common retinal response to ischaemia. In slow flow retinopathy marked asymmetry in retinal involvement is frequent and large blot haemorrhages may be prominent. In central retinal vein occlusion conspicuous hamorrhages and nerve fibre layer infarcts (cotton wool spots) cause a 'blood and thunder retina' (Duker and Brown, 1989; Duker *et al.*, 1990). The CRA pressure is often very low and ophthalmoscopy may reveal either spontaneous arterial pulsation or readily induced pulsation on the lightest pressure applied to the patient's eye. There is no specific therapy but spontaneous resolution can occur when the underlying cause of retinal hypoxia is relieved (Knox, 1965; Chawluk *et al.*, 1988; Carter, 1985; Ross-Russell and Ikeda, 1986; Russell and Page 1983).

Typically there is occlusion of at least one, and marked stenosis of the remaining, common carotid or vertebral arteries as collateral circulations to the ophthalmic artery via the circle of Willis and even the external carotid can provide adequate supply. Aortic arch and distal internal carotid atherosclerotic lesions are typical. In such patients a steal phenomenon whereby blood is redirected away from the eye to brain may contribute to the clinical picture. When neovascularization develops, retinal ablation therapy may be indicated to try to prevent the development of thrombotic (rubeotic) glaucoma. The visual prognosis in established ischaemic oculopathy is very poor, and the role of extracranial and extracranial–intracranial surgical bypass procedures to improve cerebral cortical perfusion remains controversial. Ischaemic uveitis is unresponsive to topical steroids.

CAROTID–CAVERNOUS FISTULAS

When communications arise between the carotid artery and the venous circulation in the cavernous sinus the venous pressure in the globe and orbit rises and the arterial perfusion pressure falls, resulting in a major drop in perfusion pressure (Kwan *et al.*, 1989). Fistulas may be classified as:

direct / indirect
traumatic / spontaneous
high flow / low flow

or by anatomical configuration on angiography:

- type A: intracavernous carotid artery — cavernous sinus
- type B: extradural branches of internal carotid — cavernous sinus
- type C: extradural branches of external — cavernous sinus
- type D: extradural branches of both internal and external carotid — cavernous sinus

Most commonly, direct fistulas (type A) have a high flow and indirect (types B-D) have low flow.

Direct carotid cavernous fistulas

Direct fistulas may be located anywhere along the course of the intracavernous carotid artery and may project anteriorly or posteriorly. The most common cause is head trauma which may be either penetrating or non-penetrating, and is not necessarily associated with basal skull fracture. Symptoms may not develop for days or weeks after the initial injury. Sometimes a fistula results from spontaneous rupture of a pre-existing aneurysm of the intracavernous carotid artery which may previously have been asymptomatic. Less commonly they arise spontaneously against a background of systemic vasculopathy such as arteriosclerosis and hypertension or fibromuscular dysplasia (Kupersmith *et al.*, 1986; Keltner *et al.*, 1987).

Clinical features

If blood escapes posteriorly through the superior and inferior petrosal sinuses the ocular signs may be minimal, although a lateral rectus palsy is frequently seen as the VIth nerve is compressed by an expanded inferior petrosal sinus. Anterior redirection of arterial blood through normal orbital venous channels leads to ocular manifestations due to raised episcleral venous pressure, reduced arterial perfusion pressure and venous stasis. The eye involved is not always ipsilateral to the site of the fistula as there are variable connections between the two cavernous sinuses and bilateral ocular signs may arise from the same lesion. Proptosis is occasionally pulsatile with associated chemosis and arterialization of the conjunctival vessels. A bruit may be heard by the patient or may only be detected on ausculation. When pulsation and a bruit are absent, the diagnosis is strongly suggested by a wide pulse pressure on applanation tonometry. Pulsatile exophthalmos is also sometimes seen in orbital arteriovenous malformations which may only be disguished from carotid cavernous fistula by neuroimaging studies. Pulsation is most evident in patients with NF1 who have congenital defects of the sphenoid bone but in this case there is no bruit or chemosis. Corneal damage may result from exposure due to proptosis, neuropathic ulceration from loss of function of the ophthalmic division of the trigeminal nerve or from anterior ocular segment hypoxia (see above).

Diplopia is common: this is a result of a number of mechanisms acting either in isolation or in combination. First, in trauma patients the ocular motor nerves may be damaged by a basal skull fracture. Second, the nerves may be compressed by the fistula in the cavernous sinus or become hypoxic due to alterations of blood flow in the vasa nervorum. Most commonly the abducens nerve is involved, probably because of its location within the cavernous sinus. Third, orbital hypoxia and oedema with venous stasis results in ophthalmoplegia due to direct myopathic effects (Leonard *et al.*, 1984). By the same mechanisms the pupil may be abnormal due to intraocular hypoxia or as a result of damage to sympathetic and parasympathetic fibres.

Visual loss is also common in patients with direct carotid-cavernous fistula (Sanders and Hoyt, 1969). Sometimes this is the result of ischaemic optic neuropathy, intracranial optic nerve compression or corneal ulceration, but typically is due to retinal ischaemia. This is due to both a reduction in retinal blood flow as a result of a drop in effective ophthalmic artery perfusion pressure together with venous stasis caused by arterialization of the orbital venous circulation. Ophthalmoscopy reveals features of a slow flow retinopathy with mild disc swelling, blot haemorrhages and microaneurysms and venous congestion and tortuosity. A picture of full-blown central retinal vein occlusion may develop; other patients have non-rhegmatogenous retinal detachments and vitreous haemorrhage.

A further mechanism for visual loss is glaucoma. This is usually due to raised episcleral venous pressure with a delayed and insidious onset, but neovascular (rubeosis) and ciliary block mechanisms may also apply in a more acute context.

Diagnosis and treatment

Untreated, most patients will have progressive ocular abnormalities and eventual blindness in one or both eyes. There are also small risks of subarachnoid and intracerebral haemorrhage. Management has been much improved by the use of selective endovascular manouvres using flow-guided detachable balloons to occlude the fistula (Figs 4.6 and 4.7). The diagnosis is ideally made by non-invasive imaging with angiography using selective arterial techniques to confirm the anatomical abnormalities and allow treatment all in the same session. A direct carotid cavernous fistula is normally clinically obvious, but pathological expansion of the superior ophthalmic vein may readily be seen on orbital ultrasound, CT and MRI. There is evidence that expansion of the superior ophthalmic vein represents a compensatory response to abnormal orbital blood flow and that patients in whom this is not seen may be at greater risk of ocular ischaemia. Colour Doppler flow mapping may be used very effectively to show flow reversal and arterialization in the superior ophthalmic vein, as well as showing that clinical deterioration may be a result of further venous obstruction from thrombosis rather than increased fistula flow.

The object of treatment is ideally to close the fistula and maintain patency of the distal carotid artery. Carotid occlusion may result in cerebral hemisphere ischaemia and in worsening ocular and orbital hypoxia ultimately resulting in ischaemic necrosis of lids, orbit and globe. Currently detachable flow-guided balloons are used to close most direct carotid cavernous fistulas. The balloon may be introduced into the cavernous sinus arterially via the internal carotid but sometimes this is not possible due to a previous surgical occlusion of the carotid or a very tortuous anatomical course. In this case the cavernous sinus may be reached by a venous route through the femoral vein and inferior petrosal sinus or via an orbitotomy and the superior ophthalmic vein. In selected cases thrombogenic coils are detached in the cavernous sinus. Following successful fistula closure ocular and orbital abnormalities will slowly reverse but may never fully resolve. Endovascular techniques may be associated with transient cerebral hemisphere

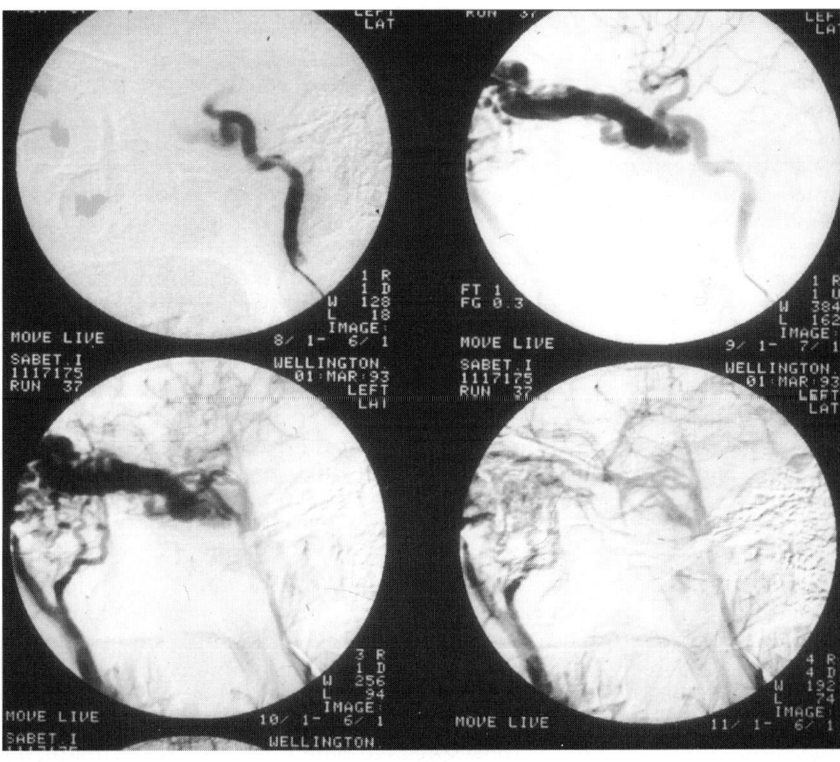

Figure 4.6 Filling of superior ophthalmic vein in direct carotid cavernous fistula on angiography.

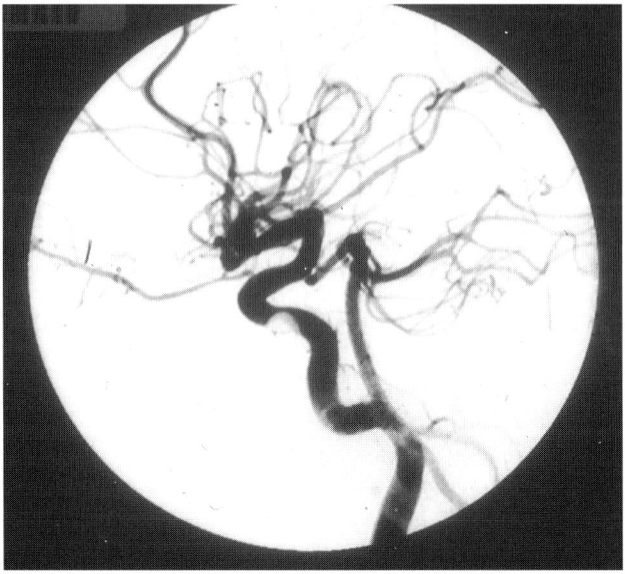

Figure 4.7 Normal appearance after endovascular occlusion.

ischaemia and a low risk of stroke but represent a great advance compared with direct surgical measures in terms of both safety and efficacy.

Indirect carotid cavernous fistulas (types B-D)

The indirect carotid cavernous fistulas are thought generally to arise from congenital arteriovenous anomalies which become symptomatic in later life in association with other vascular disorders such as hypertension and atherosclerosis. The clinical manifestations again depend on whether drainage from the cavernous sinus is mainly posterior or anterior. Posterior drainage into the petrosal sinuses results in cranial neuropathies; anterior drainage into the orbital circulation produces a syndrome similar to that of direct fistula but in a milder form. There may be no bruit, but mild proptosis and lid swelling, arterialization of the conjunctival vessels, and an abducens nerve palsy strongly suggest the diagnosis. Intraocular pressure is raised due to raised episcleral venous pressure and fundoscopy shows mild retinal vein dilation. In more advanced cases with higher flow rates, the clinical picture becomes indistinguishable from a direct fistula.

Between 20 and 50% of dural carotid cavernous fistulas close spontaneously — and sometimes after angiography. In those with a persistent fistula there may be eventual visual loss due to glaucoma or to retinal vasculopathy. Sometimes the clinical picture of orbital congestion may dramatically worsen but this does not necessarily indicate increased flow and may instead reflect thrombosis of the superior ophthalmic vein, demonstrable on MRI or with colour Doppler flow-mapping techniques. Treatment is therefore indicated in selected cases only. Because indirect fistulas most commonly have feeder vessels from both internal and external carotid arteries, either unilaterally or bilaterally, endovascular therapy is most effective when performed in conjunction with selective arteriography of both internal and external carotids bilaterally (Kupersmith *et al.*, 1988). Some patients with slow flow shunts and gross orbital ischaemia may defy interventional angiographic treatment.

REFERENCES

Acheson JF, Gregson R, Merry P and Schulenburg WE (1991). Vaso-occlusive retinopathy in the primary anti-phospholipid antibody syndrome. *Eye* **5**: 48–55.

Alexander KR, Fishman GA, Peachey NS *et al.* (1992). On response defect in paraneoplastic night blindness and cutaneous malignant melanoma. *Invest Ophthalmol Vis Sci* **33**, 477–483.

Altman NR, Purser RK and Post MDJ (1988). Tuberous sclerosis: Characteristics at CT and MR imaging. *Radiology* **167**: 527–532.

Barnes CG (1984). Behçet's syndrome. *J R Soc Med* **77**: 816–818.

Berson EL and Lessell S (1988). Paraneoplastic night blindness with malignant melanoma. *Am J Ophthalmol* **106**: 307–311.

Brod RD (1990). Presumed sarcoid choroidopathy mimicking birdshot retinochoroidopathy. *Am J Ophthalmol* **109**: 357–358.

Carter JE (1985). Chronic ocular ischaemia and carotid vascular disease. *Stroke* **16**: 721–728.

Chan CC (1988). Relationship between sympathetic ophthalmia, phacoanaphylactic endophthalmitis, and Vogt-Koyanagic-Harada disease. *Ophthalmology* **95**: 619–624.

Chawluk JB, Kushner MJ, Bank WJ *et al.* (1988). Atherosclerotic carotid artery disease in patients with retinal ischaemic syndromes. *Neurology* **38**: 858–863.

Chung SM and Selhorst JB (1992). Cancer associated retinopathy. In *Neuro-Ophthalmology in Systemic Disease* (ed. B Katz), Ophthalmology Clinics of North America, Vol. 5(3), pp. 587–596. Philadelphia: WB Saunders.

Crofts JW, Bachynski BN and Odel JG (1988). Visual paraneoplastic syndrome associated with undifferentiated enometrial carcinoma. *Can J Ophthalmol* **23**: 128–232.

Delanaey P (1977). Neurologic manifestations in sarcoidosis: review of the literature, with a report of 23 cases. *Ann Intern Med* **87**: 336–345.

Duker JS and Brown GC (1989). Neovascularisation of the optic disc associated with obstruction of the central retinal artery. *Ophthalmology* **96**: 87–91.

Duker JS, Margaral LE and Stubbs GW (1990). Quadrantic venous-stasis retinopathy secondary to an embolic branch retinal artery obstruction. *Ophthalmology* **97**: 167–170.

Easton JD and Wilterdink JL (1994). Carotid endarterectomy: Trials and tribulations *Ann Neurol* **25**: 5–17.

Enevoldsen TP, Sanders MD and Harding AE (1994). Autosomal dominant cerebellar ataxia with pigmentary macular dystrophy. *Brain* **117**: 445–460.

European Carotid Surgery Trialist Collaborative Group MRC European Carotid Surgery Trial (1991). Interim results for symptomatic patients with severe (70–99%) or mild (0–29%) carotid stenosis. *Lancet* **337**: 1235–1243.

Fletcher WA, Imes RK, Goodman D and Hoyt WF (1988). Acute idiopathic blind spot enlargement: a big blind spot syndrome without disc oedema. *Arch Ophthalmol* **106**: 44–49.

Frohman LP, Klung R, Bileory L *et al.* (1987). Acute posterior multifocal placoid pigment epitheliopathy with unilateral retinal lesions and bilateral disc edema. *Am J Ophthalmol* **104**: 548–550.

Furlan AJ, Whisnant JP and Kearns TP (1979). Unilateral visual loss in bright light. An unusual symptom of carotid artery occlusive disease. *Arch Neurol* **36**: 675–676.

Gass JDM (1989). Retinal causes of the big blind spot syndrome (editorial). *J Clin Neuro-Ophthalmol* **9**: 144–145.

Gass JDM (1993). Acute zonal occult outer retinopathy. *J Clin Neuro-Ophthalmol* **13**: 79–97.

Gass JDM and Olson CL (1976). Sarcoidosis with optic nerve and retinal involvement. *Arch Ophthalmol* **94**: 945–950.

Gass JDM, Tiedeman J and Thomas MA (1986). Idiopathic recurrent branch retinal arterial occlusions. *Ophthalmology* **93**: 1148–1157.

Greaves M (1993). Coagulation abnormalities and cerebral infarction. *J Neurol Neurosurg Psychiat* **56**: 433–439.

Grouw LG, Digre KB, Harris CP *et al.* (1944). Autosomal dominant cerebellar ataxia with retinal degeneration: Clinical, neuropathologic and genetic analysis of a large kindred. *Neurology* **44**: 1441–1447.

Gutman DH and Collins FS (1992). Recent progress toward the understanding the molecular biology of Von Recklinghausen neurofibromatosis. *Ann Neurol* **31**: 555–561.

Hamed LM, Glaser JS, Gass JDM and Schatz NJ (1989). Protracted enlargement of the blind spot in multiple evansecent white dot syndrome. *Arch Ophthalmol* **107**: 194–198.

Hankey GJ, Slattery JM and Warlow CP (1991). Prognosis and prognostic factors of retinal infarction: A prospective cohort study. *Br Med J* **302**: 499–504.

Harding AE (1993). The DNA laboratory and neurological practice. *J Neurol Neurosurg Psychiat* **56**: 229–233.

Hass WK, Easton JD and Adams HP Jr (1989). Ticlopidine aspirin stroke study group: A randomised trial comparing ticlopidine hydrochloride with aspirin for the prevention of stroke in high risk patients. *New Engl J Med* **321**: 501–505.

Heier JS, Dragoo RA, Enzhauer RW and Waterhouse WJ (1994). Screening for ocular toxicity in asymptomatic patients treated with tamoxifen. *Am J Ophthalmol* **117**: 772–775.

Holt IJ, Harding AE, Petty RKH *et al.* (1990). A new mitochondrial disease associated with mitochondrial DNA heteroplasmy. *Am J Hum Genet* **46**: 428–433.

Howard RS and Russell RWR (1987). Prognosis of patients with retinal embolism. *J Neurol Neurosurg Psychiat* **50**: 1142–1147.

International study group. (1990). Criteria for diagnosis of Behçet's disease. *Lancet* **335**: 1078–1080.

Jabs DA and Johns CJ (1986). Ocular involvement in chronic sarcoidosis. *Am J Ophthalmol*; **102**: 297–301.

Jacobson DM, Thirkill CE and Tipping SJ (1990). A clinical triad to diagnose paraneoplastic retinopathy. *Ann Neurol* **28**: 162–167.

Johnson CA and Teitelbaum CS (1990). Magnetic resonance imaging in Vogt-Koyanagi-Harada syndrome. *Arch Ophthalmol* **108**: 783–784.

Johnson MW, Thomley ML, Huang SS and Gass JDM (1994). Idiopathic recurrent branch retinal artery occlusion: natural history and laboratory evaluation. *Ophthalmology* **101**: 480–489.

Johnson WG and Gomez MR eds. (1991). Tuberose sclerosis and allied disorders. *Ann NY Acad Sci* **615**: 1–7; 17–25.

Keltner JL, Satterfield D, Dublin AB and Lee BCP (1987). Dural and carotid cavernous fistulas: Diagnosis, management and complications. *Ophthalmology* **94**: 1585–1600.

Kirkham TH, ffytche TJ and Sanders MD (1972). Placoid pigment epitheliopathy with retinal vasculitis and papillitis. *Br J Ophthalmol* **56**: 875–880.

Klötzsch C, Janssen G and Berlit P (1994). Transoesophageal echocardiography and contrast TCD in the detection of a patent foramen ovale: experiences in 111 patients, *Neurology* **44**: 160–166.

Knox DL (1965). Ischemic ocular inflammation. *Am J Ophthalmol* **60**: 995–1002.

Kupersmith MJ, Berenstein A, Flamm and Ransohoff J (1986). Neuro-ophthalmologic abnormalities and intravascular therapy of traumatic carotid-cavernous fistulas. *Ophthalmology* **93**: 906–912.

Kupersmith MJ, Berenstein A, Choi IS *et al.* (1988). Management of nontraumatic vascular shunts involving the cavernous sinus. *Ophthalmology* **95**: 121–130.

Kwan E, Hieshima GB, Higashida RT *et al.* (1989). Interventional radiology in neuro-ophthalmology. *J Clin Neuro-Ophthalmol* **9**: 83–97.

Leonard TJK, Moseley IF and Sanders MD (1984). Ophthalmoplegia in carotid-cavernous fistula. *Br J Ophthalmol* **68**: 128–134.

Lueck CJ, Pires M, McCartney ACE and Graham EM (1993). Ocular and neurological Behçet's disease without urogenital ulceration? *J Neurol Neurosurg Psychiat* **56**: 505–508.

Maher ER, Yates JR, Harries R *et al.* (1990). Clinical features and natural history of von Hippel–Lindau disease. *Q J Med* **77**: 1151–1163.

Maher ER, Bentley E, Yates JRW *et al.* (1991). Mapping of the von Hippel–Lindau disease locu to a small region of chromosome 3p by genetic linkage analysis. *Genomics* **10**: 957–960.

Mann ES and Katz B (1992). The uveo-meningeal syndromes, In *Neuro-Ophthalmology in Systemic Disease* (ed. B Katz), Ophthalmology Clinics of North America, Vol. 5(3), pp. 577–586. WB Saunders. Philadelphia.

Miller NR (1977). The big blind spot syndrome: Unilateral optic disc edema without visual loss or increased intracranial pressure. In *Neuro-ophthalmology Update,* (ed. JL Smith), pp. 163–169. New York: Masson.

Moadel K, Yannuzzi LA, Ho AC and Arsekar A (1994). Retinal vascular occlusive diseáse in a child with neurofibromatosis. *Arch Ophthalmol* **112**: 1021–1023.

Moore AT, Maher ER, Rosen P *et al.* (1991). Ophthalmological screening for von Hippel–Lindau disease. *Eye* **5**: 723–728.

Moorsman CDG *et al.* (1990). Screening for hydroxychloroquine retinal toxicity; is it necessary? *Eye* **4**: 572–576.

Moorthy RS, Inomata H and Rao NA (1995). Vogt-Koyanagi-Harada syndrome. *Surv Ophthalmol* **39**: 265–292.

Mullie MA, Harding AE, Petty RKH *et al.* (1985). The retinal manifestations of mitochondrial myopathy: a study of 22 cases. *Arch Ophthalmol* **103**: 1825–1830.

Narod SA, Parry DM, Parboosingh J *et al.* (1992). Neurofibromatosis type 2 appears to be a genetically homogeneous disease. *Am J Hum Genet* **51**: 486–496.

Newsome DA (ed) (1988). *Retinal Dystrophies and Degenerations.* New York: Raven Press.

North American Symptomatic Carotid Endarterectomy Trail Collaborators (1991). Beneficial effect of carotid endarterectomy in symptomatic patients with high-grade carotid stenosis. *New Engl J Med* **325**: 445–453.

Pagon RA (1988). Retinitis pigmentosa. *Surv Ophthalmol* **33**: 137–177.

Poole CJM and Russell RWR (1985). Mortality and stroke after amaurosis fugax. *J Neurol Neurosurg Psychiat* **48**: 902–905.

Ragge NK (1993). Clinical and genetic patterns of neurofibromatosis 1 and 2. *Br J Ophthalmol* **77**: 662–672.

Ripps H, Noble KG, Greenstein VC *et al.* (1987). Progressive cone dystrophy. *Ophthalmology* **94**: 1401–1409.

Richards EM, Maher ER, Latif F *et al.* (1993). Detailed mapping of the VHL disease tumour suppressor gene. *J Med Genet* **30**: 104–107.

Riordan-Eva P, Restori M, Hamilton AMP and Levy I (1994). Orbital ultrasound in the ocular ischaemic syndrome. *Eye* **8**: 93–96.

Rosenfeld PJ, McKusick VA, Amberger JS and Dryja TP (1994). Recent advances in the gene map of inherited eye disorders; primary heriditary diseases of retina, choroid and vitreous. *J Med Genet* **31**: 903–915.

Rosenbaum JT (1989). Uveitis: an internist's view. *Arch Intern Med* **149**: 1173–1176.

Ross-Russell RW and Ikeda H (1986). Clinical and electrophysiological observations in patients with low pressure retinopathy. *Br J Ophthalmol* **70**: 651–656.

Russell RWR and Page NGR (1983). Critical perfusion of eye and brain. *Brain* **106**: 419–434.

Sanders MD (1987). Retinal arteritis, retinal vasculitis and autoimmune retinal vasculitis. *Eye* 1 : 441–465.

Sanders MD and Hoyt WF (1969). Hypoxic ocular sequelae of carotid-cavernous fistulae: study of the causes of visual failure before and after neurosurgical treatment in a series of 25 cases. *Br J Ophthalmol* **53**: 82–97.

Savino PJ, Glaser JS and Luxemberg MN (1977a). Pulsating enophthalmos and choroidal hamartomas. Two rare stigmata of neurofibromatosis. *Br J Ophthalmol* **61**: 483–488.

Savino PJ, Glaser JS and Cassady J (1977b). Retinal stroke. Is the patient at risk? *Arch Ophthalmol* **95**: 1185–1189.

Sawyer RA, Selhorst JB, Zimmerman LE and Hoyt WF (1976). Blindness caused by photoreceptor degeneration as a remote effect of cancer. *Am J Ophthalmol* **81**: 606–613.

Schroeder R, Mets MB and Maumenee IH (1987). Leber's congenital amaurosis. Retrospective review of 43 cases and a new fundus finding in two cases. *Arch Ophthalmol* **105**: 356–359.

Shimizu T, Ehrlich GE, Inaba G *et al.* (1979). Uveo-meningitis. *Sem Arth Rheum* **8**: 223–260.

Sigismund DA, Weleber RG, Pillers D-A *et al.* (1994). Characterisation of the ocular phenotype of Duchenne and Becker muscular dystrophy. *Ophthalmology* **101**: 856–865.

Singh K, de Frank MP, Schults WT and Watzke RC (1991). Acute idiopathtic blind spot enlargement: a spectrum of disease. *Ophthalmology* **98**: 497–502.

Spalton DJ, Taylor DSI and Sanders MD (1980). Juvenile Batten's disease; an ophthalmological assessment of 26 patients. *Br J Ophthalmol* **64**: 720–732.

Stern BJ, Krumbolz A, Johns C *et al.* (1985). Sarcoidosis and its neurologic manifestations. *Arch Neurol* **42**: 909–917.

Streifler JY, Eliasziw M, Benavente OR *et al.* (1995). The risk of stroke in patients with first ever retinal vs hemispheric transient ischaemic attacks and high-grade carotid stenosis. *Arch Neurol* **52**: 246–249.

Sullivan TJ, Clarke MP, Morin JD (1992). The ocular manifestations of Sturge–Weber syndrome. *J Paed Ophthalmol Strabismus* **29**: 349–356.

Susac JO (1994). Susac's syndrome: The triad of microangiopathy of the brain and retina with hearing loss in young women. *Neurology* **44**: 591–593.

Thirkill CE, Roth AM and Keltner JL (1987). Cancer associated retinopathy. *Arch Ophthalmol* **105**: 372–375.

Trobe JD (1987). Carotid endarterectomy: Who needs it? *Ophthalmology* **94**: 725–730.

Warlow C (1984). Carotid endarterectomy: Does it work? *Stroke* **15**: 1068–1076.

Wilkinson IM, Russell RW (1972). Arteries of the head and neck in giant cell arteritis: a pathological study to show the pattern of arterial involvement. *Arch Neurol* **27**: 378–392.

Winterkorn JM, Kupersmith MJ, Wirtschafter JD and Forman S (1993). Brief report: treatment of vasospastic amaurosis fugax with calcium-channel blockers. *New Engl J Med* **329**: 396–398.

Wray SH (1982). Retinopathy associated with defects in metabolism. *Duane's Clinical Ophthalmology* Vol 3, pp. 1–38. Philadelphia: Harper and Row.

Wray SH (1993). The management of acute visual failure. *J Neurol Neurosurg Psychiat* **56**: 234–240.

Wright BE, Bird AC and Hamilton AM (1978). Placoid pigment epitheliopathy and Harada disease. *Br J Ophthalmol* **62**: 609–621.

Zimmer Galler IE and Robertson DM (1995). Tuberose sclerosis: long term observation of retinal lesions in tuberose sclerosis. *Am J Ophthalmol* **119**: 318–324.

5

Optic nerve disorders

PATHOPHYSIOLOGY OF OPTIC NERVE DISEASE AND THE SWOLLEN OPTIC DISC

GENERAL CLINICAL PRINCIPLES

Clinical pathophysiology of optic nerve disease

Optic disc swelling and optic atrophy

Experimental work by Hayreh has established a model of pathological disc swelling in which the common feature is stasis of the fast and slow elements of retrograde axoplasmic transport. This results in axonal distension which is ophthalmoscopically visible at the level of the prelaminar optic nerve as a swollen disc (Hayreh 1964). The actual mechanism resulting in impaired axoplasmic transport varies from disease to disease: in raised intracranial pressure, the intrasheath cerebrospinal fluid (CSF) pressure of the anterior optic nerve also rises leading to compromise of axonal function at the lamina cribrosa (Hayreh 1977a, b). In ischaemic optic neuropathy, vascular insufficiency of branches of the short posterior ciliary vessels which supply the retro laminar and laminar portions of the optic nerve head leads to axonal damage (McLeod *et al.*, 1980). In demyelinating optic neuritis, perivascular inflammatory cellular infiltration and interstitial oedema results in axonal compression and disc oedema (Rao, 1981). This can be observed when the demyelinating plaque occurs in the distal optic nerve on MRI with STIR sequences.

With the exception therefore of primary retinal vascular disease (such as central retinal vein occlusion), axonal distension always precedes the vascular changes which form an important element of the clinical features. These secondary vascular changes include capillary dilation, microaneurysms, haemorrhages and cotton wool spots on the disc and neighbouring retina in the distribution of the long radial peripapillary arteries as well as dilation and venous stasis of the prelaminar capillaries, and obstruction with dilation of the central retinal vein.

In optic atrophy, a lethal insult (compression, ischaemia, inflammation, toxins, genetic defects) to the retinal ganglion cells or to the axons results in death of both structures. Astroglia migrate into the space formerly occupied by axons and blood vessels are reduced in numbers. It is the reduction in the volume of the capillary bed that accounts for ophthalmoscopic pallor, together with loss of tissue volume and astrocytic proliferation (Quigley and Anderson, 1977).

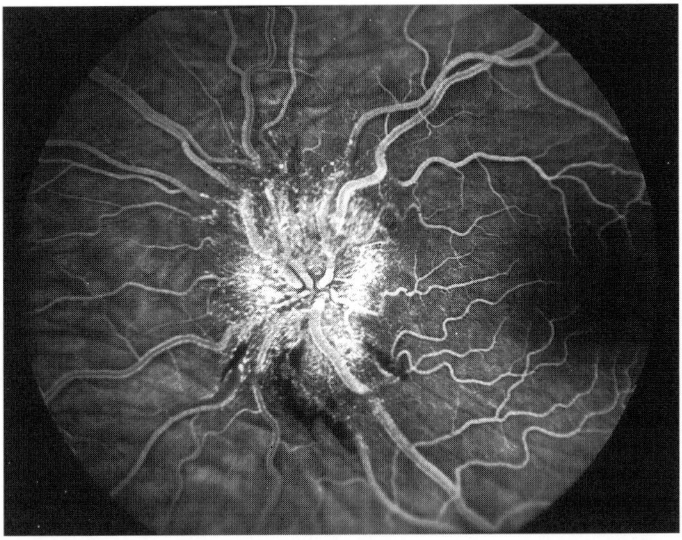

Figure 5.1

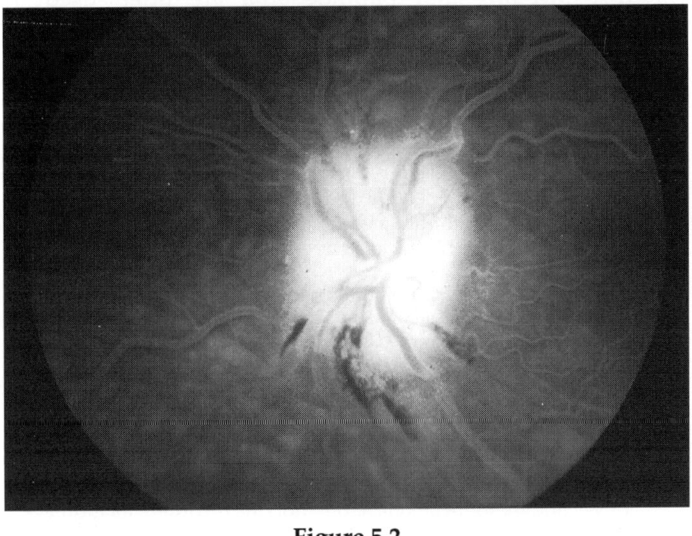

Figure 5.2

Figures 5.1, 5.2 Fluorescein angiograms showing early dilatation of prepapillary capillaries and late leakage of fluorscein in acute disc swelling.

Recovery of function after surgical decompression of extrinsic tumours of the anterior visual pathways
Loss of optic nerve function in extrinsic compression is the result of a combination of loss of nerve fibres from wallerian aronal degeneration, conduction block from demyelination, and 'physiological block' in ischaemic fibres that would be able to conduct if they were not compressed. Following surgical decompression, the early rapid phase of recovery is

probably due to the restoration of function in physiologically blocked fibres: further delayed recovery can be accounted for by remyelination of demyelinated fibres and by a degree of recovery after wallerian axonal degeneration (Kayan and Earl, 1975; McDonald, 1982).

Patterns of visual loss in optic nerve disease

The hallmark of visual loss due to acquired optic nerve disease is a central scotoma, because axons serving macular vision appear to be differentially sensitive to disease processes throughout the course of the nerve. Exceptions to this principle have diagnostic implications: an altitudinal field defect suggests infarction of the retrolaminar portion of the optic nerve head, a centrocaecal scotoma suggests heredofamilial or toxic damage to the fibres of the maculopapillar bundle in the anterior optic nerve (Plant, 1990), and a constricted field with preserved acuity suggests either post-papilloedema optic atrophy or a retinal dystrophy. When there is acute loss of function with a normal optic nerve head on fundoscopy, the term retrobulbar optic neuropathy is used. When visual loss is associated with disc swelling, the terms papillitis or papillopathy are often used. Optic atrophy may follow both variants after about 6 weeks.

Differential diagnosis of the swollen optic disc

Classification

The terms optic disc swelling and papilloedema are often used interchangeably irrespective of aetiology. However, current convention has simplified matters by

Table 5.1 Causes of optic disc swelling due to raised intracranial pressure

- Intracranial mass
- Obstructed cranial venous outflow
  - Dural venous sinus thrombosis
  - Dural venous sinus infiltration
  - Jugular vein compression
  - Dural venous sinus arteriovenous malformation
- Increased CSF production
  - Choroid plexus papilloma
- Reduced CSF outflow
  - Obstructive hydrocephalus
  - Ruptured aneurysm
  - Meningitis — infective, inflammatory and neoplastic
  - Pseudotumour cerebri syndromes
    - a) Idiopathic ('benign') intracranial hypertension
    - b) Secondary to metabolic and endocrine disorders including
      - hypoparathyroidism
      - diabetic ketoacidosis
      - thyrotoxicosis
      - Addison's disease
      - chronic uraemia
    - c) Secondary to toxic causes
      - hypervitaminosis A
      - nalidixic acid
      - tetracycline
      - steroid therapy
      - steroid withdrawal
      - lithium
      - recombinant human growth hormone

reserving the term papilloedema for the combination of pathological disc swelling with raised intracranial pressure. The remainder of cases are designated either as disc swelling arising from a local (i.e. in the eye or orbit) lesion or as pseudopapilloedema when the appearance arises as a congenital anomaly. This classification may help the clinician to think clearly when appproaching the differential diagnosis (Tables 5.1, 5.2, 5.3).

The first task is to determine whether the underlying pathology is intracranial or local to the swollen disc itself. In papilloedema due to raised intracranial pressure the disc swelling is usually but not always bilateral and symmetrical. Over a period of time, the clinical features evolve through a sequence of stages: in early papilloedema there is simply blurring of the disc margins as axons swell, together with loss of spontaneous venous pulsation.

In the acute full-blown picture there are also features of secondary vascular changes with haemorrhages, hard exudates and cotton wool spots. Symptoms include momentary fading of vision (obscurations) associated with postural changes or on the Valsalva manoeuvre reflecting vascular compromise. At this point, perimetry shows blindspot enlargement as swollen axons overlap peripapillary photoreceptors. Visual acuity and colour vision remain normal. In longstanding, chronic papilloedema, compensatory mechanisms lead to the resolution of the vascular abnormalities leaving axonal swelling with signs of mild vascular congestion in the form of dilation of the prepapillary

Table 5.2 Causes of optic disc swelling due to local disease

A. Intrinsic optic nerve disease
- Inflammatory
  - optic neuritis
  - granulomatous infiltration
- Ischaemic
  - arteritic
  - non-arteritic – including
    accelerated hypertension
    diabetes mellitus
  - other circulatory disorders including
    congenital cyanotic heart disease
    respiratory failure
    hyperviscosity syndromes
- Neoplastic
  - optic glioma
  - secondary neoplastic infiltration
- Toxic
  - methanol
  - heavy metal poisoning

B. Extrinsic optic nerve disease
- Neoplastic
  - meningiomas
  - intraconal and extraconal masses
- Inflammatory
  - dysthyroid eye disease
  - idiopathic orbital inflammatory disease (orbital pseudotumours)

C. Intraocular disease
- central retinal vein occlusion
- chronic uveitis
- hypotony
- neuroretinitis
- retinitis pigmentosa

Table 5.3 Causes of pseudopapilloedema

Buried disc drusen (hyaline bodies)
Simple hypermetropia (small discs)
Dysplastic tilted optic discs
Optic disc hamartomas

capillaries. Later, in vintage papilloedema involutional changes can be seen in the form of early disc pallor and the appearance of white refractile bodies on the disc surface – corpora amylacea. Finally in chronic atrophic papilloedema axonal loss is conspicuous leading to loss of supporting glial and vascular elements and flattening of the disc with retinal vascular attenuation. It is only in longstanding papilloedema that visual acuity loss is seen, either as a result of axonal loss, or occasionally because of adjacent retinal vascular changes which damage the macula (Sanders, 1970).

By contrast, disc oedema due to local optic nerve disease is normally associated with early loss of acuity and colour vision, together with central, arcuate or altitudinal field defects. In contrast to papilloedema, involvement is usually unilateral and consequently there is a relative afferent pupil defect. Other fundal abnormalities often yield diagnostic clues: for example retinal vascular sheathing in optic neuritis, peripheral retinal haemorrhages in retinal vein occlusions, or choroidal folds in posterior scleritis or a retrobulbar mass. A careful history is important as an acute onset of symptoms with pain on eye movements suggests inflammatory optic neuritis, while an acute onset in older adults without associated pain is typical of ischaemic optic neuropathy and a long insidious history may raise the possibility of a primary optic nerve tumour.

The appearance of 'pseudopapilloedema' mimicking true papilloedema of raised intracranial pressure may cause difficulties. All too frequently the patient with headaches is wrongly thought to have raised intracranial pressure from the fundoscopic finding of elevated discs, with important consequences for further investigation and management. A systematic approach is essential to resolve this difficulty. First, does the headache have the features of raised pressure (more severe on awakening, exacerbated by coughing)? Second, what is the approximate refraction of the eye? Hypermetropes typically have small, crowded elevated discs which are a normal variant. Similarly, myopes frequently have dysverted or tilted discs with an elevated indistinct margin superonasally. Third, what can be can be learnt on careful fundoscopy? In true papilloedema secondary vascular changes are usually prominent with prepapillary capillary dilation, haemorrhages and exudates as well as axonal swelling. Spontaneous pulsation of the central retinal vein is not always observed in the normal subject, but when seen raised intracranial pressure is highly unlikely. Superficial disc drusen appear as refractile bodies on the disc surface causing abnormal elevation, and hamartomas produce a mass effect without these vascular changes. Buried disc drusen result in an indistinct disc margin often with an anomalous retinal vascular pattern with trifurcations of the first order vessels. Sometimes further investigations are required. Intrapapillary calcification of drusen can be seen on CT scanning and ultrasound. Fundus fluorescein angiography shows an absence of any vascular dilation or late leakage from the prepapillary capillaries: typically the disc shows late staining with fluorescein but not hyperfluorescence. Sometimes the diagnosis can be made before fluorescein injection as disc drusen have the property of autofluorescence when illuminated with blue light.

Visual loss secondary to chronic raised intracranial pressure
The management of chronic raised intracranial pressure depends upon the careful separation of truly idiopathic cases from those in which there is an identifiable cause requiring specific treatment. Because idiopathic intracranial hypertension is typically a disease of obese young females, the same syndrome in normal weight males in particular requires the careful exclusion of specific CSF outflow abnormalities. Magnetic resonance angiography is adequate to exclude dural sinus thrombosis or arteriovenous malformations involving the sinuses in most cases, but formal cerebral angiography may still be required on occasion. Sinus thrombosis indicates the need to search for occult abnormalities of thrombosis and haemostasis regulation such as the procoagulant defects of protein C and S, the presence of anti-cardiolipin antibodies or an undetected neoplasm, and anticoagulation may be indicated. Arteriovenous malformations may be specifically amenable to endovascular embolization techniques, reducing the risk of haemorrhage as well as the risk of visual loss from chronic raised intracranial pressure (Corbett, 1983).

Whilst idiopathic intracranial hypertension (pseudotumour cerebri, benign intracranial hypertension) may carry a good prognosis for life when compared with many other diseases causing papilloedema, the condition is far from benign in terms of visual function (Gu *et al.*, 1995). More than 80% of patients have been shown to eventually develop some degree of visual loss, and up to 10% have significant field defects and acuity loss rather than simply obscurations and blindspot enlargement, and careful follow-up is required (Wall and George, 1987, 1991; Corbett *et al.*, 1982; Orcutt *et al.*, 1984). Medical measures to control headache and visual symptoms in chronic raised intracranial pressure may be both ineffective and poorly tolerated. These include weight loss, carbonic anhydrase inhibitors, corticosteroids and serial lumbar punctures. Surgical CSF diversion procedures are more effective but conventional shunting is associated with a high rate of either failure or of low-pressure headache, and visual loss has sometimes been shown to progress even after the establishment of a successful shunt (Rosenberg *et al.*, 1993). Specific measures to protect vision take the form of optic nerve sheath

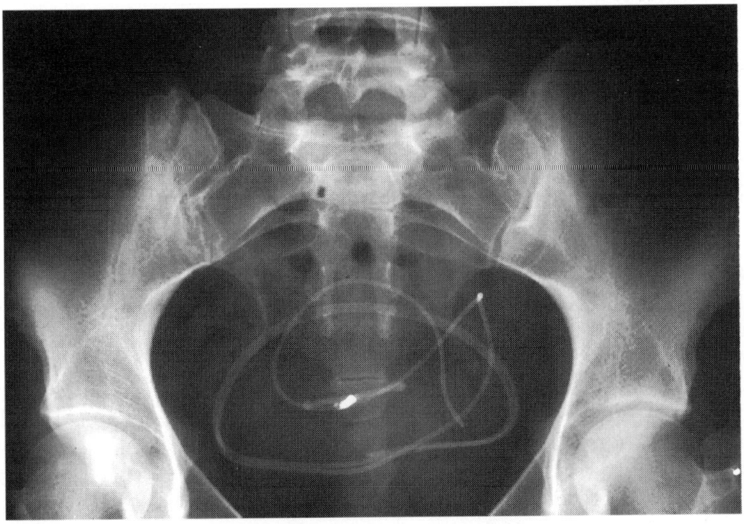

Figure 5.3 Disconnected lumbar peritoneal shunt with both ends within peritoneal cavity on plain pelvic X-ray. (Courtesy of Dr G Plant.)

decompression (ONSD) or fenestration. Fashioning a window in the retrolaminar optic nerve sheath may reduce the intrasheath pressure and relieve the axoplasmic stasis and eventual axonal loss which results from chronic raised intracranial pressure. In some cases vision dramatically improves following this procedure – other patients are simply protected from insidious progressive loss.

The theoretical basis for ONSD is incompletely understood. Vision is improved or protected in the short term but exactly how the operation continues to work over a period of time remains speculative. Headaches and contralateral disc swelling are relieved in some patients suggesting that there is a prolonged lowering of intracranial pressure via a persistent orbital fistula. However, in other cases the operation only achieves a local effect and the headaches and contralateral papilloedema deteriorate even if the ipsilateral disc and visual function improve. Reparative fibrosis at the site of fenestration may prevent transmission of raised intracranial pressure past the subarachnoid scars and protect the ipsilateral optic nerve but not reduce the intracranial pressure (Corbett, 1983; Keltner, 1988; Liu 1993; Liu and Michon, 1995). A CSF filled cyst may form in the orbit at the site of sheath decompression. However, accurate direct measurement of intrasheath CSF pressure *in vivo* has yet to be achieved and so the functional significance of these arachnoid cysts remains unclear.

The relationship between ONSD and other CSF-diversion procedures (lumbo-peritoneal shunt and ventriculoperitoneal shunt) is of interest and awaits clarification. Shunts may fail because of disconnection or obstruction and the main consequences may be visual rather than exacerbated headaches. Sometimes ONSD does reduce headaches, intracranial pressure and contralateral disc swelling, and sometimes effective shunting may relieve headaches and intracranial pressure but not papilloedema and visual loss. Therefore it may not be correct to assume that the intracranial and intrasheath subarachnoid spaces are all in continuity with one another. Arachnoid trabeculations in the optic nerve sheaths may allow the sequestration of CSF and modulate the results of ONSD. As experience grows it may be possible to recommend shunting as the procedure of choice in cases only where headache is the dominant complaint, and ONSD initially when visual failure is prominent (Acheson *et al.*, 1994).

DEVELOPMENTAL ABNORMALITIES

HYPOPLASIA

Hypoplasia of the optic disc may be unilateral or bilateral, obvious or subtle and may be associated with both good and poor visual function. There is a subnormal number of axons within the affected nerve although the mesodermal elements and glial supporting cells are both normal (Lambert *et al.*, 1987).

The diagnosis is normally made on the basis of marked reduction of disc substance. This typically leaves an area of bare exposed sclera which coincides with a gap between the retinal pigment epithelial border and the point to which a normal disc should have extended. The retinal nerve fibre layer is thinned. In less marked cases diagnosis becomes more difficult and photographic methods to evaluate the ratio of the disc diameter to the centre disc/fovea distance may be valuable: a ratio of more than 3.0 is considered to be diagnostic. Field defects are variable and may reflect more extensive visual pathway anomalies: as a general rule the smaller the disc, the worse the visual acuity (Apple *et al.*, 1982).

Optic nerve hypoplasia may occur as an isolated defect or in association with a wide range of facial, ocular and intracranial anomalies reflecting the embryological derivation from the forebrain. These include albinism, aniridia, ocular colobomas, Duane's syndrome, Klippel–Trenauney–Weber syndrome, Goldenhar's syndrome, blepharophimosis and hemifacial atrophy (Zeki *et al.*, 1992). There are also interesting associations with intracranial developmental anomalies which are often referred to as septo-optic dysplasia (de Morsier's syndrome). Clinically there is short stature and frequent nystagmus. Imaging shows as single anterior ventricle (holoprosencephaly) without a midline partition by the septum pellucidum. Associated neuroendocrine dysfunction results in growth hormone deficiency which is treatable. Cases of bilateral hypoplasia should therefore undergo imaging and endocrine assessment. Unilateral cases should have careful developmental and growth monitoring as well as ophthalmic treatment for any superadded visual loss due to strabismus or amblyopia. More extensive brain malformations are also possible (Kaufman *et al.*, 1989; Brodsky and Glaser, 1993). Patients with congenital cerebral hemisphere lesions may undergo transsynaptic degeneration of the anterior visual pathways resulting in bow-tie or homonymous hemioptic hypoplasia. There is a further association between optic nerve hypoplasia and congenital suprasellar tumours such as infantile craniopharyngioma (Novakovic *et al.*, 1988; Taylor, 1982).

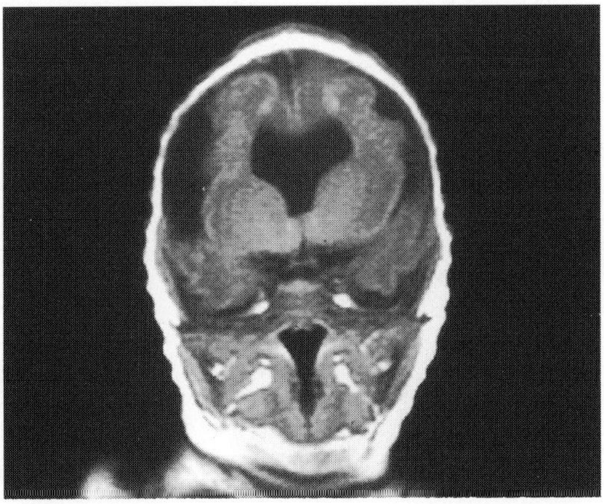

Figure 5.4 MRI brain scan – coronal view – of infant with bilateral optic nerve hypoplasia to show associated single ventricle.

No single cause has been identified but there is an association with the fetal alcohol syndrome and maternal crack cocaine use as well as with phenytoin, lysergic acid diethylamide (LSD) and quinine. The observation in normal optic nerve embryogenesis, that there is a decline in the number of axons from a peak of over 3 million at 16–17 weeks gestation to 1.1 million at 31 weeks is significant, as this suggests that optic nerve hypoplasia may be the result of an exaggeration of a normal developmental process, rather than a simple failure of neuronal development in the first place. It also indicates that the timing of the teratogenic insult need not be confined to the first trimester of pregancy (Hoyt and Good, 1992).

OTHER CONGENITAL DISC ANOMALIES

Colobomas and pits

In contrast to optic nerve hypoplasia, optic disc colobomas and pits are thought to arise as a consequence of faulty closure of the embryonic fetal fissure of the optic stalk and cup. Other colobomas involving the lens, iris and choroid are frequently seen in association. A variety of forms may occur, and each may be associated with acuity loss or field defects: enlarged discs with deep excavation which may be mistaken for glaucomatous cupping; enlarged discs in which the central excavation is filled with embryonic vascular and glial remnants ('morning glory disc'); excavated discs contiguous with retinochoroidal colobomas and slightly enlarged discs containing pits within the borders of the nerve head. In addition to being mistaken for glaucoma, two associations are important: first, congenital forebrain anomalies including basal encephalocoeles which must be considered in the differential diagnosis of masses in the orbit and nasopharynx; second with central serous retinal detachment in which fluid is believed to flow from the vitreous cavity through the pit and then beneath the temporal juxtapapillary neurosensory retina to cause reduced vision (Apple *et al.*, 1982).

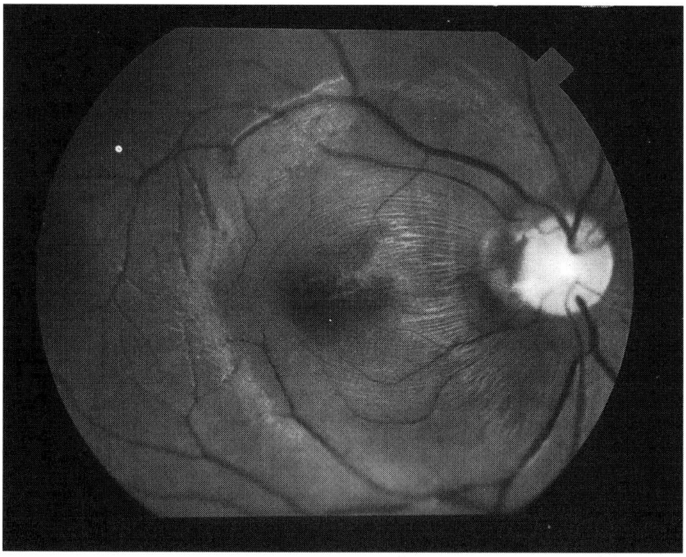

Figure 5.5 Red free fundus photograph of congenital optic disc pit with associated serous retinal detachment.

Dysversions, crescents and situs inversus

Congenital tilted discs arise when the optic nerve enters the globe at an extremely oblique angle and the associated crescent is seen when there is a disparity between the scleral and retinal openings. The term situs inversus describes the apparent origin of the retinal vessels from the temporal side of the disc rather than the nasal: the disc itself may in addition be hypoplastic. This anomaly is important clinically for two reasons. First, the oblique entry of the optic nerve into the globe means that often the inferonasal margin of the disc is deficient with associated retinal nerve fibre layer defects in this quadrant. Temporal field defects may result and the patient may be mistakenly thought to have chiasmal compression. However, in this situation, careful perimetry shows that the temporal field defect is sloping and does not respect the vertical meridian. Second, the opposite, healthy side of the disc – usually the superotemporal aspect – is frequently elevated resulting in the incorrect diagnosis of pathological disc swelling (Apple *et al.*, 1982; Dorrell, 1978).

Anomalous disc elevation, pseudopapilloedema and hyaline bodies (disc drusen)

In some cases anomalous elevation of the optic nerve head may closely resemble pathological optic disc swelling with important diagnostic implications especially in children and young adults who have headaches but no other features of raised intracranial pressure (Rosenberg *et al.*, 1979). These distinctions are crucial if a large range of unnecessary neurological investigations are to be avoided. After tilted discs with asymmetrical elevation mentioned above, and physiologically elevated discs in hypermetropic eyes, the most important entity to consider is disc drusen or hyaline bodies (Tso, 1981).

Disc drusen (not to be confused with the much commoner drusen of the retinal pigment epithelium which form part of the spectrum of macular degeneration) are acellular concretions of material thought to derive from axoplasmic derivatives of degenerating nerve fibres disrupted because of a congenitally narrowed scleral canal. Drusen initially are buried within the optic nerve head and slowly become more visible at the optic disc margins and surface as time passes. When buried, the disc is simply elevated, but clues to their presence are found in associated anomalous vascular bifurcations, and an absent central optic disc cup. Furthermore, the absence of prepapillary capillary dilation, haemorrhages or cotton wool spots help to distiguish pathological from anomalous disc elevation. Finally, in anomalous disc elevation due to buried disc drusen, spontaneous venous pulsation will be present (Sanders and ffytche, 1967).

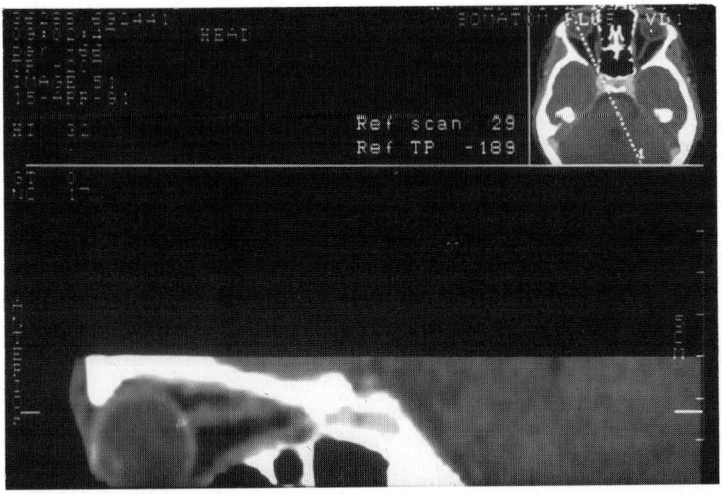

Figure 5.6 CT scan of optic nerve head showing calcification indicating optic disc drusen.

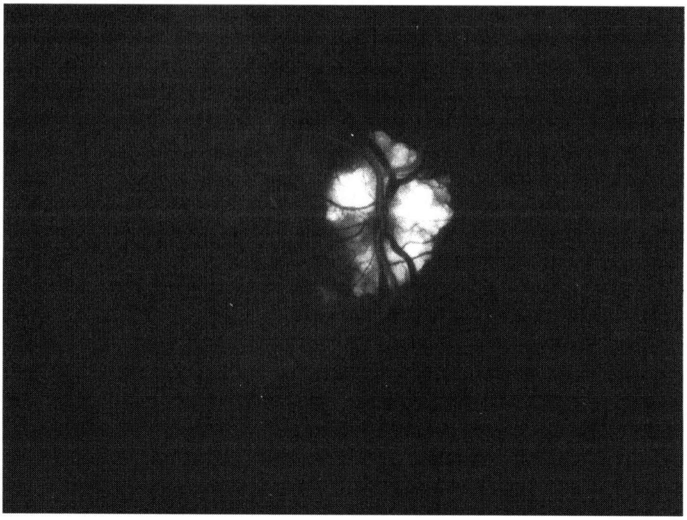

Figure 5.7 Autofluorescent optic disc drusen.

Disc drusen may be calcified, giving rise to diagnostic appearances on CT scanning and standard echography, and may show the property of autofluorescence on fundus photography with cobalt blue light. There is an association between disc drusen and retinitis pigmentosa, in which case the drusen are typically seen in the peripapillary zone rather than on the disc surface (Novack and Foos, 1987; Mullie and Sanders, 1984, 1985).

In addition to causing confusion with acquired pathological disc swelling, disc drusen may in themselves be associated with visual loss (Sarkies and Sanders, 1987; Savino *et al.*, 1979). Usually this takes the form of peripheral field loss, sector defects, arcuate scotomas or concentric narrowing. Central visual loss is exceptional and may be the result of superadded anterior ischaemic optic neuropathy in an optic nerve head with abnormal vasculature. Slow progression of field loss is more typical, but it remains to be established whether the mechanism is mechanical axonal compression or associated circulatory disturbance, or both. Disc and peripapillary haemorrhages may be seen: these are not in themselves thought to cause visual loss unless there is the associated formation of a juxtapapillary subretinal neovascular membrane which may directly damage macular function (Sanders *et al.*, 1971).

HEREDO-FAMILIAL OPTIC NEUROPATHIES

LEBER'S HEREDITARY OPTIC NEUROPATHY (LHON) AND OTHER MITOCHONDRIAL DISEASES ASSOCIATED WITH OPTIC ATROPHY

Leber's disease is readily distinguished from other hereditary optic neuropathies by its characteristic clinical presentation: sudden central visual loss in the second to third decade of life, usually in males. Weeks, months or sometimes years later the second eye is involved, although bilateral simultaneous visual loss may occur. Colour vision is severely affected, and perimetry shows a large central scotoma.

Unlike optic neuritis, there is no pain on eye movements and recovery is both exceptional and delayed by months or even years when it occurs. During the acute phase of visual loss, hyperaemia of the optic nerve head may be seen, together with tortuosity of retinal vessels and circumpapillary telangectatic microangiopathy with nerve fibre layer thickening. The presence of retinal haemorrhages in a small percentage (10%) adds credence to the theory that pathological changes are occurring at the retinal neural and microcirculatory level. Fundus fluorescein angiography does not, however, show leakage from the disc, distinguishing these appearances from those due to true optic disc swelling. These fundus appearances are also sometimes observed in maternal relatives suggesting an increased risk for subsequent visual loss. However, the absence of these features does not exclude the diagnosis in an individual who loses vision, nor does it exclude the possibility of future visual loss in a maternal relative. Eventually optic atrophy with retinal nerve fibre layer defects develops which is particularly obvious in the papillomacular bundle. On magnetic resonance imaging (MRI) increased signal can be demonstrated in the optic nerves on STIR sequences, probably reflecting localized wallerian degeneration and gliosis. In distinction to many cases of clinically isolated optic neuritis, multiple cerebral white matter changes are not normally seen (Riordan-Eva *et al.*, 1995; Nikoskelainen *et al.*, 1982, 1984).

Generally the visual loss occurs in isolation, but in some pedigrees there are associated cardiac dysrhythmias (pre-excitation syndromes). Where they are found, these additional abnormalities are often referred to as 'Leber's plus'. A maternal line of inheritance has been established for many years, pointing to the possibility of transmission through the extrachromosomal DNA residing in the female gamete. This has now been shown to be due to one of a number of point mutations in mitochondrial DNA, most commonly occurring at the 11778 location with the substitution of adenine for guanine. This mutation has not been found in control subjects. As a consequence, histidine rather than arginine is coded for in subunit 4 of Complex I in the respiratory chain (Parker *et al.*, 1989). Why axons of the papillomacular bundle of the optic nerves should be selectively vulnerable is not understood. However, heteroplasmy — the coexistence of mutant and normal mitochondrial (mt) DNA within the same individual — has been demonstrated and the relative content of mutant mtDNA within the tissues of the same individual may influence phenotypic expression. About 50% of patients with a clinical picture of LHON and a pathogenic mtDNA mutation do not have a history of similarly affected relatives, and in these cases the detection of specific mutations is of great diagnostic value. Although LHON is primarily a disease of young males, among those patients in the UK with the 11778 mutation, over 25% of patients are female and an overlap syndrome with multiple sclerosis has been described (Singh *et al.*, 1989; Newman *et al.*, 1991; Harding *et al.*, 1992).

There are now reports of an association in some pedigrees with other mutations at other sites, the most important of which are at 3460 and 14484. This information carries important prognostic implications. The visual recovery rate may only be 4% in patients with the 11778 mutation, but up to 37% of those with a defect at site 14484 may recover. Female involvement in these mutations appears to be rare. The microangiopathy of LHON is less likely to be present in patients with the 14484 mutation. The association of LHON with mutations at other sites has been reported, including 15257, 15812 and 4160, but the clinical significance of these accounts is unclear as the same defects may occur in healthy unrelated controls (Johns *et al.*, 1992, 1993a,b; Huoponen *et al.*, 1991).

In Europe, the 11778 and 3460 mutations account for at least 90% of families with this disease as defined by a subacute optic neuropathy with a positive maternal family history. Before these modern genetic insights were available, the hypothesis that Leber's disease might somehow reflect the effects of cynanide toxicity in predisposed individuals who could have had deficiencies in detoxification enzymes was put forward and used to support the use of hydroxycobalamin in treatment. Although this treatment never enjoyed great success, it is of great interest that recently tobacco and alcohol have been reported to play a role in the phenotypic expression of the 3460 and 14484 mutations. This would explain the association between Leber's disease and heavy tobacco consumption,

Table 5.4 Primary mtDNA mutations associated with Leber's hereditary optic neuropathy

Primary mutation	Frequency in N Europe (%)	Recovery rate (%)
11778	50–60	2–17
3460	15–30	20–40
14484	10	37–50

Table 5.5 History of alcohol and tobacco consumption in patients with Leber's hereditary optic neuropathy by mutation

	Tobacco (%)	Alcohol (%)	Both (%)
11778 (n = 37)	49	14	11
3460 (n = 7)	86	50	50
14484 (n = 12)	67	67	58

perhaps in nutritionally deficient patients. In addition, it raises the intriguing possibility that other toxic optic neuropathies such as those resulting from ethambutol or isoniazide therapy might only occur in patients with an as yet unidentified mtDNA mutation (Mackey, 1994).

It is also becoming evident that atypical cases of LHON also arise in which there is a subclinical or chronic course. This is particularly important in children who present with unexplained optic atrophy. Further typical cases with an acute onset do not harbour a primary mtDNA base substitution.

Peripheral blood samples are adequate for mtDNA analysis in LHON: the neurogenetics laboratory at the Institute of Neurology, London (Harding, 1993) normally requires 20ml of fresh blood in EDTA tubes, but where this is not practical, DNA in blood spots collected on Guthrie cards may be amplified using polymerase chain reaction techniques with minimal biohazard risks and storage and transport costs (Mackey, 1993).

An effective treatment for Leber's disease remains to be found: the use of vitamin B_{12} is unproved and probably ineffective but it may be valuable to counsel individuals at risk (after first eye involvement, or unaffected maternal relatives) against tobacco and alcohol use and on the benefits of a balanced diet.

OTHER MITOCHONDRIAL DISEASES AND OPTIC ATROPHY

Other mitochondrial disorders with clinical presentations quite different from LHON may demonstrate optic atrophy as a variable mainfestation of the disease. Examples include cases of myoclonic epilepsy and ragged red fibres (MERFF); mitochondrial myopathy, encephalopathy and stroke-like episodes (MELAS); chronic progressive external ophthalmoplegia (CPEO) and Leigh's disease. In these diseases the optic atrophy is an infrequently noted and a variable finding (Newman, 1992).

AUTOSOMAL RECESSIVE OPTIC ATROPHY

Simple

This entity is occasionally noted in the neonate and termed congenital, but more usually is discovered in infancy before the age of 3 or 4 years. Severe but stable visual impairment is the rule and associated nystagmus is variable. Disc pallor and retinal arterial attenuation may suggest a retinal dystrophy such as Leber's congenital amaurosis, but the flash electroretinogram is normal indicating retention of normal retinal photoreceptor function (Heher *et al.*, 1992).

Complex

The association of infantile recessive optic atrophy spinocerebellar degenerations and cerebellar ataxia is known as Behr's syndrome. There may be an overlap with Charcot–Marie–Tooth disease. Another association is with *D*iabetes *I*nsipidis, *D*iabetes *M*ellitus (*O*ptic *A*trophy) and sensori-neural *D*eafness (DIDMOAD, or Wolfram's syndrome) (Barrett *et al.*, 1995).

AUTOSOMAL DOMINANT OPTIC ATROPHY

Following the pattern of many genetic disorders, the dominant form of optic atrophy is less severe than the recessive, and is also seen more frequently. The diagnosis can normally be established by applying the following clinical criteria: a dominant mode of inheritance; insidious visual loss between the ages of 4 and 8 years; moderate visual acuity reduction in the range of 6/12 to 6/24 (rarely as poor as 6/60) with possible asymmetry; temporal disc pallor with thinning of the papillomacular bundle; centrocaecal blindspot enlargement with full peripheral fields to white targets; acquired blue-yellow dyschromatopsia. The clinical course is normally mildy progressive and usually the child can manage at a normal school and take up most occupations. Normally the deficit occurs in isolation, but some cases of associated hearing loss and nystagmus have been reported (Hoyt, 1980; Kline and Glaser, 1979). Several groups have isolated the gene defect to chromosome 3, and precise mapping is likely in the near future.

Table 5.6 Classification by aetiology

Typical
Idiopathic
Multiple sclerosis
Atypical
Infectious, postviral and parainfectious, granulomatous
Autoimmune, contiguous inflammation of sinuses, meninges or orbit

INFLAMMATORY OPTIC NEUROPATHIES (OPTIC NEURITIS)

The term optic neuritis simply conveys the inflammatory component in an optic neuropathy and the differential diagnosis includes a wide range of immune related, granulomatous and infective disorders in addition to the common idiopathic form. Most frequently the disc is not swollen in which case the term retrobulbar neuritis is used: cases in which disc swelling is seen are sometimes referred to as papillitis. The distinction between optic neuropathies causing disc swelling and visual loss and papilloedema due to raised intracranial pressure is discussed in the section on papilloedema.

TYPICAL OPTIC NEURITIS

Clinical features

In a typical episode of optic neuritis there is an acute or subacute onset of visual loss progressing over hours or a few days with function reaching its nadir by one week.

Unilateral involvement is usual – the less common bilateral disease is a characteristic of the postviral form especially in children (Parkin *et al.*, 1984). Pain on eye movements and mild tenderness of the globe are characteristic in the early stages. Visual loss may range from field and contrast defects with maintained acuity to profound acuity loss with no perception of light. Formal perimetry may show a variety of defects ranging from generalized depression to a central scotoma or altitudinal and nerve fibre layer defects and severe ipsilateral headache or orbital ache may precede the onset of visual symptoms. The combination of pain on eye movements with visual loss may also be seen in granulomatous optic neuropathy, scleritis, sphenoid sinus mucocoele and malignant optochiasmal glioma.

The occipital pattern evoked potential (PVEP) shows marked latency changes with small amplitude reductions which simply reflect the degree of acuity loss. This is in contrast to other optic nerve diseases in which the visual loss in primarily due to axonal fallout (for example acute visual loss due to toxic, compressive, or ischaemic conditions) when there are marked amplitude reductions. The latency changes may be greater than can be accounted for by demyelination and conduction block in the optic nerve: there may a contribution to this delay from both cortical and retinal elements. The Pattern electroretinogram (PERG) may also show abnormalities even though the lesion is apparently upstream in the optic nerve. This is interpreted to mean that the PERG is generated in the inner retina and that in optic neuritis inner retinal function may be abnormal electrophysiologically if not clinically. After clinical recovery latency changes in the PVEP also improve: this is thought to reflect recovery from that component of the conduction block which is due to oedema and the acute inflammatory response: remyelination plays little role in the mature central nervous system (McDonald, 1983).

Usually vision begins to recover after 2–3 weeks and stabilizes by 5–6 weeks. Many patients experience virtually complete restoration of acuity but persistent subtle residual defects of colour vision, contrast sensitivity, depth perception and evoked potential latency changes are nearly always demonstrable. In some individuals acuity only makes a partial recovery: rarely there is no recovery whatsoever. In retrobulbar neuritis, the fundus is by definition normal at the time of onset but subsequently disc pallor may be marked. The final degree of optic atrophy does not correlate closely with the level of visual recovery. This is particularly striking in children where marked optic atrophy and retinal nerve fibre layer loss may follow optic neuritis, but the visual acuity returns to normal. There is evidence that central adaptive mechanisms may contribute to this effect, as there are no alternative anterior visual pathways. In some instances there is intraocular inflammation – the two most important patterns being neuroretinitis and retinal periphlebitis. In neuroretinitis there is marked swelling not only of the disc but also the posterior retinal nerve fibre layer with the formation of retinal exudates in Henlé's layer around the fovea (macular star) together with inflammatory cells in the vitreous. In retinal periphlebitis sheathing around peripheral retinal veins can be observed together with other evidence of inner blood–retinal barrier dysfunction such as cystoid macular oedema. Sometimes this can be purely subclinical and only detectable on fluorescein angiography but periphlebitis is of considerable clinical significance because of the implications for the subsequent development of multiple sclerosis (see below) and an association with other central nervous system (CNS) inflammatory diseases including sarcoidosis, syphilis, tuberculosis and Behçet's disease (Lightman *et al.*, 1987; Graham *et al.*, 1989; Vine, 1992).

In clinical assessment it is important to establish whether the optic neuritis is isolated or taking place in the context of a systemic illness. The history focuses on other possible CNS lesions by inquiring about paraesthesia, diplopia or unsteadiness; or on preceding infective episodes especially in the respiratory and gastrointestinal systems. A typical attack occurs in childhood or adults below the age of 50 years with mild ocular ache and/or pain on eye movements which may reflect the movement of the inflamed nerve within the meninges. The absence of pain may indicate intracanicular or intracranial demyelination while failure to follow the typical time course of evolution and recovery of visual loss prompts the careful search for other optic neuropathies, either atypical inflammatory lesions, compression by tumours or ischaemia. The possibility of central visual loss being due, not to optic nerve, but to retinal disease affecting the macula should never be forgotten (see Chapter 2).

Most patients with multiple sclerosis (MS) develop optic neuritis at some stage but not all patients with clinically isolated optic neuritis go on to develop MS. Subclinical abnormalities of contrast sensitivity and evoked potentials in the fellow eye at the time of acute symptoms imply disseminated white matter lesions in space and time and a diagnosis of MS. Recurrent attacks in the same eye occurs in 20–30% of cases but the predictive significance of this for subsequent MS is uncertain. Patients with a clinical picture of neuroretinitis are less likely to develop MS than those with typical optic neuritis: the origins of this variant are more likely to be clearly postviral. It has now become clear that, in a northern European population, up to 75% of these patients will eventually develop MS and that specific risk factors include female sex, haplotypes DR-2 and DR-3, retinal periphlebitis and a winter onset of initial symptoms. This figure is based on life table studies based on at least 15-year follow-up periods and does not contain any indication of eventual severity of involvement (McDonald, 1983; Francis *et al.*, 1987; Miller *et al.*, 1988a; Rizzo and Lessell, 1988; Comptson *et al.*, 1978).

Important insights into optic neuritis have been offered by MRI. Increased signal which is believed to correspond to the site of acute demyelination with oedema can be identified within the optic nerve on short tau inversion sequences (STIR). It has been shown that disc swelling not only occurs with lesions in the anterior optic nerve, but also with lesions in the optic canal, and that a poor visual recovery may be correlated with both lesion length as well as a canal location (Miller, 1988b). In some cases the lesion may appear to extend to more than 2 cm. Poor recovery rates in canal lesions may reflect severe axonal compression due to oedema in a confined space during the acute episode. In addition, gadolinium enhancement of optic nerve lesions appears in the acute stages correlating with the level of visual loss measured clinically and degree of conduction block measured electrophysiologically. This reversible change presumably correlates with localized breakdown of the blood–brain barrier and an acute inflammatory infiltrate with demyelination (Youll *et al.*, 1991). Clinical recovery occurs as the blood–brain barrier is restored and oedema resolves corresponding to disappearance of gadolinium enhancement. It is also evident that up to 70% of patients with clinically isolated optic neuritis will have MRI lesions elsewhere in the brain, most frequently in the periventricular regions of the cortex, subcortical white matter and pons (Morrisey *et al.*, 1993). This observation was first made in 1985, but the predictive significance for subsequent clinical MS is only now being clarified, most notably by the Optic Neuritis Treatment Trial (ONTT).

THE OPTIC NEURITIS TREATMENT TRIAL

The multicentre prospective ONTT of the effect of corticosteroids has recently published results with important implications for investigation and management of typical cases between the ages of 18 and 45 years old. Patients were randomized into three treatment categories: intravenous (i.v.) methyl prednisolone plus oral prednisolone, oral prednisolone alone and oral placebo. There was no i.v. placebo group. The results (Beck, 1992; Beck and Cleary, 1993a,b; Beck *et al.*, 1993a,b) may be summarized as follows:

1. All patients with typical optic neuritis underwent MRI brain scanning, chest X-ray, syphilis serology and antinuclear antibody tests. In all 457 cases the blood tests were normal and in only one case did the imaging reveal a compressive lesion mimicking optic neuritis. It was concluded that no ancillary testing is required to support the clinical diagnosis of typical optic neuritis.

2. Patients receiving oral prednisolone did not recover any more quickly or achieve a better final acuity than those given oral placebo. Those given i.v. methyl prednisolone did, however, show a more rapid visual recovery, but did not have a higher likelihood of good final vision.

3. After a 2-year follow-up period, the rate of recurrent episodes of optic neuritis was significantly higher in the group given oral prednisolone than in the group given either oral placebo or i.v. methyl prednisolone. However, this higher rate (30%) was still little different from that of untreated patients in other series, so the significance of this is unclear.

4. Of 389 patients who did not have MS at study entry, 10 (7.5%) of the 134 intravenously treated patients developed at least one further CNS lesion within 2 years compared with 21 (16.7%) of 126 placebo treated patients. Patients treated with oral prednisolone had a similar incidence to those treated with placebo. By 4 years of follow-up, little clinical difference in the rate for developing MS was apparent.

5. At presentation with optic neuritis MRI may predict the development of MS; 36% of placebo treated patients whose study entry MRI scans revealed two or more periventricular signal abnormalities of a least 3-mm diameter developed definite MS within 2 years, compared with only 3% of those in whom MRI scans were normal. In another study, progression to clinical MS (defined by the Posen criteria) occured in 82% of patients presenting with optic neuritis and an abnormal brain MRI compared with 8% of those with a normal MRI.

In our hospital, it is current practice to treat with high dose steroids only those patients with acute optic neuritis who have poor vision in the fellow eye due to some other disease process and who have bilateral acute involvement.

It is also prudent to be cautious in offering prognostic advise to patients presenting with optic neuritis for two following reasons. First, MRI abnormalities are due to changes in the water content of CNS lesions and do not correlate with clinical effects or eventual disease burden. Second, the likelihood of developing MS does not correlate closely with the likelihood of neurological disability

OPTIC NEURITIS IN MULTIPLE SCLEROSIS VARIANTS

Devic's disease (neuromyelitis optica)

The association of acute or subacute visual loss due to an optic neuropathy in one or both eyes preceded or followed by transverse or ascending myelitis is known as Devic's disease. In contrast to MS, neuromyelitis optica tends to occur as a single episode without recurrences (Leys *et al.*, 1987).

Acute disseminated encephalomyelitis (ADEM)

Optic neuritis which is bilateral and simultaneous may form part of a monophasic syndrome of coma or drowsiness, seizures and multifocal neurological signs indicating damage to cerebral hemispheres, cerebellum, spinal cord and optic nerves. A hypersensitivity or immune response to myelin is thought to underlie the pathogenesis, sometimes triggered by overt viral infection and exceptionally following vaccination.

Chronic progressive optic neuritis

Unilateral or bilateral visual loss that progresses may occur in MS. However, the diagnosis can only be made after exhaustive efforts to exclude granulomatous, infiltrative and mass lesions. All these conditions can respond to corticosteroids in the short term (Ormerod and McDonald, 1984).

ATYPICAL OPTIC NEURITIS

Autoimmune

The association between optic neuritis and systemic lupus erythematosis (SLE) and related diseases has suggested that elements within the optic nerve may be susceptible to autoantibody-mediated attack. However, it may be more accurate to ascribe the optic neuropathy to small vessel occlusive disease arising either as a consequence of circulating immune complex deposition or to the direct effects of associated anticardiolipin or antiphospholipid antibodies on vascular endothelium (Cordeiro *et al.*, 1994; Scott and Brillman, 1994). In other instances, such as in Sjörgren's syndrome and the vasculitides, (polyarteritis nodosa, Churg-Strauss syndrome) primary vessel wall inflammation leads to an ischaemic rather than to a purely inflammatory optic neuropathy. Similarly, in Behçet's disease, acute disc swelling is more likely to be due to intracranial venous thrombosis and raised intracranial pressure, or an ischaemic process in the optic nerve head than an inflammatory mechanism. Other reported causes of 'immune' optic neuritis include therapy with interleukin-2, interferon -α, bee-stings (Berrios, 1994) and the trivalent (MMR) vaccine (Jabs *et al.*, 1986; Kazerian and Gager, 1978).

Postviral, parainfectious and infective optic neuropathy

Optic neuritis may follow clinically and laboratory confirmed viral illness: in particular chickenpox, rubella, infectious mononucleosis, and mumps usually at an interval of 7 to 10 days and with full spontaneous recovery (Anderson, 1994). This is the category into which many children with optic neuritis fit, when involvement is frequently bilateral and simultaneous. Postinfective immune mechanisms are suggested by the time course except in herpes zoster ophthalmicus where the mechanism is more likely to be an associated vasculitis involving the short posterior ciliary vessels (Miller *et al.*, 1986; Selbst *et al.*, 1983; Hamed *et al.*, 1993).

Primary infection of the optic nerve is rare outside the context of immunosupression and/or infectious intraocular disease. In acquired immunodeficiency syndrome (AIDS), the differential diagnosis of infectious optic neuritis includes acute retinal necrosis (herpes viruses), cytomegalovirus and hepatitis B, as well as granulomatous perineuritis due to tuberculosis, cryptococcus, aspergillus or syphilis. Although acute retinal necrosis does arise in immunocompetent individuals, extension into the optic nerve appears more likely in association with immunosuppression. Management is generally the control of the underlying medical condition, but there are reports of benefit from specific surgical measures. For example, optic nerve sheath decompression may bring at least short-term visual benefits in cryptococcal optic neuropathy. Human immunodeficiency virus (HIV/HTLV III) has been implicated in retrobulbar neuritis together with disseminated CNS lesions. Rarely, Lyme disease, toxoplasmosis and toxocariasis may cause optic neuritis, but not without other features of intraocular inflammation (Cohen and Glasgow, 1993; Newman and Lessell, 1992; Tomsak *et al.*, 1992; Winward *et al.*, 1989; Jacobson *et al.*, 1991).

Granulomatous and 'steroid dependent' optic neuropathy: differential diagnosis of perineuritis and sarcoidosis

In granulomatous optic neuropathy, there is visual loss and disc swelling either as a result of infiltration of the intraorbital nerve sheath or of the nerve itself. The differential diagnosis includes syphilis, cryptococcus, tuberculosis, sarcoidosis and idiopathic granulomatous meningeal disease. The clinical presentation may be acute or chronic.

Secondary syphilis may result in papillitis, neuroretinitis and choroiditis while optic atrophy complicates the taboparetic forms of tertiary disease. A typical attack of retrobulbar optic neuritis is extremely rare in syphilis but a primary involvement of the optic nerve sheath (perineuritis) may occur. In this instance, peripheral field is lost with disc swelling and relative preservation of central acuity. Imaging shows marked thickening of the intraorbital optic nerve meninges.

In sarcoidosis, granulomatous inflammation may involve the ocular adnexae, uveal tract and retina as well as the optic nerve. Ocular abnormalities are the presenting feature of sarcoidosis in 20% of patients, 60–70% of which are accounted for by anterior uveitis. Posterior ocular segment disease includes vitreous infiltrates, retinal vasculitis, and choroidal lesions as well as optic nerve disease. Clinically it is important to distinguish between optic disc swelling which may be a non-specific feature of posterior uveitis as a result of local blood–ocular barrier breakdown, and disc swelling as a manifestation of nerve or nerve sheath granulomatous infiltration (Graham *et al.*, 1986; Westlake *et al.*, 1995). This is not difficult if the rules for discriminating causes of visual loss due to retinal disease from those due to optic nerve disease (see Chapter 2) are applied (Beardsley *et al.*, 1984; DeBroff and Donahue, 1993).

A total of 20% of patients with sarcoidosis and posterior uveitis also have CNS disease: in addition to optic neuropathy there may be disseminated white matter lesions, aseptic meningitis and cranial polyneuropathy. In some cases of sarcoidosis diagnostic difficulties arise because there do not appear to be any obvious lesions outside the eye and CNS, leading to a close resemblance to MS. This is made harder by the fact that although in MS intraocular inflammation usually takes the form of asymptomatic vitritis and periphlebitis, sometimes eye involvement is much more severe with vitreous infiltration, retinal neovascularization and macular oedema all of which also point towards sarcoidosis. Choroidal infiltrates appear to be unique to sarcoidosis.

A further diagnostic possibility in patients with inflammatory eye disease associated with relapsing neurological disease is Behçet's disease. In these cases, retinal infiltrates and branch vein and smaller venous occlusions are characteristic. In these difficult cases, experience indicates that CSF oligoclonal bands and angiotensin converting enzyme

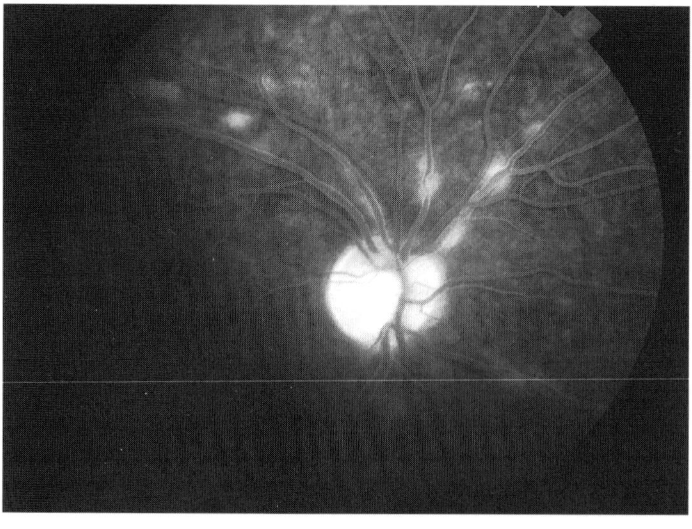

Figure 5.8 Fluorescein angiogram showing retinal venous leakage (periphlebitis) in sarcoidosis.

levels are uninformative and that careful systemic evaluation is mandatory. The search will include the use of plain chest radiographs, lung function tests, serum angiotensin converting enzyme levels, serum and urinary calcium, cutaneous anergy to tuberculin and a positive Kveim test. Gallium scanning may show increased uptake at sites of involvement and bronchio-alveolar lavage may yield a typical lymphocyte/neutrophil ratio and a high CD4+/CD8+ T-lymphocyte ratio. Endobronchial biopsy and liver biopsy may be helpful in finding non-caseating granulomas when the Kveim test is unavailable or yields equivocal results. It is helpful to remember that sarcoid granulomas may be very simply demonstrated on conjunctival or lacrimal gland biopsy in cases when there is only mild clinical involvement of these structures. Some cases cannot be characterized and must be treated symptomatically with steroid-sparing immunosuppressive regimes.

Occasionally, meningeal granulomatous disease arises in clinical isolation causing visual loss with an entirely negative systemic medical evaluation. In these cases the diagnosis may only be confirmed on biopsy, usually of the nerve sheath of the blind eye when the fellow eye is involved. The clinical course and radiological picture may mimic a primary optic nerve sheath meningioma although pain on eye movements would be expected in any inflammatory nerve sheath disease, and meningiomas often show dystrophic sheath calcification on CT.

Steroid dependent optic neuropathy
Another mimic of optic neuritis is neoplastic disease. Mechanisms are direct infiltration of the optic nerve head in leukaemia causing disc swelling, meningeal involvement by non-Hodgkin's lymphoma or metastatic carcinoma of breast and lung, and paraneoplastic optic neuropathy in oat-cell carcinoma of the bronchus. The term 'steroid dependent' optic neuropathy is sometimes used in this context, referring to the fact that unlike typical optic neuritis, vision usually drops again when systemic steroid therapy is withdrawn. Occasionally, the patient with steroid dependent optic neuropathy is found to have a collagen vascular disease such as SLE, in which case the mechanism may be one of small vessels occlusive disease at the optic nerve head. Steroid-sparing immmunosuppressive therapies may be required; usually the underlying general medical abnormality becomes evident after sufficient follow-up.

Contiguous inflammation and optic neuritis
A period of only 40 years separates current clinical thinking from a time when virtually all optic neuritis was held to be associated with paranasal sinus disease, and the association with contiguous inflammatory sinuses retains a reduced but nonetheless still important place in the differential diagnosis.

The question of whether a typical attack of retrobulbar neuritis may be due to sinusitis has probably been resolved by studies showing the virtual universality of radiographic evidence of sinus disease in the asymptomatic population, meaning that on its own mucosal inflammation within the sinus is an insufficient explanation for optic neuritis. However, contiguous inflammation in sinusitis may be important: the bony wall of the optic canal is often defective medially leaving the nerve sheath in direct anatomical relationship with the sphenoid sinus. As a result therefore mucocoeles and pyomucocoeles of the posterior ethmoid and sphenoid sinus may result in optic nerve compression. When orbital cellulitis complicates sinus disease, optic nerve function may fail because of diffuse orbital interstitial pressure rise and intraorbital and subperiosteal absess formation. Only in a minority of cases is it necessary to postulate infective endarteritis obliterans of the intracanalicular nerve sheath to explain visual loss in contiguous sinus disease (Slavin and Glaser, 1987; Casteels *et al.*, 1992).

Idiopathic orbital inflammatory disease may also be associated with visual loss due to optic nerve failure. The terms orbital pseudotumour and Tolosa-Hunt syndrome are

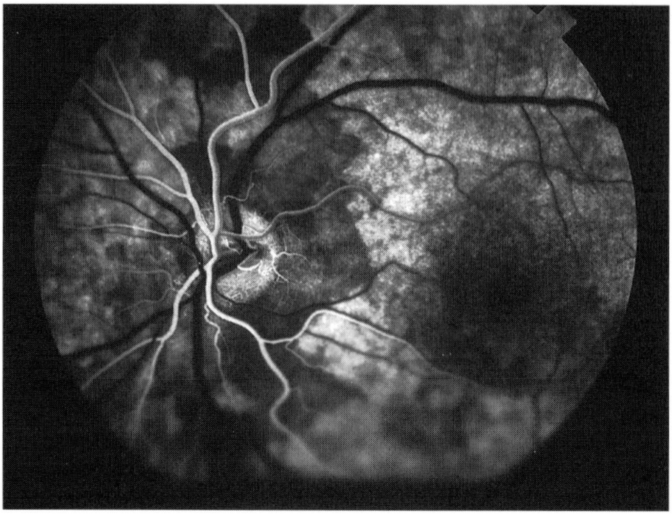

Figure 5.9

sometimes used in this context. A range of structures may be involved by inflammatory infiltration or by loss of function arising from the local mass effect of inflammatory tissue. Tissues are involved either singly or in combination from the sclera, orbital fat, lacrimal gland optic nerve sheath and extraocular muscles in the anterior orbit, to the crowded neurovascular structures of the superior orbital fissure and cavernous sinus posteriorly (Margo *et al.*, 1989; Dutton and Anderson, 1985).

Diagnosis and management are best based on tissue diagnosis, as a spectrum of histological entities may be found. These range from benign and neoplastic lymphoproliferative processes to granulomatous and vasculitic lesions. Merging with the granulomatous lesions are the specific disorders of syphilis, sarcoidosis and tuberculosis as well as granulomatous vasculitis (systemic and localized versions of Wegener's disease). Most frequently however, the disorder does appear to be isolated and neither infective nor neoplastic. The clinical picture varies from acute onset with pain and signs of orbital inflammation (proptosis, ophthalmoplegia, conjunctival and scleral injection) which may settle rapidly with systemic steroid therapy, to a more chronic indolent clinical picture which is refractory to treatment and in which the tissue damage is influenced by the degree of reparative fibrosis in chronically inflamed tissue.

ISCHAEMIC OPTIC NEUROPATHY

Anterior ischaemic optic neuropathy (AION) due to infarction of the optic nerve head is a common cause of visual loss in patients past middle age. Posterior ION is extremely rare: the term refers to infarction of the retrobulbar optic nerve without disc swelling, which makes this a difficult and speculative diagnosis.

The blood supply of the optic nerve head is primarily derived from choroidal and posterior ciliary branches of the ophthalmic artery. The posterior ciliary arteries arise independently from the ophthalmic artery and may number from two to four. Usually

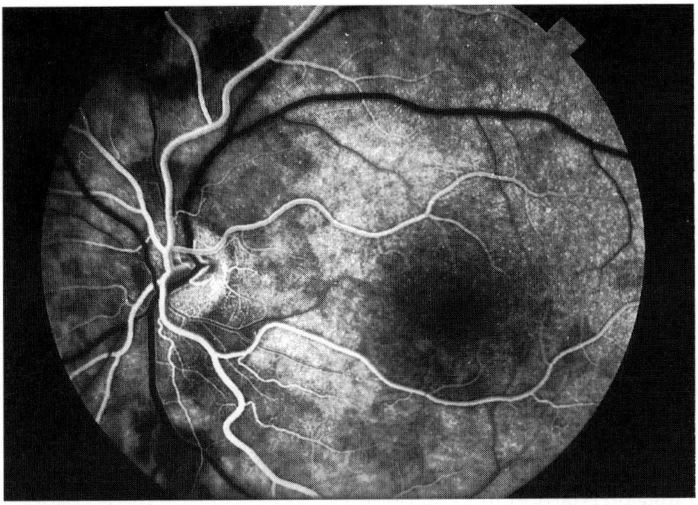

Figure 5.10

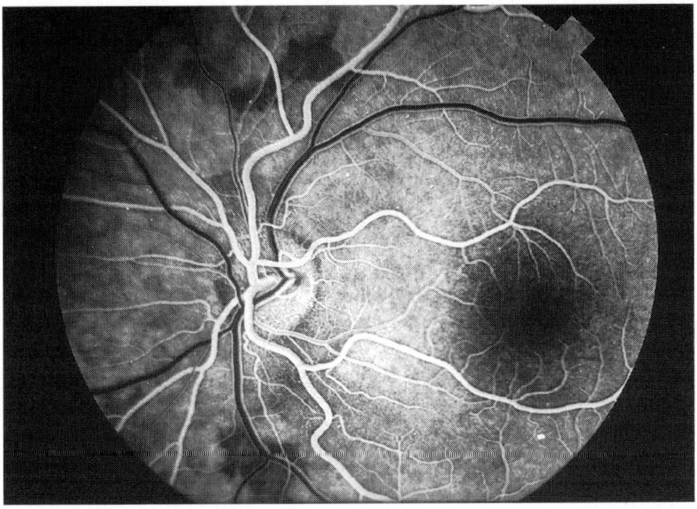

Figure 5.11

Figures 5.9–5.11 Fluorescein angiograms showing watershed zone of slower filling of the choroidal circulation between the medial and lateral short posterior ciliary vascular territories.

they form medial and lateral groups, and because they are end arteries a watershed zone is formed between territory perfused by the medial group and territory perfused by the lateral group (Olver *et al.*, 1994). When the watershed zone traverses the optic nerve head, this structure is particularly vulnerable to haemodynamic disturbance resulting in infarction and a permanent visual deficit (Hayreh, 1970; Hayreh, 1974; Williamson *et al.*, 1993).

AION occurs in two forms: non-arteritic and arteritic, usually due to giant cell arteritis.

NON-ARTERITIC ION

In a typical attack, there is a painless loss of acuity and field (usually in an altitudinal pattern) in a patient aged between 50 and 70 years. The onset is acute, first being noticed on awakening, although some patients experience progressive step-wise visual loss over the period of 1–2 weeks. The lack of pain and the age of onset help to distinguish ION from inflammatory optic neuritis. A relative afferent pupil defect indicates that the visual loss is of neuroretinal origin and fundoscopy reveals pallid optic disc swelling which may be sectoral rather than general, often with one or more splinter haemorrhages at the disc margin (Eagling *et al.*, 1974; Boghen and Glaser, 1975; Sawle *et al.*, 1990).

Rheological abnormalities are frequently identified in patients with non-arteritic ION. These include the three components making up Virchow's triad for conditions predisposing to thrombosis: disorders of the vessel wall — arteriosclerosis, diabetes, hypertension, migraine (McDonald and Sanders, 1971; Hayreh *et al.*, 1994), disorders of blood flow — haemodynamic shock, emboli (Tomsak, 1985), carotid artery occlusion, and disorders of blood constituents — hyperviscosity states and acquired defects of thrombosis and haemostasis regulation (Acheson and Sanders, 1994; Hayreh, 1987). In addition to these vascular considerations, there is evidence of an anatomical predisposition as hypermetropic eyes with small optic discs with low cup-disc ratios ('the disc at risk') are especially vulnerable (Burde, 1993; Beck *et al.*, 1987a). This association also exists in rare cases of ION in the young. For this reason clinicians should be guarded about making the diagnosis in a myopic eye where the requisite crowding of neurovascular structures into a tight scleral canal does not exist. Buried optic disc drusen may also contribute a risk factor (Beck *et al.*, 1987b). The fellow eye is eventually involved in up to 40% of cases (Beri *et al.*, 1987), but surprisingly, recent reports indicate that spontaneous recovery may be more common than previously supposed (Aiello *et al.*, 1992; Barratt *et al.*, 1992).

ARTERITIC ION

In giant cell arteritis (GCA), systemic symptoms of anorexia, malaise, proximal arthralgia and myalgia (polymyalgia rheumatica), together with headache, scalp tenderness and jaw claudication usually precede visual loss. The visual deficit is often severe, with pallid swelling of the entire optic disc and an additional retinal cherry red spot when ophthalmic artery disease results in a combined posterior ciliary and central retinal artery occlusion (Hinzpeter and Naumann 1976; Liu *et al.*, 1994). Giant cell arteritis is a vasculitis of large and mid-sized arteries containing an elastic lamina. Such vessels are only found extradurally, but cerebral infarction may result from vertebrobasilar and carotid involvement in the neck. Aortic arch and coronary vessels may also be occluded. The diagnosis is based on the findings of a typical history supported by an elevated ESR and C-reactive protein and fibrinogen levels together with a positive superficial temporal artery biopsy. Because the disease characteristically causes focal vascular involvement (skip lesions) biopsy may be negative, and less commonly, the ESR may be normal (Jacobson and Slamovits, 1987). A high index of suspicion is required to make the diagnosis and without adequate treatment the incidence of second eye involvement reaches 80%. In younger patients, arteritic ION may occur as part of other systemic vasculitides including polyarteritis nodosa, Churg–Strauss syndrome (Acheson *et al.*, 1993) and Sjögren's disease.

THE MANAGEMENT OF ACUTE ION

The management of acute ION consists of:

1) Increase optic nerve head perfusion pressure by measures such as oral Diamox® and (in selected cases with second eye involvement) posturing the patient flat.
2) High dose corticosteroids and temporal artery biopsy in suspected giant cell arteritis. As a minimum, this comprises 80 mg prednisolone daily plus 200 mg i.v. hydrocortisone immediately. When the patient presents with second eye involvement, or the ESR does not fall rapidly after commencing oral steroids, a 3-day course of pulse i.v. methyl prednisolone 10 mg/kg is given. A delay of up to 48 hours will not affect the biopsy result after the patient has started corticosteroids. Anti-platelet agents (ticlopidine) or low dose heparin may also be of value in cases of progressive visual failure.
3) Identification and treatment of systemic vascular risk factors in non-arteritic ION (carotid disease, hypertension, diabetes, pro-thrombotic states) to reduce the risk of subsequent stroke.
4) After several years of controversy, optic nerve sheath decompression has now been shown not be of value in the management of this condition (Jablons *et al.*, 1993; The Ischaemic Optic Neuropathy Decompression Trial Research Group, 1995), even in those cases with progressive visual loss.

TUMOURS AND THE OPTIC NERVE

PRIMARY OPTIC NERVE TUMOURS

Meningiomas

Optic nerve function may be directly impaired by meningiomas arising from the optic nerve sheath, usually in the orbital portions of the nerve. More commonly however, optic nerve sheath meningiomas arise secondarily from the sphenoid wing, tuberculum sellae or olfactory groove which subsequently invade the optic canal and orbit. Intracranial extension of primary optic nerve sheath meningiomas may also occur. Meningiomas spread along lines of least resistance in the subarachnoid space and are usually encapsulated by intact dura and arachnoid. When adjacent to bone the Haversian canals are often invaded giving rise to hyperostosis and bone proliferation. Growth is typically indolent over many years and may be initiated or accelerated by pregnancy. In the optic nerve, compression results in axonal transport obstruction, disc swelling and eventual demyelination. Obliteration of the pial blood supply contributes to eventual optic atrophy. Meningiomas arise from meningothelial cells which are present in arachnoid villi at multiple sites in the middle cranial fossa and uniformly along the intracanalicular and intraorbital optic nerve. Histologically there are two common types: a meningothelial or syncitial type and a transitional pattern which is associated with psammoma bodies and dystrophic calcification (Boniuk *et al.*, 1985; Karp *et al.*, 1974; Dutton, 1992).

Primary optic nerve sheath meningiomas, in common with the same tumour at other sites, most frequently develop in middle aged females. Most tumours are unilateral, but bilateral and multifocal cases exist raising the possibility of an association with central neurofibromatosis (NF2) (Cunliffe *et al.*, 1992). Clinically there are features of a slowly progressive optic neuropathy with loss of acuity, colour vision and a central scotoma. Less commonly, there is abrupt visual loss as the central retinal artery and/or vein are compressed, or there is a history of transient visual obscurations. Cases of gaze-evoked amaurosis have been reported where movement of the eye in a particular direction (usually abduction) results in compression of the tumour and reversible impairment of ocular blood flow. Fundoscopy reveals either simple optic atrophy, or atrophy in association with chronic disc oedema. Optociliary (retino-choroidal anastomoses) venous shunt vessels indicating chronic central retinal vein obstruction may appear. Axial proptosis reflecting an intraconal orbital mass is usual in the later stages.

Meningiomas arising from the sphenoid and tuberculum sellae may cause visual failure either by compression of the intracranial portions of the optic nerve or chiasm, or by intracanalicular and intraorbital extension. In addition, a large inner sphenoid wing meningioma may cause visual loss and anosmia on one side and disc oedema contralaterally (Foster-Kennedy syndrome) as a result of raised intracranial pressure or nerve compression or by a combination of both mechanisms. Tumours arising at this location commonly give rise to ophthalmoplegia, Horner's syndrome and trigeminal sensory loss as a result of parasellar and superior orbital fissure involvement. Orbital fissure involvement is generally also associated with proptosis (Sarkies, 1987).

Imaging reveals a number of specific features in meningiomas of the orbit. Sphenoid hyperostosis and contrast enhancement on CT are seen in orbital extension of an intracranial mass. In primary optic nerve sheath tumours, tramline calcification of the orbital optic nerve sheath is a characteristic feature, which will be seen on CT but not on MRI. Commonly there is diffuse tubular expansion of the orbital nerve-sheath complex with a degree of anterior or posterior expansion. Less commonly there is marked central orbital fusiform enlargment in which case the appearances may be confused with a glioma. These points of uncertainty have been clarified by MRI, especially when fat suppression and gadolinium enhancement techniques are available: where a meningioma causes fusiform enlargement of the nerve-sheath complex the nerve and sheath components can readily be distinguished. By contrast, in primary optic glioma the mass can clearly be shown to arise from the optic nerve. In addition, the early detection of intracanalicular and early intracranial extension of primary nerve sheath tumours is possible (Lindblom *et al.* 1992; Zimmerman *et al.*, 1990).

The treatment of orbital meningiomas remains controversial. In sphenoid wing tumours which principally have an intracranial component, surgical resection is the treatment of choice. However, because of the intimate relationship of these tumours to the anterior visual pathways, superior orbital fissure and optic canal, and to the frontal and temporal lobes, excision is frequently incomplete. In the elderly, slowly progressive proptosis may be adequately treated by oculoplastic measures designed to cover an exposed cornea for example by upper and lower eyelid retractor recession, and by lateral and medial canthotomy. Radiotherapy requires large doses (50–200 Gy) because of the slow growing nature of the tumour and is associated with risks of radiation damage to the optic nerve, retina, lacrimal glands and lens. Endocrine therapy represents a new alternative. Meningiomas typically have hormonal receptors which explains why they are more common in females than males and why growth may be markedly influenced by pregnancy. Both progesterone antagonists such as mefipristone (and RU486) and oestrogen antagonists such as tamoxifen may be helpful depending on the exact receptor population in a particular tumour. Early clinical experience with mefipristone has indicated modest tumour shrinkage in some cases but the side-effect profile of nausea, fatigue, hot flushes, alopecia and gynaecomastia are prominent. Further evaluation continues in the hope of finding satisfactory medical therapy in cases where surgical resection is incomplete, but in the meantime, radiotherapy offers the only effective remedy when progressive disease is clearly documented (Rose, 1993; Wright *et al.*, 1980a).

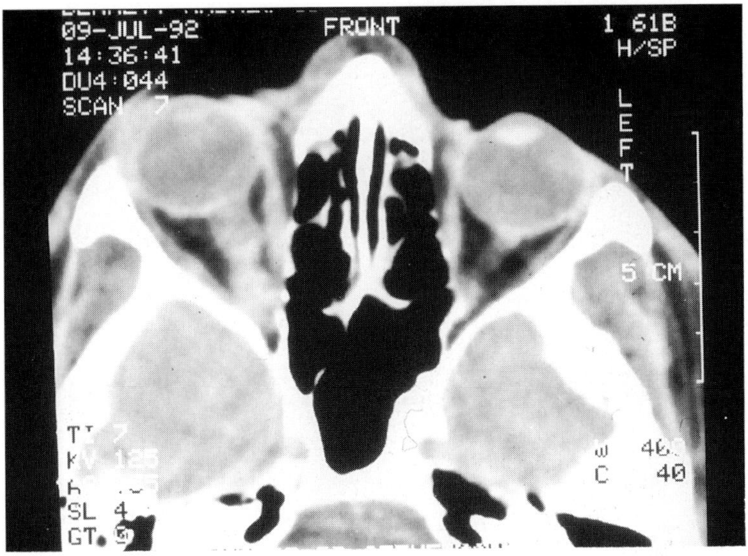

Figure 5.12

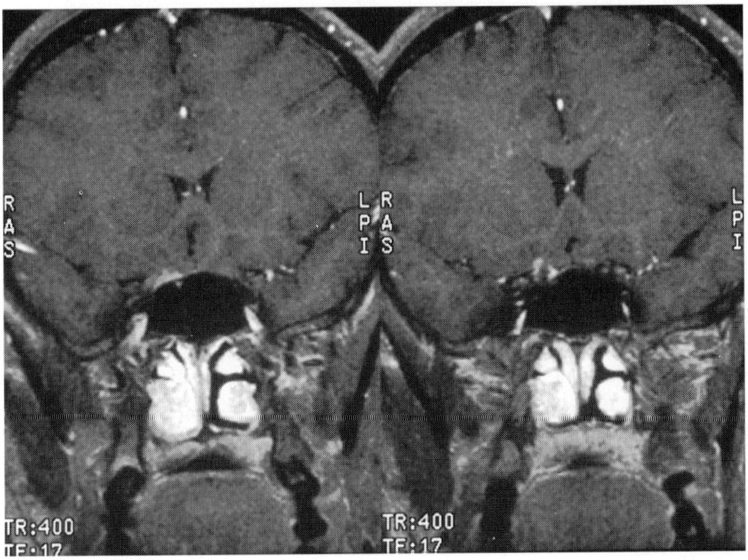

Figure 5.13

Figures 5.12, 5.13 Primary optic nerve sheath meningioma on standard imaging: contrast enhanced MRI shows intracranial extension.

By contrast, in primary optic nerve sheath meningiomas the surgical approach is not mandatory. No patient is reported to have died from this tumour even after the event of intracranial spread, and the prognosis for vision in affected eye is very poor regardless of therapy. There are cases in which, following visual loss from a primary intraorbital lesion,

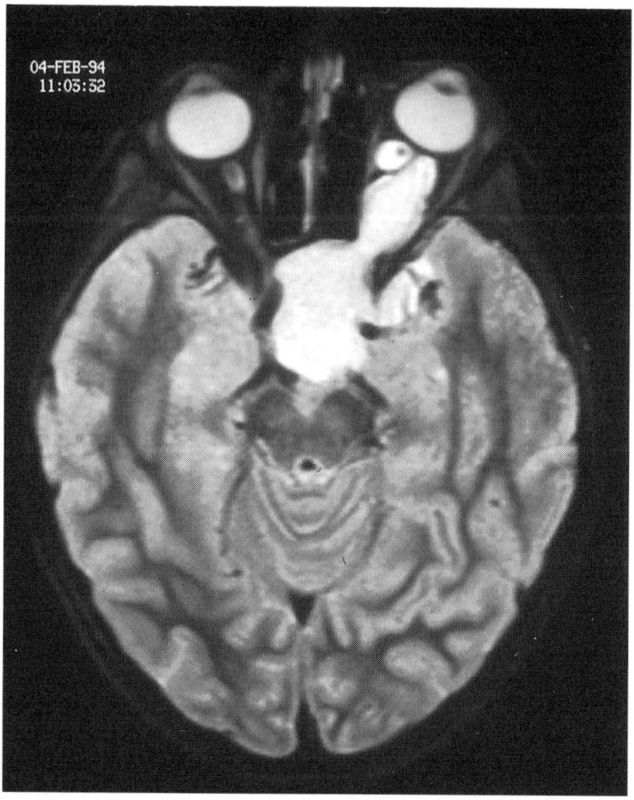

Figure 5.14 MRI study of optochiasmal glioma.

intracranial spread appears be the next development and radical resection appears to be logical. However, total excision of meninges around the canal is almost impossible, and removal of the dura and optic nerve removes a physical barrier to tumour spread. It is also important to consider that involvement of the contralateral optic nerve due to spread via the planum sphenoidale has never been clearly documented and surgery is therefore unlikely to influence the likelihood of bilaterality. Bilateral optic nerve sheath meningiomas are thought in fact to arise *de novo*. A further factor which may temper surgical enthusiasm is that modern imaging with contrast enhanced MRI and fat suppression techniques may show evidence of intracranial extension at presentation even in tumours thought to be confined to the orbit on CT. The object of surgery is to control the rare case of aggressive local disease and this generally requires a combined neurosurgical orbitocranial approach. This is more likely to apply to younger adults and children. Radiotherapy may result in temporary visual improvement but the benefits have not been reported to be sustained; there are as yet no reports of endocrine therapy in primary optic nerve sheath meningioma.

Optic and optochiasmal glioma

Primary glial tumours of the anterior visual pathways (optic glioma) are seen in two fundamentally different forms. First, there are benign gliomas of childhood and second there is the rare malignant glioblastoma of adulthood. These are discussed as separate entities, even though they may both present with visual loss and orbital mass effects. Involvement may be of one optic nerve, intraorbital or intracranial, of both optic nerves, of the optic chiasm and of the hypothalamus or thalamus. Malignant optic gliomas of adulthood do not arise from indolent childhood tumours (Dutton, 1994).

Benign optic gliomas of childhood may cause insidious proptosis and visual loss when confined to the orbit. The optic disc may be swollen and / or atrophic and sensory strabismus frequently accompanies visual loss (Repka and Miller, 1988). Progressive proptosis does not necessarily indicate tumour growth, haemorrhage or necrosis: arachnoid hyperplasia and the extracellular accumulation of PAS-positive mucopolysaccharide material are characteristic and visual function may fluctuate or even improve spontaneously in some cases. The presence of arachnoid hyperplasia may result in diagnostic confusion with meningioma on biopsy, and it is only with modern fat suppression contrast enhanced MRI that the glioma itself can clearly be distinguished from surrounding tissue changes. The absence of mitotic figures and the capacity for childhood gliomas to grow without any tumour cell division has raised the possibility that these lesions are in fact hamartomas and not true neoplasms at all. This pathological evidence together with the variable clinical course mitigates in favour of conservative management in most cases. Generally speaking, patients with optic glioma do not appear to be predisposed towards the development of other intracranial tumours (Glaser *et al.*, 1971).

The association of optic glioma with peripheral neurofibromatosis (NF1) is well known although figures for this vary widely between 10 and 70%. Any child with diminished vision and an optic neuropathy requires a search for the cutaneous stigmata of NF1 – axillary freckles, café-au-lait spots, peripheral nerve tumours and iris hamartomas. A detailed family history may also be helpful. Recent imaging evidence suggests an association between downwards kinking of the mid-orbital portion of the optic nerve and a characteristic tubular thickening pattern of arachnoid proliferation in cases with NF1 (Imez and Hoyt, 1991).

Chiasmal optic gliomas of childhood are more common than those confined to one optic nerve. Cases present with visual loss, visual field defects and nystagmus.

The visual loss is generally bilateral and field analysis may show either central scotomas or temporal hemianopic defects. Nystagmus may be horizontal or rotatory, sometimes with head-nodding mimicking spasmus nutans. A see-saw pattern may also be observed. In addition features of hypothalamic or thalamic involvement may be present. The diencephalic syndrome of childhood includes emaciation and dwarfism in spite of adequate nutrition, skin pallor without anaemia, sleep disturbance and sexual precosity. In addition hydrocephalus and signs of raised intracranial pressure may develop and leptomeningeal spread has also been reported (McDonnell and Miller, 1983; Bruggers *et al.*, 1991). In other instances, spontaneous regression has been reported (Brzoski *et al.*, 1992).

Nowadays, the diagnosis can normally be made securely with neuroimaging without the need for biopsy which may itself cause further visual loss. Typical features on CT scanning include a smoothly expanded optic canal and a suprasellar mass flattening the floor of the third ventricle. The suprasellar mass is contiguous to an expanded chiasm or optic nerves or may show spread into the optic tract. Sometimes, tubular expansion of the chiasm and optic nerves alone is seen, without any suprasellar mass. In addition MRI may reveal posterior extension into the basal ganglia, cortex and cerebellum (Imes and Hoyt, 1991).

The management of optic glioma has a different emphasis depending on whether the disease is thought be purely orbital or intracranial. In intraorbital tumours the role of surgery remains undefined: incomplete resection is not associated with recurrence or malignant transformation, but evidence of extension of an optic nerve glioma to involve the chiasm subsequently is very scanty. Symptoms in the fellow eye may simply reflect progressive effects from tumour residing in the chiasm from the outset. Therefore, surgery is generally reserved for palliative treatment in cosmetically unacceptable blind eyes, and the remainder of patients may best be treated conservatively. When surgery is undertaken, a healthy globe can be preserved when care is taken to preserve the short and long posterior ciliary branches of the ophthalmic artery and the branches of oculomotor, trochlear, trigeminal, and abducens nerves as they pass through the superior ophthalmic fissure (Wright *et al.*, 1980b).

In chiasmal glioma, surgical resection is not associated with improved vision or prolonged life. However, surgical intervention may be required for hydrocephalus, decompression of an intraneural cyst or for biopsy when imaging leaves diagnostic doubt. The weight of evidence is now in favour of regarding chiasmal glioma as a benign pilocytic astrocytoma with little tendency to grow. Where growth is clearly documented, radiotherapy may result in tumour shrinkage and visual improvement. However, the benefits must be weighed against the risks of radionecrosis and demyelination both at local and remote sites in an immature brain. Interstitial stereotactic radiosurgery may offer advantages to external beam radiotherapy where available. Sometimes posterior tumour extension results in obstructive hydrocephalus, requiring shunting. Chemotherapy has also been employed but may be hard to justify in such an indolent tumour (Imes and Hoyt, 1986; Hoyt and Bagdassarian 1969).

By complete contrast, primary malignant gliomas of the optic nerve have been documented in childhood but generally arise in males aged 40–60 years. Patients present with symptoms and signs that may mimic optic neuritis with rapid monocular visual loss, retrobulbar pain, disc oedema and transient improvement on corticosteroids, but within several weeks complete blindness and contralateral visual loss ensues. The fundus may show features of central retinal vein or artery occlusion as a result of vascular compression. Radiotherapy and combination chemotherapy may be of some value but death usually ensues within months and therefore the disease represents the occurrence of a relatively common brain tumour at an uncommon site (Hoyt *et al.*, 1973).

THE OPTIC NERVE IN SYSTEMIC CANCER

Infiltration of the meninges by systemic cancer may sometimes result in painless progressive visual loss due to retrobulbar optic neuropathy (Mansour *et al.*, 1993). Adenocarcinoma of the breast and lung are the common causes of this syndrome which may be diagnosed by demonstrating meningeal contrast enhancement on MRI together with cytological findings of neoplastic cells in the CSF (Little *et al.*, 1974; Olson *et al.*, 1974). Paraneoplastic optic neuropathy has also been described in patients with oat-cell carcinoma of the bronchus (Malik *et al.*, 1992; Boghen *et al.*, 1988). In lymphoproliferative disorders (certain leukaemias, non-Hodkin's lymphomas and related conditions) the optic nerve may be involved by direct tumour infiltration, typically with optic disc swelling (Horton *et al.*, 1992; Kattah *et al.*, 1993; Kay, 1986; Zaman *et al.*, 1993). A similar clinical picture can present in sarcoidosis and a careful systemic evaluation is required in all cases of 'atypical optic neuritis'.

COMPRESSIVE OPTIC NEUROPATHIES

Thyroid ophthalmopathy

Patients with thyroid ophthalmopathy (Graves' disease, dysthyroid eye disease, thyroid eye disease, TED) show signs of orbital congestion, proptosis and ophthalmoplegia in varying degrees. The extraocular muscles and orbital fat are expanded by inflammatory infiltrate, mucopolysaccharide deposition and, later in the disease process, by fibrotic tissue. The optic nerve may become compressed by swollen muscles and fat at the confined space of the orbital apex. Visual failure most commonly occurs in the inactive, fibrotic phase of the disease, often without conspicuous features of anterior orbital disease such as

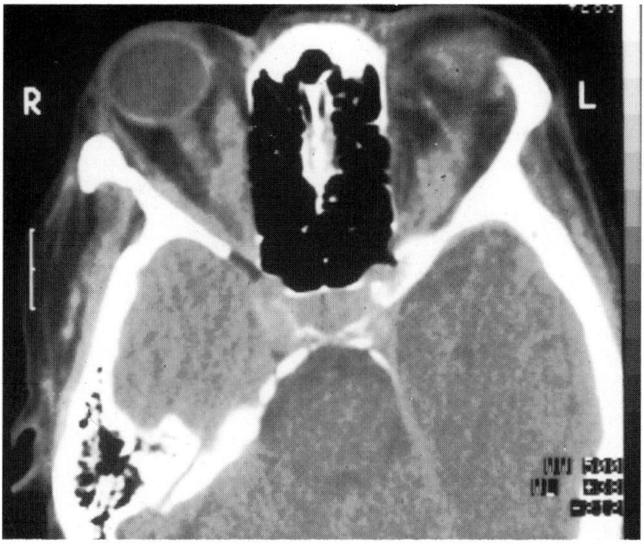

Figure 5.15 Extraocular muscle enlargement causing compressive optic neuropathy in dysthyroid eye disease.

proptosis (Neigel *et al.*, 1988; Trobe *et al.*, 1978; Guy *et al.*, 1989; Ravin *et al.*, 1975). However, in some cases, optic nerve compression forms part of the presenting, acute inflammatory phase, in which case chemosis and conjunctival injection particularly at the sites of insertion of the rectus muscles is conspicuous. Dyschromatopsia, choroidal folds and optic disc swelling support the diagnosis, but often fundoscopy is normal. Visual function is best monitored by serial measures of acuity and fields. Colour contrast sensitivity measurements over time may be a useful test for deteriorating function (Tanner *et al.* 1995).

Imaging shows characteristic swelling of the extraocular muscles posteriorly, and excludes other causes of optic nerve compression (Anderson *et al.*, 1989; Feldon *et al.*, 1984). In addition MRI may show increased signal from inflamed muscle as opposed to fibrotic muscle (Hoh *et al.*, 1994; Mourits *et al.*, 1989), allowing the more selective rational use of high dose immunosuppression only for those patients with features of inflammation. Additional measures to save vision include radiotherapy and surgical orbital decompression.

Aneurysms and orbital tumours

The intracranial portion of the optic nerve is intimately related to the major arteries that form the anterior aspect of the basal circle of Willis: the anterior cerebral and anterior communicating arteries, the ophthalmic artery, and the supraclinoid portion of the internal carotid artery itself. Saccular aneurysms may cause a variety of compressive syndromes of the anterior visual pathways including ipsilateral and contralateral optic neuropathy and/or chiasmal dysfunction (see Chapter 6). Fusiform aneurysms (ectatic dilatation) of the internal carotid artery may be a common incidental asymptomatic finding on high resolution imaging, but in certain cases have been proposed as a mechanism for the progressive optic neuropathy of normal-tension glaucoma (Kalenak *et al.*, 1992; Gutman *et al.*, 1993; Hilton and Hoyt, 1966).

Within the orbit, ophthalmic artery aneurysms are seen in the context of trauma; other masses which commonly result in the syndrome of optic neuropathy, ophthalmoplegia and proptosis include vascular tumours (cavernous haemangioma), and inflammatory pseudotumours (see Chapter 8).

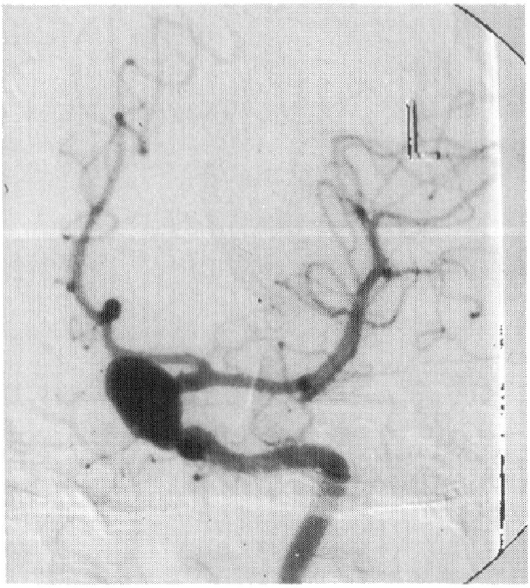

Figure 5.16

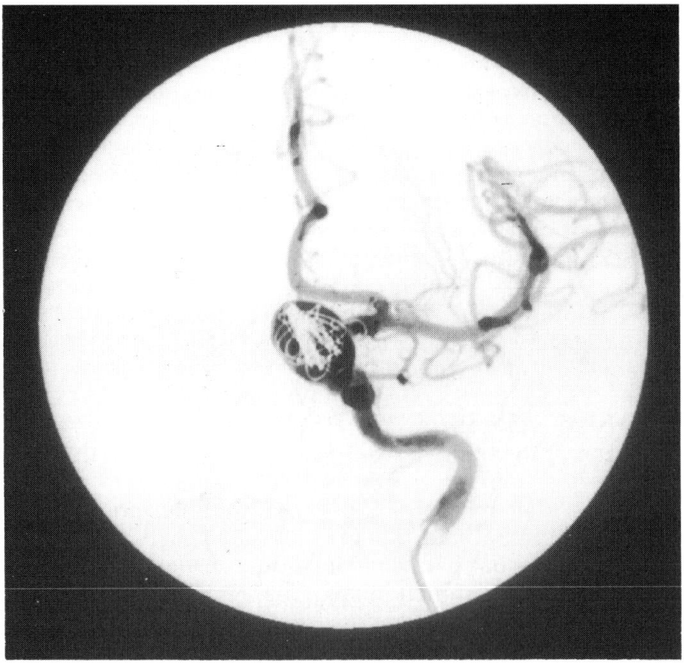

Figure 5.17

Figures 5.16, 5.17 Giant supraclinoid internal carotid aneurysm causing compressive optic neuropathy, treated by endovascular coil occlusion.

TOXIC, NUTRITIONAL AND TRAUMATIC OPTIC NEUROPATHIES

Slowly progressive bilateral visual loss with central or centrocaecal scotomata and loss of colour vision always suggests the possibility of optic nerve failure due to a toxic cause or nutritional deficiency. A careful family history will exclude heredofamilial disease. In Caucasian patients the toxic-nutritional optic neuropathies are usually due to a multifactorial combination of dietary B_1 and B_2 vitamin complex deficiency, ethanol abuse

Table 5.7 Drugs and toxins implicated in toxic optic neuropathy

Category	Agent	Notes
Antibiotics and related agents	Ethambutol	Visual loss may be reversible if identified early. Unlikely to occur in doses of < 15mg/kg/day
	Isoniazid	
	Streptomycin	
	Metronidazole	
	Amantadine	
Cytotoxic agents	Chlorambucil	
	Vincristine	
	Ara-C	
	Cis-platinum	
Cardiovascular drugs	Amiodarone	
	Digitalis	
Immunotherapeutic agents	OKT-3	
	MMR (trivalent vaccine)	
	Alpha-interferon 2B	
	Cyclosporine	
Drugs acting on the CNS	Vigabactrin	
	Chlorpromazine	
Metabolic agents	Chlorpropamide	
	Disulfiram	
	Clomiphene	
	Omeprazole	
	Lanzoprazole	
Industrial exposure	Cobalt	
	Lead	
	Carbon disulphide	
	Carbon tetrachloride	
	Chlorodinitrobenzene	
	Toluene	
	Styrene	
Miscellaneous	Aconite	(in oriental herbal remedies)
	Hexachlorphene (pHisohex)	
	Methyl alcohol	
	Ethylene glycol	
Others	Clomiphene	
	Vigabactrin	
	Cyproterone	
	Cobalt	

Note: about 40 agents are listed by Grant (1974) as possibly causing toxic optic neuropathy. Many of these, such as the arsenicals, have passed out of current clinical usage in the UK. Those agents which are listed in the 1995 British National Formulary together with some more recent additions to the literature are included in this table.

and high levels of tobacco consumption. Less commonly, malabsorbtion and vitamin B_{12} deficiency states produce the same picture. There is a possible relationship between the phenotypic expression of the Leber's hereditary optic neuropathy and these environmental factors.

In other patient populations, additional associations exist. Social dislocation amongst refugee groups in Africa is associated with consumption of uncooked cassava which contains high levels of cyanide. Adequate detoxification mechanisms may be defective when there is an additional B_{12}-deficiency state. HTLV-1 retrovirus infection has been implicated in the syndrome of combined spastic paraparesis and optic neuropathy in African–Americans (Cockerell, 1993). A recent epidemic of optic neuropathy in Cuba has been extensively investigated from the point of view of both genetic and environmental factors. Multiple dietary deficiencies have been identified as the probable cause (Sadun *et al.*, 1994).

Drug-induced and toxic causes of bilateral optic neuropathy may need careful enquiry to elucidate. Drug-induced disease may be dose-dependent (ethambutol, halogenated hydroxyquinolones and isoniazid), or idiosyncratic (disulfiram, vincristine). Toxins which have been implicated in optic neuropathies include methanol, volatile hydrocarbons and heavy metals encountered in the course of unprotected occupational exposure or recreational substance abuse (Table 5.7).

TRAUMATIC OPTIC NEUROPATHY

Mechanical injury

Mechanical injury to the optic nerve may be direct (penetrating orbitocranial trauma) or indirect. Direct injuries arise from missiles or perfecting stab wounds to the orbit. Visual loss is usually instantaneous with impact. Indirect injury is associated with deceleration injuries to the orbital margin or globe which may result in disruption of pial blood supply to the intracanicular nerve even in the absence of a fracture (Anderson *et al.*, 1982; Lessell, 1989). Typically the visual acuity is reduced to CF (20/400) or less with a dense relative afferent pupil defect. In less than 10% of cases, the onset of visual loss appears to be delayed, possibly due to the evolution of an intrasheath haematoma. Fundoscopy may reveal haemorrhage when there is optic nerve avulsion or orbital vascular injury, but may also be normal when the site of insult is at the intracanalicular or intracranial portion of the nerve. A CT scan will demonstrate a subperiosteal haematoma and is superior to MRI for delineating fractures which may impinge on the nerve within the optic canal, but MRI may be required to reveal intrasheath haematoma formation.

Extrapolation of experimental and clinical evidence from acute spinal cord injury has suggested a role for very high doses of corticosteroids in the management of acute optic neuropathy if given soon (within 8 hours) after the injury. An additional role for surgical decompression of the optic canal by the transethmoidal route has been proposed to relieve presumed axonal swelling within a confined space. This procedure may be indicated in those patients whose general condition permits and in whom there has been no response to intravenous methyl prednisolone after 48 hours. In practice however, surgical intervention is usually confined to those cases where there is a tense orbit requiring lateral canthotomy, a subperiosteal haematoma requiring orbital exploration and drainage, or an intrasheath haematoma requiring optic nerve sheath decompression (Joseph *et al.*, 1990; Levin *et al.*, 1994; Seiff, 1990; Steinsapir and Goldberg, 1994).

Radiation injury to the optic nerve and anterior visual pathways

See Chapter 6.

REFERENCES

Acheson JF and Sanders MD (1994). Coagulation abnormalities in ischaemic optic neuropathy. *Eye* **8**: 89–92.

Acheson JF, Cockerell C, Bentley C and Sanders MD (1993). Allergic vasculitis (Churg-Strauss syndrome) presenting as bilateral sequential optic neuropathy. *Br J Ophthalmol* **77**: 118–119.

Acheson JF, Green WT and Sanders MD (1994). Optic nerve sheath decompression for the treatment of visual failure in chronic raised intracranial pressure. *J Neurol Neurosurg Psychiat* **57**: 1426–1429.

Aiello AL, Sadun AA and Feldon SE (1992). Spontaneous improvement of progressive ischaemic optic neuropathy: report of two cases. *Arch Ophthalmol* **110**: 1197–1199.

Albers GW, Hoyt WF, Forno LS *et al.* (1988). Treatment response in malignant optic glioma of adulthood. *Neurology* **38**: 1071–1074.

Anderson RL, Panje WR and Gross CE (1982). Optic nerve blindness following blunt forehead trauma. *Ophthalmology* **89**: 445–455.

Anderson RL, Tweeten JP, Patrinely JR *et al.* (1989). Dysthyroid optic neuropathy without extraocular muscle involvement. *Ophthalmic Surg* **20**: 568–574.

Apple DJ, Rabb MF and Walsh PM (1982). Congenital anomalies of the optic disc. *Surv Ophthalmol* **27**: 3.

Barrett DA, Glaser JS, Schatz NJ and Winterkorn JMS (1992). Spontaneous recovery of vision in progressive anterior ischaemic optic neuropathy. *J Clin Neuro-Ophthlamol* **12**: 219–225.

Barrett TG, Bundley SE and Macleod AF (1995). Neurodegeneration and diabetes: UK nationwide study of Wolfram (DIDMOAD) syndrome. *Lancet* **346**: 1458–1462.

Beardsley TL, Brown SVL, Sydnor DF *et al.* (1984). Eleven cases of sarcoidosis of the optic nerve. *Am J Ophthalmol* **97**: 62–77.

Beck RW and ONTT study group (1992). A randomised, controlled trial of corticosteroids in the treatment of acute optic neuritis. *New Engl J Med* **326**: 581–588.

Beck RW, Cleary PA (1993a). Optic Neuritis Study Group. Optic Neuritis Treatment Trial: one year follow-up results. *Arch Ophthalmol* **111**: 73–75.

Beck RW and Cleary PA (1993b). Optic Neuritis Study Group. Recovery from severe visual loss in optic neuritis. (Letter) *Arch Ophthalmol* **111**: 300.

Beck RW, Corbett JJ, Thompson HS and Sergott RC (1987a). Decreased visual acuity from optic disc drusen. *Arch Ophthalmol* **71**: 537–539.

Beck RW, Servais GE and Hayreh SS (1987b). Acute ischaemic optic neuropathy IX. Cup-disc ratio and its role in the pathogenesis of acute ischaemic optic neuropathy. *Ophthalmology* **94**: 1503–1508.

Beck RW, Kupersmith MJ, Cleary PA *et al.*, and the Optic Neuritis Study Group (1993a). The effects of corticosteroids for acute optic neuritis on the subsequent development of multiple sclerosis. *New Engl J Med* **329**: 1764–1769.

Beck RW, Arrington J, Murtagh FR *et al.* (1993b). Brain magnetic resonance imaging in acute optic neuritis: experience of the optic neuritis study group. *Arch Neurol* **50**: 841–846.

Beri M, Klugman MR, Kohler JA and Hayreh SS (1987). Acute ischaemic optic neuropathy VII. Incidence of bilaterality and various influencing factors. *Ophthalmology* **94**: 1020–1028.

Boghen DR and Glaser JS (1975). Ischaemic optic neuropathy: the clinical profile and natural history. *Brain* **98**: 689–708.

Boghen D, Sebag M and Michaud J (1988). Paraneoplastic optic neuritis and encephalomyelitis. Report of a case. *Arch Neurol* **45**: 353–356.

Boniuk M, Messmer EP and Font RL (1985). Hemangiopericytoma of the meninges of the optic nerve. A clinicopathologic report including electron microscopic observations. *Ophthalmology* **92**: 1780–1787.

Brodsky MC and Glaser CM (1993). Optic nerve hypoplasia: clinical significance of associated central nervous system abnormalities on magnetic resonance imaging. *Arch Ophthalmol* **111**: 66–74.

Bruggers CS, Friedman HS, Philips PC *et al.* (1991). Leptomeningeal dissemination of optic pathway gliomas in three children. *Am J Ophthalmol* **111**: 719–723.

Brzowski AE, Bazan CI, Mumma JV and Ryan SG (1992). Spontaneous regression of optic glioma in a patient with neurofibromatosis. *Neurology* **42**: 679–681.

Burde RM (1993). Optic disc risk factors for nonarteritic anterior ischaemic optic neuropathy. *Am J Ophthalmol* **115**: 759–763.

Casteels I, De Loof E, Brock P *et al.* (1992). Sudden blindness in a child: presenting symptom of a sphenoid sinus mucocoele. *Br J Ophthalmol* **76**: 502–504.

Cohen DB and Glasgow BJ (1993). Bilateral optic nerve cryptococcosis in sudden blindness in patients with acquired immune deficiency syndrome. *Am J Ophthalmol* **116**: 721–727.

Compston DAS, Batchelor JR, Earl CJ *et al.* (1978). Factors influencing the risk of multiple sclerosis developing in patients with optic neuritis. *Brain* **101**: 495–511.

Corbett JJ (1983). Problems in the diagnosis and treatment of pseudotumor cerebri. *Can J Neurol Sci* **10**: 221–229.

Corbett JJ, Savino P, Thompson HS *et al.* (1982). Visual loss in pseudotumour cerebri; follow-up of 57 patients from 5 to 41 years and a profile of 14 patients with permanent severe visual loss. *Arch Neurol* **39**: 461–474.

Corbett JJ, Nerad JA, Tse DT *et al.* (1988). results of optic nerve sheath fenestration for pseudotumor cerebri. The lateral orbitotomy approach. *Arch Ophthalmol* **106**: 1391–1397.

Cordeiro MJ, Lloyd ME, Spalton DJ and Hughes GR (1994). Ischaemic optic neuropathy, transverse myelitis and epilepsy in an antiphospholipid positive patient with systemic lupus erythematosis. *J Neurol Neurosurg Psychiat* **57**: 1142–1143.

Cunliffe IA, Moffat DA, Hardy DG and Moore AT (1992). Bilateral optic nerve sheath meningiomas in a patient with neurofibromatosis type 2. *Br J Ophthalmol* **76**: 310–312.

DeBroff BM and Donahue SP (1993). Bilateral optic neuropathy as the initial manifestation of systemic sarcoidosis. *Am J Ophthalmol* **116**: 108–111.

Dorrell D (1978). The tilted disc. *Br J Ophthalmol* **62**: 16–20.

Dutton JJ (1992). Optic nerve sheath meningiomas. *Surv Ophthalmol* **37**: 167–183.

Dutton JJ (1994). Gliomas of the anterior visual pathway. *Surv Ophthalmol* **38**: 427–452.

Dutton JJ and Anderson RL (1985). Idiopathic inflammatory perioptic neuritis simulating optic sheath meningioma. *Am J Ophthalmol* **11**: 424–430.

Eagling EM, Sanders MD and Miller SJ (1974). Ischaemic papillopathy. *Br J Ophthalmol* **58**: 990–1008.

Feldon SC, Muramatsu S and Weiner J (1984). Clinical classification of Grave's ophthalmopathy: identification of risk factors for optic neuropathy. *Arch Ophthalmol* **102**: 1469–1472.

Fletcher WA, Imes RK and Hoyt WF (1986). Chiasmal gliomas: Appearance and long-term changes demonstrated by computerized tomography. *J Neurosurg* **65**: 154.

Francis DA, Compston DAS, Batchcor JR *et al.* (1987). A reassessment of the risk of multiple scerosis developing in patients with optic neuritis after extended follow up. *J Neurol Neurosurg Psychiat* **50**: 758–765.

Glaser JS, Hoyt WF and Corbett J (1971). Visual morbidity with chiasmal glioma: long term studies of visual fields in untreated and irradiated cases. *Arch Ophthalmol* **85**: 3.

Graham EM, Ellis CJK, Sanders MD and McDonald WI (1986). Optic neuropathy in sarcoidosis. *J Neurol Neurosurg Psychiat* **49**: 756–763.

Graham EM, Francis DA, Sanders MD and Rudge P (1989). Ocular inflammatory changes in established multiple sclerosis. *J Neurol Neurosurg Psychiat* **52**: 1360–1363.

Grant WM (1974). *Toxicology of the Eye* 2nd edn. Springfield Il: CC Thomas.

Gu XZ, Tsai JC, Waall M and Sadun AA (1995). Pattern of axonal loss in longstanding papilledema due to idiopathic intracranial hypertension. *Curr Eye Res* **14**: 173–180.

Gutman I, Melamed S, Ashkenazi I and Blumenthal M (1993). Optic nerve compression by carotid arteries in low-tension glaucoma. *Graefe's Arch Clin Exp Ophthalmol* **231**: 711–717.

Guy JR, Fagien S, Donovan JP *et al.* (1989). Methyl prednisolone pulse therapy in severe dysthyroid optic neuropathy. *Ophthalmology* **96**: 1048–1053.

Hamed LM, Silbiger J, Guy J *et al.* (1993). Parainfectious optic neuritis and encephalomyeltis: a report of two cases with thalamic invovement. *J Clin Neuro-Ophthalmol* **13**: 18–23.

Harding AE (1993). The DNA laboratory and neurological practice. *J Neurol Neurosurg Psychiat* **56**: 229–233.

Harding AE, Sweeney MG, Miller DH *et al.* (1992). Occurrence of a multople sclerosis-like illness in women who have a Leber's hereditary optic neuropathy mitochondrial DNA mutation. *Brain* **115**: 979–989.

Hayreh SS (1964) Pathogenesis of oedema of the optic disc (papilloedema); a preliminary report. *Br J Ophthalmol* **48**: 522–543.

Hayreh SS (1974). Acute ischaemic optic neuropathy I. Terminology and pathogenesis. *Br J Ophthalmol* **58**: 955–963.

Hayreh SS (1977a). Optic disc edema in raised intracranial pressure-V. Pathogenesis. *Arch Ophthalmol* **95:** 1553–1565.

Hayreh SS (1977b). Optic disc edema in raised intracranial pressure-VI. Associated visual disturbances and their pathogenesis. *Arch Ophthalmol* **95:** 1566–1579.

Hayreh SS (1987). Acute ischaemic optic neuropathy VIII. Clinical features and pathogenesis of post-haemorrhagic amaurosis. *Ophthalmology* **94**: 1488–1502.

Hayreh SS, Joos KM, Podhajsky PA and Long CR (1994). Systemic diseases associated with nonarteritic anterior ischaemic optic neuropathy. *Am J Ophthalmol* **118**: 766–780.

Heher KL, Traboulsi EI and Maumenee IH (1992). The natural history of Leber's congenital amaurosis. *J Ped Ophthalmol Strab* **99**: 241–245.

Henkind P, Charles NC and Pearson J (1970). Histopathology of ischaemic optic neuropathy. *Am J Ophthalmol* **69**: 78–90.

Hilton GF and Hoyt WF (1966). An arteriosclerotic chiasmal syndrome: Bitemporal hemianopia associated with fusiform dilatation of the anterior cerebral arteries. *J Am Med Assoc* **196**: 1018.

Hinzpeter EN and Naumann G (1976). Ischaemic papillopathy in giant cell arteritis. *Arch Ophthalmol* **94**: 624–628.

Horton JC, Garcia EG and Becker EK (1992). Magnetic resonance imaging of leukaemic invasion of the optic nerve. *Arch Ophthalmol* **110**: 1207–1208.

Hoh B, Laitt R, Wakeley CJ *et al.* (1994). The value of STIR sequence in magnetic resonance imaging of thyroid eye disease. *Eye* **8**: 506–510.

Hoyt CS (1980). Autosomal dominant optic atrophy. A spectrum of disability. *Ophthalmology* 87: 245.

Hoyt WF and Bagdassarian SA (1969). Optic glioma of childhood: natural history and rationale for conservative management. *Br J Ophthalmol* **53**: 793–798.

Hoyt CS and Good WV (1992). Do we really understand the difference between optic nerve hypoplasia and optic atrophy? *Eye* **6**: 201–204.

Hoyt WF, Meshel LG, Lessels S *et al.* (1973). Malignant optic glioma of adulthood. *Brain* **96**: 121–132.

Hughes RAC (1992). Pathogenesis of multiple sclerosis. *J R Soc Med* **85**: 373–375.
Huoponen K, Vilkki J, Aula P *et al.* (1991). A new mtDNA mutation associated with Leber optic neuroretinopthy. *Am J Hum Genet* **48**: 1147–1153.
Imes RK and Hoyt WF (1986). Childhood chiasmal gliomas: update on the fate of patients in the 1969 San Francisco study. *Br J Ophthalmol* **70**: 179–182.
Imes RK and Hoyt WF (1991). Magnetic resonance imaging signs of optic nerve gliomas in neurofibromatosis 1. *Am J Ophthalmol* **111**: 729–734.
The Ischemic Optic Neuropathy Decompression Trial Research Group (1995). Optic nerve decompression surgery for nonarteric anterior ischaemic optic neuropathy (NAION) is not effective and may be harmful. *J Am Med Assoc* **273**: 625–632.
Jablons MM, Glaser JS, Schatz NJ *et al.* (1993). Optic nerve sheath fenestration for treatment of progressive ischemic optic neuropathy: results in 26 patients. *Arch Ophthalmol* **111**: 84–87.
Jabs DA, Miller NR, Newman SA *et al.* (1986). Optic neuropathy in systemic lupus erythematosus. *Arch Ophthalmol* **104**: 564–568.
Jacobson DM and Slamovits TL (1987). The ESR and its relationship to haematocrit in giant cell arteritis. *Arch Ophthalmol* **105**: 965–967.
Jacobson DM, Marx JJ and Diesk A (1991). Frequency and clinical significance of Lyme seropositivity in patients with isolated optic neuritis. *Neurology* **41**: 706–711.
Johns DR, Smith KH and Miller NR (1992). Leber's hereditary optic neuropathy: Clinical manifestations of the 3460 mutation. *Arch Ophthalmol* **110**: 1577–1581.
Johns DR, Smith KH, Savino PJ and Miller NR (1993a). Leber's hereditary optic neuropathy: clinical manifestations of the 15257 mutation. *Ophthalmology* **100**: 981–986.
Johns DR, Heher K, Miller NR and Smith KH (1993b). Leber's hereditary optic neuropathy: Clinical manifestations of the 14484 mutation. *Arch Ophthalmol* **111**: 495–498.
Joseph MP, Lessell S, Rizzo J and Momose KJ (1990). Extracranial optic nerve decompression for traumatic optic neuropathy. *Arch Ophthalmol* **108**: 1091–1093.
Kalenak JW, Kosmorsky GS and Hassenbusch G (1992). Compression of the intracranial optic nerve mimicking unilateral normal-pressure glaucoma. *J Clin Neuro-Ophthalmol* **12**: 230–235.
Karp LA, Zimmerman Le Borit A *et al.* (1974). Primary intraorbital meningiomas. *Arch Ophthalmol* **91**: 24–28.
Kattah JC, Chrousos GC, Roberts J *et al.* (1993). Metastatic prostate cancer to the optic canal. *Ophthalmology* **100**: 1711–1715.
Kaufman LM, Miller MT and Mafee MF (1989). Magnetic resonance imaging of pituitary stalk hypoplasia: a discrete midline anomaly associated with endocrine abnormalities in septo-optic dysplasia. *Arch Ophthalmol* **107**: 1485–1489.
Kay MC (1986). Optic neuropathy secondary to lymphoma. *J Clin Neuro-Ophthalmol* **6**: 31.
Kayan A and Earl CJ (1975). Compressive lesions of the optic nerves and chiasm. Pattern of recovery of vision following surgical treatment. *Brain* **98**: 13–28.
Kazarian EL and Gager WE (1978). Optic neuritis complicating measles, mumps, and rubella vaccination. *Am J Ophthalmol* **86**: 544.
Keltner JL (1988). Optic nerve sheath decompression. How does it work? Has its time come? *Arch Ophthalmol* **106**: 1365–1369.
Keltner JL, Johnson CA, Spurr JO *et al.* (1993). Baseline visual field profile of optic neuritis: the experience of the Optic Neuritis Treatment Trial. *Arch Ophthalmol* **111**: 231–234.
Kline LB and Glaser JS (1979). Dominant optic atrophy: the clinical profile. *Arch Ophthalmol* **97**: 1680.
Lambert SR, Hoyt CS and Narahara MH (1987). Optic nerve hypoplasia. *Surv Ophthalmolol* 32; 1–9.
Lessell S (1989). Indirect optic nerve trauma. *Arch Ophthalmol* **107**: 382–386.
Lessell S, (1992). Pediatric pseudotumour cerebri (idiopathic intracranial hypertension). *Surv Ophthalmol* **37**: 155–156.
Levin LA, Joseph MP, Rizzo JF III and Lessell S (1994). Optic canal decompression in indirect optic nerve trauma. *Ophthalmology* **101**: 566–569.
Leys D, Petit H, Block AM *et al.* (1987). Neuromyelitis optica (Devic's disease). Four cases. *Rev Neurol (Paris)* **143**: 722–728.
Lightman S, McDonald WI, Bird AC *et al.* (1987). Retinal venous sheathing in optic neuritis: its significance for pathogenesis of multiple sclerosis. *Brain* **100**: 405–414.
Lindblom B, Truwit CL and Hoyt WF (1992). Optic nerve sheath meningioma: definition of intraorbital, intracanalicular and intracranial components with magnetic resonance imaging. *Ophthalmology* **99**: 560–566.
Little JR, Dale AJD and Okazaki H (1974), meningeal carcinomatosis: Clinical manifestations. *Arch Neurol* **30**: 138–143.
Liu D and Kahn M (1993). Measurement and relationship of subarachnoid pressure of the optic nerve to intracranial pressure in fresh cadavers. *Am J Ophthalmol* **116**: 548–556.
Liu GT and Lessel S (1992). Spontaneous visual improvement in chiasmal gliomas. *Am J Ophthlamol* **114**: 193–201.
Liu D and Michon J (1995). Measurement of sub-arachnoid pressure of the optic nerve in human subjects. *Am J Ophthalmol* **119**: 81–85.
Liu GT, Glaser JS, Shatz NJ and Smith JL (1994). Visual morbidity in giant cell arteritis: Clinical characteristics and prognosis for vision. *Ophthalmology* **101**: 1779–1785.
Mackey D, Nasioulas S and Forrest S (1993). Finger prick blood testing in Leber hereditary optic neuropathy. *Br J Ophthalmol* **77**: 311–312.

Mackey DA (1994). Three subgroups of patients from the United Kingdom with Leber hereditary optic neuropathy. *Eye* **8**: 431–436.
McDonald WI (1982). The symptomatology of tumours of the anterior visual pathways. *Can J Neurol Sci* **9**: 381–390.
McDonald WI (1983). The significance of optic neuritis. *Trans Ophthalmol Soc UK* **103**: 230–245.
McDonald WI and Sanders MD (1971). Migraine complicated by ischaemic optic neuropathy. *Lancet* **ii**: 521–523.
McDonnell P and Miller NR (1983). Chiasmal and hypothalamic extension of optic nerve glioma. *Arch Ophthalmol* **101**: 1412–1415.
McLeod D, Marshall J and Kohner EM (1980). Role of axoplasmic transport in pathophysiology of ischaemic disc swelling. *Br J Ophthalmol* **64**: 247–261.
Malik A, Furlan AJ, Sweeney PJ *et al.* (1992). Optic neuropathy: a rare paraneoplastic syndrome. *J Clin Neuro-Ophthalmol* **12**: 137–141.
Mansour AM, Dinowitz K, Chaljub G and Guinto FC (1993). Metastatic lesion of the optic nerve. *J Clin Neuro-Ophthalmol* **13**: 102–104.
Margo CE, Levy MH and Beck RW (1989). Bilateral idiopathic inflammation of the optic nerve sheaths. *Ophthalmology* **96**: 200–206.
Miller DH, Kay R, Schon F *et al.* (1986). Optic neuritis following chickenpox in adults. *J Neurol* **233**: 182.
Miller DH, Ormerod IEC, McDonald WI *et al.* (1988a). The early risk of multiple sclerosis after optic neuritis. *J Neurol Neurosurg Psychiat* **51**: 1569–1571.
Miller DH, Newton MR, Van der Poel JC *et al.* (1988b). Magnetic resonance imaging of the optic nerve in optic neuritis. *Neurology* **38**: 175–179.
Morrissey SP, Miller DH, Kendall BE *et al.* (1993). The significance of brain magnetic resonance imaging abnormalities at presentation with clinically isolated syndromes suggestive of multiple sclerosis. *Brain* **116**: 135–146.
Mourits MP, Koorneef LK, Wiersinga WM *et al.* (1989). Clinical criteria for the assessment of disease activity in Grave's ophthalmopathy: a novel approach. *Br J Ophthalmol* **73**: 639–644.
Mullie MA and Sanders MD (1984). Scleral canal size and optic nerve head drusen. *Am J Ophthalmol* **99**: 356–359.
Mullie MA and Sanders MD (1985). Computed tomographic diagnosis of buried drusen of the optic nerve head. *Can J Ophthalmol* **20**: 114–117.
Neigel JM, Rootman J, Belkin RI *et al.* (1988). Dysthyroid optic neuropathy. The crowded orbital apex syndrome. *Ophthalmology* **95**: 1515–1521.
Newman NJ (1992). Mitochondrial disease and the eye. *Int Ophthalmol Clin Am* **5**: 405–424.
Newman NJ and Lessell S (1992). Bilateral optic neuropathies with remission in two HIV-positive men, *J Clin Neuro-Ophthalmol* **12**: 1–5.
Newman NJ, Lott MT and Wallace DC (1991). The clinical characteristics of pedigrees of Leber's hereditary optic neuropathy with the 11778 mutation. *Am J Ophthalmol* **111**: 750–762.
Nikoskelainen E, Hoyt WF and Nummelin K (1982). Ophthalmoscopic findings in patients with Leber's hereditary optic neuropathy. I. Fundus findings in asymptomatic family members. *Arch Ophthalmol* **100**: 1597–1602.
Nikoskelainen E, Hoyt WF, Nummelin K *et al.* (1984). Fundus findings in Leber's hereditary optic neuroretinopathy. III. Fluorescein angiographic studies. *Arch Ophthalmol* **102**: 981–989.
Novack RL and Foos RY (1987). Drusen of the optic disc in retinitis pigmentosa. *Am J Ophthalmol* **103**: 44–47.
Novakovic P, Taylor DSI and Hoyt WF (1988). Localising patterns of optic nerve hypoplasia – retina to optic disc. *Br J Ophthalmol* **72**: 176–182.
Olver JM, Spalton DJ and McCartney ACE (1994). Quantitative morphology of human retrolaminar optic nerve vasculature. *Inv Ophthalmol Vis Sci* **35**: 3858–3866.
Olson ME, Chernik NL and Posner JB (1974). Infiltration of the leptomeninges by systemic cancer: A clinical and pathologic study. *Arch Neurol* **30**: 122–137.
Optic Neuritis Study Group (1991). The clinical profile of optic neuritis. Experience of the Optic Neuritis Treatment Trial. *Arch Ophthalmol* **109**: 1673–1678.
Orcutt JC, Page NGR and Sanders MD (1984). Factors affecting visual loss in benign intracranial hypertension. *Ophthalmology* **91**: 1303–1312.
Ormerod IEC and McDonald WI (1984). Multiple sclerosis presenting with progressive visual failure. *J Neurol Neurosurg Psychiat* **47**: 943–946.
Parker WD Jr, Oley CA and Parks JK. A defect in mitochondrial electron transport activity (NADH-conenzyme Q oxidoreductase) in Leber's hereditary optic neuropathy. *New Engl J Med* **320**: 1331–1333.
Parkin PJ, Hierons R and McDonald WI (1984). Bilateral optic neuritis. A long-term follow-up. *Brain* **197**: 951.
Pearson PA, Baker RS, Khorram D and Smith TJ (1991). Evaluation of optic nerve sheath fenestration in pseudotumour cerebri using automated perimetry. *Ophthalmology* **98**: 99–105.
Plant GT and Perry VH (1990). The anatomical basis of the caecocentral scotoma. New observations and a review. *Brain* **113**: 1441–1457.
Quigley HA, Anderson DR (1977). The histological basis of optic disc pallor *Am J Ophthalmol* **83**: 709–717.
Rao NA (1981). Chronic experimental allergic optic neuritis. *Invest Ophthalmol Vis Sci* **20**: 159–172.
Ravin JG, Sisson JC and Knapp WT (1975). Orbital radiation for the ocular changes of Graves' disease. *Am J Ophthalmol* **179**: 285-288.
Repka MX and Miller NR (1988). Optic atrophy in children. *Am J Ophthalmol* **106**: 191–193.

Riordan-Eva P, Sanders MD, Govan GG *et al.* (1995). The clinical features of Leber's hereditary optic neuropathy defined by the presence of a pathogenic mitochondrial DNA mutation. *Brain* **118**: 319–337.

Rizzo JF and Lessell S (1988). Risk of developing multiple sclerosis after uncomplicated optic neuritis: a long-term prospective study. *Neurology* **38**: 185–190.

Rose GE (1993). Orbital meningiomas: surgery, radiotherapy or hormones? *Br J Ophthalmol* **77**: 313–314.

Rosenberg MA, Savino PJ, Glaser JS (1979). A clinical analysis of pseudopapilledema. I. Population, laterality, acuity, refractive error, ophthalmoscopic characteristics, and coincident disease. *Arch Ophthalmol* **97**: 65.

Rosenberg MA, Smith C, Beck R *et al.* (1993). Cerebrospinal fluid diversion procedures in pseudotumour cerebri. *Neurology* **43**: 1071–1072.

Sanders MD (1970). A classification of papilloedema based on a fluorescein angiographic study of 69 cases. *Trans Ophthalmol Soc UK* **89**: 177–197.

Sanders MD and ffytche TJ (1967). Fluorescein angiography in the diagnosis of drusen of the disc. *Trans Ophthalmol Soc UK* **87**: 457–468.

Sanders MD and Flaconer MA (1964). Optic nerve compression by an intracanalicular meningioma. *Br J Ophthalmol* **48**: 13–18.

Sanders MD, Gay AJ, Newman M (1971). Hemorrhagic complications of drusen of the optic disc. *Am J Ophthalmol* **71**: 204–217.

Sarkies NJC (1987). Optic nerve sheath meningiomas: diagnostic features and therapeutic alternatives. *Eye* **1**: 597–602.

Sarkies NJC and Sanders MD (1987). Optic disc drusen and episodic visual loss. *Br J Ophthalmol* **71**: 537–539.

Savino PJ, Glaser JS and Rosenberg MA (1979). A clinical analysis of pseudopapilloedema: II. Visual field defects. *Arch Ophthalmol* **97**: 71–75.

Sawle GV, James CB and Russell RW (1990). The natural history of nonarteritic anterior ischaemic optic neuropathy. *J Neurol Neurosurg Psychiat* **53**: 830–833.

Scott TF, Hess D and Brillman J (1994). Antiphospholipid antibody syndrome mimicking multiple sclerosis clinically and by magnetic resonance imaging. *Arch Intern Med* **154**: 917–920.

Seiff SR (1990). High dose corticosteroids for treatment of vision loss due to indirect injury to the optic nerve. *Ophthal Surg* **21**: 389–395.

Selbst RG, Selhorst JB, Harbison JW *et al.* (1983). Para-infectious optic neuritis. *Arch Neurol* **40**: 347–350.

Singh G, Lott MT and Wallace DC (1989). A mitochondrial DNA mutation as a cause of Leber's hereditary optic neuropathy. *New Engl J Med* **320**: 1300–1305.

Slavin ML (1986). Acute, severe, symmetric visual loss with caecocentral scotomas due to olfactory groove meningioma. *J Clin Neuro-Ophthalmol* **6**: 224–227.

Slavin M, Glaser JS (1987). Acute severe irreversible visual loss with sphenoethmoiditis – 'posterior' orbital cellulitis. *Arch Ophthalmol* **105**: 345–348.

Steinsapir KD and Goldberg RA (1994). Traumatic optic neuropathy. *Surv Ophthalmol* **38**: 478–517.

Tanner V, Tregear SJ, Ripley LG and Vickers SF (1995). Automated contrast sensitivity testing in dysthyroid eye disease. *Eye* **9**: 352–357.

Taylor D (1982). Congenital tumours of the anterior visual system with dysplasia of the optic disc. *Br J Ophthalmol* **66**: 455–463.

Tomsak RL (1985). Ischemic optic neuropathy associated with retinal embolism. *Am J Ophthalmol* **99**: 590–592.

Tomsak RL, Lystad LD, Katirji MB and Bussel TC (1992). Rapid response of syphilitic optic neuritis to posterior sub-Tenon's steroid injection. *J Clin Neuro-Ophthalmol* **12**: 6–7.

Trobe JD, Glaser JS and Laflamme P (1978). Dysthyroid optic neuropathy. Clinical profile and rationale for management. *Arch Ophthalmol* **96**: 1199–1209.

Tso MO (1981). Pathology and pathogenesis of drusen of the optic nerve head. *Ophthalmology* **88**: 1066–1080.

Vine AK (1992). Severe periphlebitis, peripheral retinal ischaemia, and preretinal neovascularisation in patients with multiple sclerosis. *Am J Ophthalmol* **113**: 28–32.

Wall M and George D (1987). Visual loss in pseudotumor cerebri. Incidence and defects related to visual field strategy. *Arch Neurol* **44**: 170–175.

Wall M and George D (1991). Idiopathic intracranial hypertension: a prospective study of 50 patients. *Brain* **114**: 155–180.

Youll BD, Turano G, Miller DH *et al.* The pathophysiology of acute optic neuritis. *Brain* **114**: 2437–2450.

Westlake WH, Heath JD and Spalton DJ (1995). Sarcoidosis involving the optic nerve and hypothalamus. *Arch Ophthalmol* **113**: 669–670.

Williamson TH, Baxter GM and Dutton GN (1993). Colour Doppler velocimetry of the optic nerve head in arterial occlusion. *Ophthalmology* **100**: 313–317.

Winward KE, Hamed LM and Glaser JS (1989). The spectrum of optic nerve disease in human immunodeficiency virus infection. *Am J Ophthalmol* **107**: 373–380.

Wright JE, Call NB and Liarcos S (1980a). Primary optic nerve meningioma. *Br J Ophthalmol* **64**: 553–558.

Wright JE, McDonald WI and Call NB (1980b). Management of optic nerve gliomas. *Br J Ophthalmol* **64**: 545–552.

Zaman AG, Graham EM and Sanders MD (1993). Anterior visual system involvement in non-Hodgkin's lymphoma. *Br J Ophthalmol* **77**: 185–187.

Zeki SM, Hollman AS and Dutton GN (1992). Neuroradiological features of patients with optic nerve hypoplasia. *J Pediat Ophthalmol Strab* **29**: 641–645.

Zimmerman CF, Schatz NJ and Glaser JS (1990). Magnetic resonance imaging of optic nerve meningiomas. *Ophthalmology* **97**: 585–591.

6

Chiasmal disease

APPLIED PHYSIOLOGY AND CLINICAL FEATURES

A bitemporal hemianopia is the clinical hallmark of chiasmal lesions, although it is not clear precisely why crossing fibres in the hemidecussation should be selectively vulnerable in both extrinsic and intrinsic disease. In some individuals the intracranial portion of the optic nerves is relatively long and the chiasm is formed in the posterior cistern (postfixed), with the consequence that expanding sellar lesions may cause optic nerve compression rather than chiasmal compression. Conversely, other individuals may have a prefixed chiasm so that mass lesions of the pituitary fossa may impinge on the optic tract (Fig. 6.1). As fibres from the optic nerve enter the chiasm, those serving the nasal and temporal hemiretinas become separated and the anterior nasal projecting fibres loop into the contralateral optic nerve as they cross the midline and pass into the optic tract (Fig. 6.2). Consequently, lesions of the anterior chiasm may result in an anterior chiasmal syndrome of a contralateral temporal hemianopic field defect and an ipsilateral central scotoma. Occasionally, a lesion anterior to the chaism will result in a unilateral hemianopia as fibres on the nasal side of the of the posterior optic nerve are damaged selectively before entry into the chiasm. Lesions at the posterior chiasmal notch may selectively involve only dorsal crossing fibres serving central vision resulting in hemianopic scotomata. There is evidence that the principle of retinotopy may not be as rigidly applied to the chiasm as was once supposed, and accurate association of fibres from corresponding points in the two retinas does not fully take place until the optic tract. Macular fibres are present throughout the chiasm and because they serve the central 5 degrees of field, and form at least 30% of all the fibres, this has two simple clinical consequences:

1) chiasmal lesions usually cause defects in central vision (e.g acuity or colour tasks) in one or both eyes
2) temporal defects respecting the vertical meridian are usually apparent when testing the central visual field only.

In some patients a distinctive bow-tie pattern of atrophy may be seen where the 3 and 9 o'clock positions on the disc are defective in nerve fibres whilst the upper and lower poles are normal. This is because the retinal representation of the hemidecussation is across the fovea. Consequently, selective loss of crossing fibres will be seen on ophthalmoscopy as a defect in fibres of the maculopapillar bundle entering the disc from the temporal side as well as fibres from the nasal retina entering the disc at its temporal margin. In practice this selective pattern may only be seen clearly in instances of traumatic chiasmal dehiscence (see below) and in developmental chiasmal dysplastic syndromes. More commonly, diffuse temporal disc pallor is seen (Hoyt and Beeston, 1966; Anderson *et al.*, 1983).

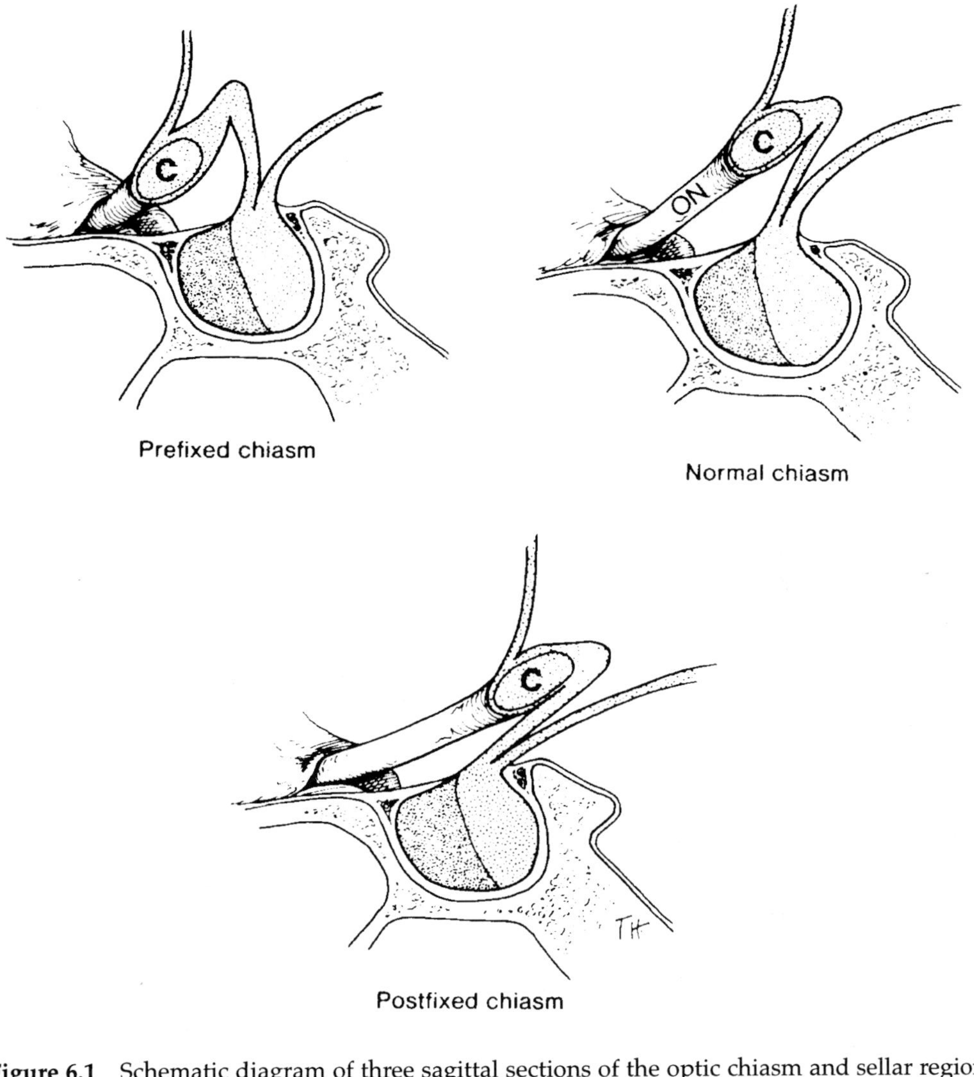

Figure 6.1 Schematic diagram of three sagittal sections of the optic chiasm and sellar region showing the positions of a prefixed chiasm above the tuberculum sellae (left), a normal chiasm above the diaphragm sellae (centre), and a postfixed chiasm above the dorsum sellae (right). (From Rhoton *et al.*, 1977, redrawn in Miller, 1982–1994.)

The functional separation of the retinogeniculate pathways in humans into parvocellular and magnocellular may have clinical importance in the context of chiasmal disease. Statokinetic dissociation may be found on perimetry in patients with chiasmal lesions, whereby fibres serving motion detection (tested in part by kinetic perimetry) are damaged earlier in certain disease processes than fibres serving purely static threshold functions.

Patients with a bitemporal hemianopia may present with double vision in the presence of apparently normal eye movements. When there are dense temporal field defects,

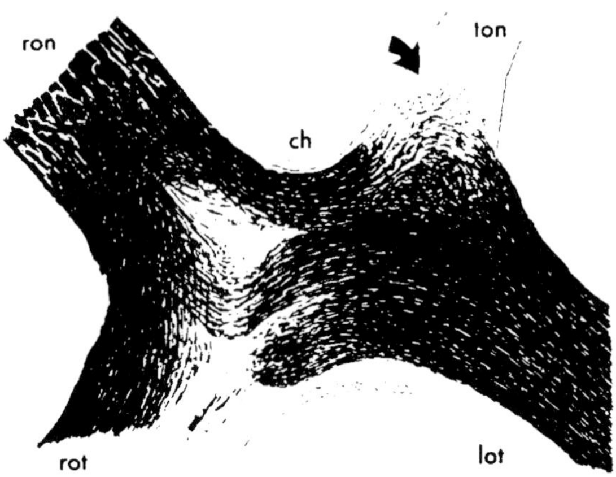

Figure 6.2 Horizontal section of the human optic chiasm stained by the Weigert method in a patient whose left eye was lost 24 years before death. The left optic nerve (lon) is completely atrophic. Fibres of the right optic nerve (ron) enter the left optic tract (lot) and right optic tract (rot). The arrow indicates the decussating fibres of von Wilbrand's knee that detour into the fellow optic nerve. (From Polyak, 1957, reproduced in Horton, 1992.)

binocular fusion is not supported by overlapping temporal hemifields in the visual cortex. As a result, latent heterophorias may readily break down leading to variable vertical or horizontal diplopia. In other instances there may be difficulties in performing tasks requiring depth perception and judgement. This reflects postfixational blindness whereby when the subject fixates on a near target, objects beyond may project onto both nasal hemiretinas and become invisible. Faulty motion perception may arise as a result of asymmetric conduction latencies (Pulfrich phenomenon).

Diplopia may also be paretic: sometimes this is due to a lateral rectus palsy complicating raised intracranial pressure as late presentation occurs with obstructive hydrocephalus. More commonly diplopia reflects parasellar involvement of one or more of the ocular motor nerves either by compression of the cavernous sinus or direct invasion.

COMMON PITFALLS IN VISUAL FIELD TESTING IN SUSPECTED CHIASMAL DISEASE

In the knowledge that the hallmark of chiasmal disease is a bitemporal hemianopia, the clinician may wrongly ascribe every case with bitemporal field loss to chiasmal disease. Bitemporal field defects are also found in:

- massive papilloedema due to blindspot enlargement
- centrocaecal scotomas
- tilted, dysplastic optic discs
- uncorrected refractive errors
- baggy overhanging upper eyelids
- bilateral nasal retinal disease (e.g. sector retinitis pigmentosa).

In practice, these errors are much more likely on confrontation field testing than on some form of quantitative or semiquantitative testing when close attention is given to ensuring accurate fixation. In this way it can be determined whether or not the defect respects the vertical meridian and thereby can correctly be attributed to a chiasmal rather than to a more anterior cause. However, automated perimetry may create its own problems; for example, fixation is checked automatically by retesting stability of the blindspot and this cannot be done in a subject with dense temporal defects. As a rule, we have found the combination of confrontation testing with red-coloured targets, tangent screen testing to a red target together with perimetry using the manual Goldmann or the automated Humphrey machines to be much more reliable than any one technique on its own.

NEUROIMAGING

Plain skull radiography is no longer performed in suspected chiasmal disease: a normal study does not rule out compression and an abnormal study must always be followed up with imaging. However, imaging must be used with care: not only are clinicians responsible to other patients for the resources they consume but inappropriate imaging may lead to a false sense of security if adequate views of relevant structures are not demonstrated. An unenhanced axial computed tomography (CT) head scan with one cut across the suprasellar region may be normal, but will not necessarily exclude chiasmal compression. The best way to use the powerful tools of high resolution fine cut CT and magnetic resonance imaging (MRI) is to apply clinical examination methods to determine whether the problem is optical, retinal, pregeniculate or retrogeniculate and then apply the best techniques available. Although CT is preferable to MRI for the demonstration of parasellar calcification in a meningioma, craniopharyngioma, aneurysm, or bony destruction and hyperostosis, MRI is superior in demonstrating the relationship of chiasm to tumour mass, showing intrinsic chiasmal lesions and the relationship with adjacent blood vessels. It is likely that magnetic resonance angiography (MRA) will replace conventional angiography in the preoperative distinction between aneurysm and tumour (Davis *et al.*, 1987).

EXTRINSIC LESIONS: TUMOURS AND OTHER MASS LESIONS

Pituitary tumours constitute some 12–15% of clinically symptomatic intracranial neoplasms and it has been estimated that up to 20% of all individuals have asymptomatic adenomas at autopsy.

CLINICAL DIAGNOSIS

Patients may present with visual symptoms as discussed above, or may develop headache and/or symptoms and signs of endocrine hypofunction such as loss of secondary sexual characteristics and impotence in men and secondary amenorrhoea in women. Uncommonly, presentation is by downward invasion into the sphenoid sinus causing epistaxis and nasal obstruction or cerebrospinal (CSF) rhinorrhoea. In functioning tumours a number of specific sydromes arise as listed. Nowadays, with the increasing use of endocrine testing in the evaluation of patients with infertility and related problems, a higher proportion of pituitary adenomas present before they cause visual failure. When patients present to the endocrinologist with a functioning tumour it is important to

Table 6.1

Clinical classification
Functional / non-functional
Microadenoma / macroadenoma
Pituitary apoplexy
Functional classification
Adenomas with clinically manifest endocrine overactivity
• growth hormone (acromegaly and giantism)
• prolactin (galactorrhoea, amenorrhoea in women)
• ACTH (Cushing's disease and Nelson's syndrome)
• TSH and FSH / LH-RH (both very rare)
• multiple hormones
Adenomas without clinically manifest overactivity
• null cell (may result in hypopituitarism)
• inactive oncocytoma
• prolactin without galactorrhoea
• hyposecretion syndromes.

ACTH: adrenocortiocotropic hormone; TSH: thyroid stimulating hormone; FSH / LH-RH: follicle stimulating hormone and luteinizing hormone releasing hormone.

determine whether or not there is suprasellar extension (a macroadenoma) so as to assess the risks of subsequent visual failure even if there is no deficit at presentation. This is best done by imaging because an adenoma must extend a full 10 mm across the normal suprasellar cistern before reaching the chiasm. At present even the best imaging may not clearly discriminate a microadenoma from adjacent healthy anterior pituitary tissue.

MEDICAL THERAPY

Prolactin and many growth hormone secreting microadenomas respond to bromocriptine and other dopaminergic agonists both in terms of reduced secretion and tumour bulk. This approach can also be used in some functioning macroadenomas even if they present with chiasmal compression. In addition, some patients with macroadenomas and normal peripheral blood hormone levels will have prolactin secreting cell types and may shrink with bromocriptine (Wass *et al.*, 1982; Spark *et al.*, 1982; Moster *et al.*, 1985).

SURGERY, RADIOTHERAPY AND TUMOUR RECURRENCE

In 75–95% of patients presenting with visual failure, there will be improvement in visual acuity and field after surgery regardless of whether transfrontal or transphenoidal techniques are used. This is often almost immediate but may continue for some months (McDonald, 1982). As one would expect, those with longstanding visual loss and optic atrophy are less likely to have a full recovery, but the prognostic significance of these features is hard to gauge in an individual patient. In those who have transfrontal surgery alone, recurrence rates may be between 7 and 35%. If combined with radiotherapy, 5-year recurrences fall to 7–13%. In patients treated by transphenoidal surgery supplemented by radiotherapy, recurrence rates are less than 10%. The low morbidity of this microsurgical operation means that it can be offered to a wider and wider range of patients including the elderly, those who cannot tolerate or do not respond to bromocriptine, and those with microadenomas. A transfrontal approach may still be required for large macroadenomas and in those with significant lateral extension.

The optimum method of follow-up to detect recurrence remains to be established. Microadenomas are unlikely to develop into lesions causing visual failure except in pregnancy but reliance on endocrine testing alone is unwise as fluctuations in prolactin or growth hormone levels may be hard to interpret. Repeat imaging is expensive and in the case of CT, exposes the patient to excess cumulative doses of radiation. In addition the functional significance of persistent suprasellar masses can only be determined by formal visual assessment. Vision testing alone is inadequate because of the possibility of tumour recurrence into a previous field defect which will not be detectable by perimetry and because vision may deteriorate without recurrence in instances of chiasmal herniation into an empty sella (Kaufman *et al.*, 1989) or anterior visual system radionecrosis. It is our current practice to use a combination of all three methods emphasizing the importance of a multidisciplinary approach to the management of these patients not only in diagnosis but also in follow-up (Teng *et al.*, 1988; Marcus *et al.*, 1991).

PITUITARY APOPLEXY

Pituitary apoplexy results from haemorrhagic infarction and necrosis of a pituitary gland containing an adenoma. In the absence of a tumour, the same event may occur after postpartum haemorrhage (Sheehans's syndrome). The difference is that in patients with a pre-existing tumour, the volume expansion will cause sudden visual loss due to chiasmal compression if it is principally in an upward direction together with external ophthalmolplegia if in a lateral direction, whereas in the absence of a tumour the consequences are generally medical from pituitary failure. Where there is ophthalmolplegia, the oculomotor nerve may be especially vulnerable, either because of mechanical compression or because its blood supply depends on meningohypophyseal branches of the internal carotid which may be disrupted. Headache, meningeal irritation and drowsiness accompany this event as a result of blood escaping into the subarachnoid space. The diagnosis is made on clinical grounds together with imaging which shows both haemorrhage and features of a pre-existing tumour. Prompt medical measures are required to support pituitary and adrenal function and visual recovery is more likely if early surgical decompression is performed (Reid *et al.*, 1985).

PITUITARY TUMOURS AND PREGNANCY

Normal pregnancy is associated with considerable increase in the volume and mass of the pituitary gland as a result of lactotroph hyperplasia. However, as the suprasellar cistern is a space separating the diaphragmae sellae and the chiasm by some 10 mm, there is an ample safety margin and it is incorrect to attribute visual loss in pregnancy to this physiological event. Visual failure in pregnancy must therefore raise the possibility of tumour growth both of adenomas and of meningiomas. In patients known to have microprolactinomas at the onset of pregnancy the risk of clinically significant complications has been quoted at 6.7% and this rises to 15% in macroadenomas. Visual defects may resolve spontaneously after delivery in these patients, but the risks of permanent visual loss can be reduced safely by the use of bromocriptine. In addition to physiological expansion, accelerated tumour growth, and peripartum haemorrhagic necrosis, the pituitary gland in pregnancy may also develop into an expanding mass as a result of lymphocytic hypophysitis (Cosman *et al.*, 1989). This mimic of pituitary tumours appears to be an autoimmune phenomenom akin to autoimmune thyroiditis and adrenalitis, and is strongly associated with pregnancy. Management is by surgical decompression of the chiasm together with corticosteroids. A frozen section biopsy at transphenoidal surgery will protect the patient from an extensive pituitary resection and an unnecessary risk of subsequent hypopituitarism (Fig. 6.3).

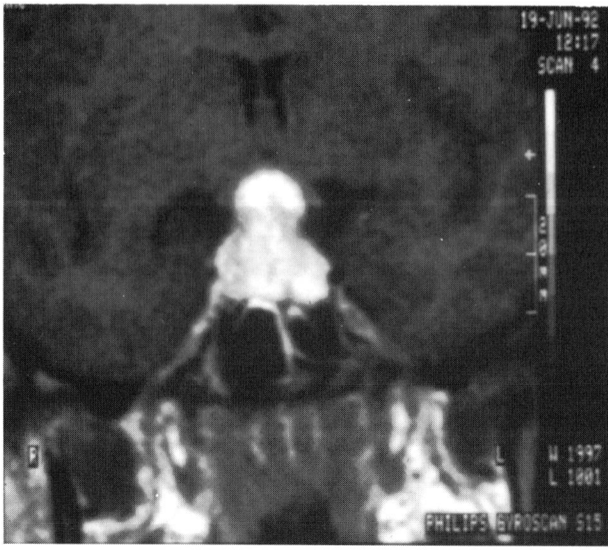

Figure 6.3A Mass in pituitary fossa with suprasellar extension and chiasmal compression due to lymphocytic adenohypophysitis.

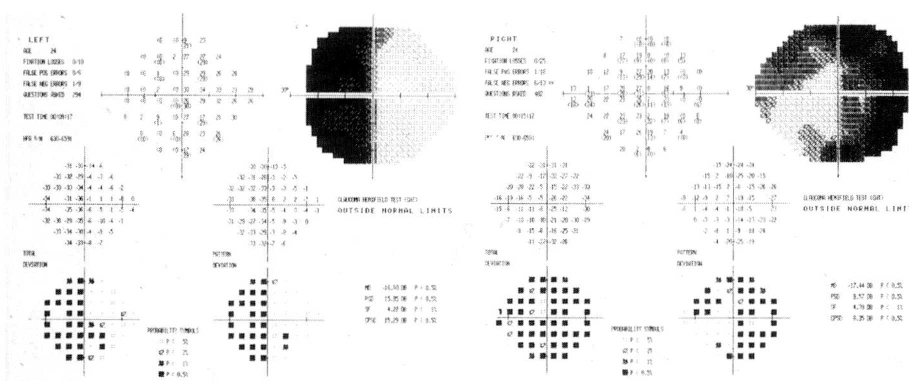

Figure 6.3B Automated perimetry in the same patient showing a bitemporal herniation.

MENINGIOMAS

Meningiomas arising from the tuberculum sellae, planum sphenoidale, inner third sphenoid ridge, optic foramen and olfactory groove may all interfere with function in the intracranial optic nerve and then the chiasm. Normally visual loss is very asymmetric reflecting the unilateral origins of these tumours and occurrence is most common in middle-aged females. Intracranial extension of perioptic meningiomas is discussed in Chapter 5. The Foster–Kennedy syndrome of optic atrophy in one eye and disc swelling in the other due to subfrontal meningioma is well known, although it must be emphasized that this combination of physical signs is much more likely to be the consequence of sequential ischaemic optic neuropathy due to microvascular disease at the optic nerve head than to any intracranial tumour. When a genuine surgical Foster–Kennedy syndrome does arise, the mechanisms may be compressive optic neuropathy leading to optic atrophy in one eye with a space-occupying lesion giving rise to raised intracranial pressure and papilloedema in the other (Watnick and Trobe, 1989). Anosmia should always be sought in patients with parasellar tumours as when present this strongly suggests a meningioma. Delayed diagnosis results in frontal lobe dysfunction with mental state changes.

Both contrast enhanced CT and MRI are sensitive to mengiomas at this site, but MRI is superior for demonstrating vascular displacement and planning surgery. Parasellar and sphenoid wing meningiomas account for over 25% of all intracranial meningiomas coming to surgery and recurrences or progression may occur in up to 20% of patients. Radiotherapy as an adjunct to surgery is commonly used, as attempted total resection may expose the patient to unwarranted risks without reducing the chances of recurrence. Only in some patients is radiotherapy recommended as as alternative to surgery, for example when major vessels are encased by tumour or there is invasion of the skull base.

Visual function improves following microsurgical dissection of the meningioma from the chiasm or optic nerve, but not as frequently as in pituitary adenoma. This may reflect permanent axonal loss due to chronic compression before diagnosis, or the inevitable interference with microvascular structures and blood supply during surgery (Petty *et al.*, 1985; Yeakly *et al.*, 1988).

CRANIOPHARYNGIOMAS AND RELATED LESIONS (RATHKE'S CLEFT CYSTS AND EPIDERMOID CYSTS)

Craniopharyngiomas, suprasellar epidermoid cysts and Rathke's cleft cysts are related tumours of embryonic origin arising from vestigial epidermoid remnants of evaginating stomatadeum and Rathke's pouch scattered in the infundibulohypophyseal region. Although predominantly arising in the suprasellar region, an intrasellar origin is also possible. In each tumour there is a mixture of solid and cystic elements, typically including fluid filled cysts (Fig. 6.4A). In at least 80% of craniopharyngiomas there is dystrophic calcification — a feature of diagnostic importance on CT scanning. Desquamated epithelium, degenerate blood, necrotic tissue and cholesterol crystals contribute to the oily cystic fluid within a craniopharyngioma. In Rathke's cleft cysts mucin-producing goblet cells produce a characteristic white fluid free of cholesterol crystals and keratinized debris, but the clinical consequences of these lesions depends entirely on their size and location rather than on histological characteristics.

Craniopharyngiomas have a bimodal age distribution of presentation with one peak in childhood and a second in late middle age. They account for some 2–4% of all intracranial tumours, and for over 50% of suprasellar masses in childhood and 20% in adults. In childhood, symptomatic visual loss usually arises quite late and presentation with hypopituitarism and diabetes insipidis or hypothalamic syndromes are typical. As the suprasellar mass enlarges, obstructive hydrocephalus with headache, vomiting and papilloedema will ensue. By contrast, adults usually present with acuity loss or field defects. Although a bitemporal pattern of field loss characterizes any chiasmal lesion, incongruous homonymous defects with asymmetric acuity loss are also typical in adult craniopharyngiomas due to optic tract compression. Other patterns of visual field defect include the anterior chiasmal syndrome of a central scotoma in one eye and a temporal defect in the other, and also unilateral and bilateral retrobulbar optic neuropathies. In both adults and children, posterior suprasellar extension may not only cause obstructive hydrocephalus, but may also cause ocular motility defects typical of ventral midbrain syndromes. These include Parinauds' syndrome of convergence retraction nystagmus,

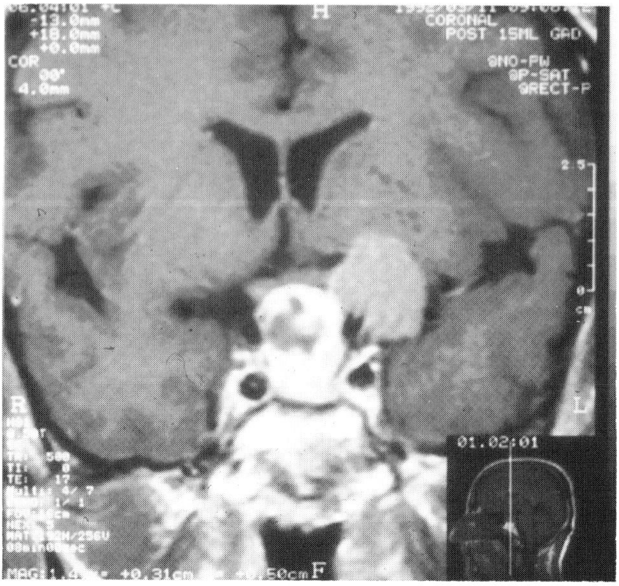

Figure 6.4A MRI scan of intrasellar and suprasellar craniopharyngioma with cystic lateral expansion.

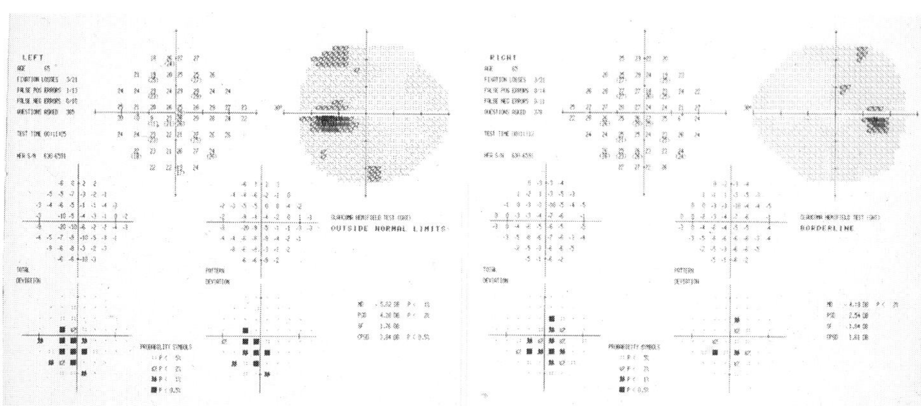

Figure 6.4B Automated perimetry of same patient showing subtle central threshold elevation in left eye.

pupillary light-near dissociation and supranuclear upgaze palsy, and also see-saw nystagmus.

The diagnosis can often be made on CT showing dystrophic calcification with cyst formation. In instances where cystic elements predominate, a craniopharyngioma may appear to be isodense with CSF on CT and MRI will more clearly delineate the tumour because of the bright signal on T2-weighted imaging sequences. In some patients the optic nerves and chiasm may appear to be thickened with extension through the optic foramen into the orbit (Brodsky *et al.*, 1988). This suggests either infiltration by craniopharyngioma or an optochiasmal glioma. However, adjacent cystic elements and bone erosion are suggestive of a craniopharyngioma.

The primary management of craniopharyngioma is always surgical, but complete resection is rarely possible. Many patients now undergo cyst aspiration, intracapsular dissection and subsequent radiotherapy. Most cases will require a frontal craniotomy, but when the craniopharyngioma arises low in the hypophyseal stalk, a transphenoidal decompression can be achieved. The visual prognosis following surgery depends, as in pituitary adenoma, on the size and duration of the compression of the visual pathways and associated optic atrophy. For this reason, it is said that adults are more likely to recover vision than children. Recurrent cyst formation may be managed by simple aspiration, further resection or by interstitial radiotherapy. Most patients will require life-long endocrine surveillance and replacement therapy following surgery (Freeman *et al.*, 1987).

DYSGERMINOMAS

Primary suprasellar dysgerminomas are rare causes of visual failure from chiasmal compression arising in children and young adults. They arise in the anterior portion of the floor of the third ventricle and although histologically resemble pineal teratomas, are in fact separate from the pineal gland. Other clinical features will include those associated with obstructive hydrocephalus and upper brain stem ocular motility syndromes. After confirming the diagnosis by biopsy (stereotactic or by craniotomy) long-term remission may be achieved by radiotherapy (Isayama *et al.* 1980).

SUPRASELLAR ANEURYSMS

Aneurysms are generally classified as saccular or fusiform. Saccular (berry) aneurysms arise from developmental defects of the arterial wall, usually at sites of bifurcation, and although not present at birth are termed congenital. Hypertension, degenerative vascular disease and elastic tissue defects such as Ehlers–Danlos syndrome may contribute to the development of saccular aneurysms and there is an association with aortic coarctation and polycystic kidney disease. The majority of saccular aneurysms arise from the carotid system on anterior communicating, middle cerebral and internal carotid arteries, or in the region of the origins of the posterior communicating arteries. Only some 5% of aneurysms arise on the vertebrobasilar system. Fusiform aneurysms are degenerative tortuous dilatations and elongations of an artery, strongly associated with atherosclerosis and commonly affect the basilar and intracranial carotid artery. Because of the close anatomical relationship between the circle of Willis and the anterior visual pathways, aneurysms frequently give rise to visual symptoms. Spontaneous rupture results in subarachnoid, intraventricular and intracerebral haemorrhage. Progressive enlargement leads to compression of adjacent structures. As a result, visual loss may be acute, fluctuating or chronic and progressive.

SACCULAR ANEURYSMS OF THE INTRACAVERNOUS CAROTID (INFRACLINOID)

These aneuryms arise in the carotid artery as it traverses the cavernous sinus. Rupture is unusual and results in a direct carotid cavernous fistula. More commonly, symptoms arise from slowly progressive compression of the motor and sensory divisions of the trigeminal nerve and the oculomotor, trochlear and abducens nerve resulting in a clinical syndrome of periocular pain and ophthalmoplegia, often with Horner's syndrome. Anterior expansion may lead to erosion of the anterior clinoid, optic foramen and superior orbital fissure producing proptosis and visual loss. Posterior expansion may erode the petrous ridge and involve structures of the cerebellar pontine angle causing facial weakness and hearing loss. Medial extension may erode the sellar simulating a pituitary tumour and inferior expansion will involve the sphenoid sinus and nasopharynx. Intracavernous carotid aneuryms may be suitable for treatment by endovascular balloon occlusion techniques, which are especially effective for pain relief.

SUPRACLINOID CAROTID ANEURYSMS

Giant (i.e. diameter > 25mm) aneurysms of the supraclinoid carotid artery represent a relatively common and treatable cause of visual loss. They may arise at the origin of the ophthalmic artery (carotid-ophthalmic) or at the bifurcation of the middle cerebral, and tend to expand upwards and forwards to compress the ipsilateral optic nerve and eventually reach the chiasm itself. In instances of prefixed chiasm, such aneurysms will impinge directly on the lateral chiasm or optic tract resulting in unilateral nasal field loss or in an incongruous homonymous hemianopia. More commonly there is visual acuity loss in one eye with a central scotoma, with eventual development of an anterior chiasmal syndrome and temporal field loss in the fellow eye. Large aneurysms at this site may therefore simulate pituitary tumours, even to the extent of producing hyperprolactinaemia, underlining the fact that MRI or arteriography is required in the evaluation of many patients with parasellar syndromes. As in infraclinoid aneurysms, giant supraclinoid aneurysms may also be suitable for endovascular therapy, but in some patients, especially the elderly, the indolent nature of the disease and the typically late presentations argue in favour of conservative management (Norwood *et al.*, 1986).

FUSIFORM ANEURYSMS OF THE CAROTID SYSTEM

A dilated or tortuous supraclinoid carotid artery may compress the optic nerve against the dura at the opening of the optic foramen. With the evolution of high resolution imaging, some instances of progressive glaucomatous optic neuropathy without raised intraocular pressure ('low-tension glaucoma') have been attributed to this cause (Gutman *et al.*, 1993). However, how this pathology could produce the pathological cupping of the optic disc which is normally associated with raised intraocular pressure is unexplained and it is possible that in many cases low tension glaucoma and degenerative intracranial carotid disease coexist in individuals harbouring the same risk factors for vascular disease.

EMPTY SELLA SYNDROME

The empty sella syndrome requires description in this section because it may both accompany and sometimes mimic pituitary disease. Anatomically, there is extension of the sub-arachnoid space through a deficient diaphragmae sellae. In patients with idiopathic intracranial hypertension, increased CSF pressure may then lead to erosion of the floor of the pituitary fossa. Empty sella syndrome may arise spontaneously and is also seen in association with arachnoidal cysts and previous pituitary infarction. An empty sella is also seen after pituitary surgery and radiotherapy.

The empty sella syndrome can mimic pituitary tumours by giving rise to moderate hyperprolactinaemia, and by leading to an expanded pituitary fossa in a patient with headaches and benign intracranial hypertension. There are also reports of secondary visual loss when, following pituitary surgery, the chiasm may herniate through the diaphragmatic defect. This may be more likely in the presence of postoperative adhesions and it has been suggested that packing, or chiasmoplexy, of the fossa after hypophysectomy may prevent this complication. There are, however, also reports of visual defects complicating excessive chiasmopexy and not all surgeons use this method (Slavin *et al.*, 1993).

INTRINSIC ABNORMALITIES

Intrinsic disease of the visual pathways at the chiasm is very much less common. Bitemporal field loss and chiasmal enhancement is occasionally seen in optic neuritis (Spector *et al.*, 1980; Reynolds *et al.*, 1982): steroids are usually indicated because of the bilaterality of visual loss but otherwise management and prognosis are similar to optic neuritis and are covered in Chapter 5 (Fig. 6.5). Optochiasmal gliomas (Fig. 6.6) are also

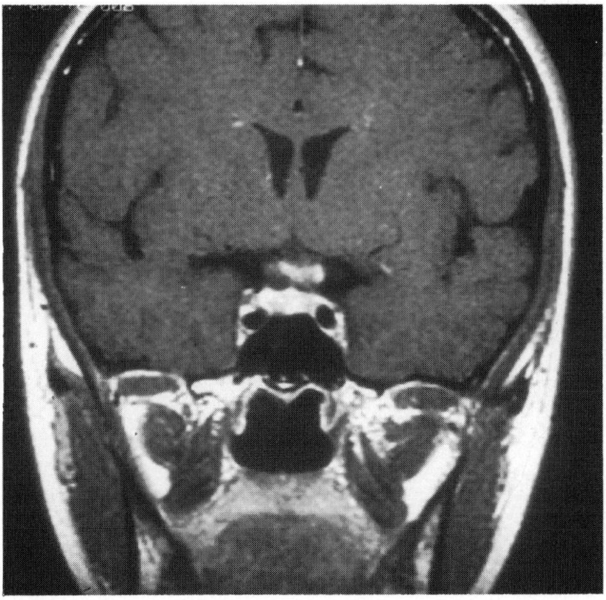

Figure 6.5A High signal on a coronal view MRI of the optic chiasm in chiasmal neuritis.

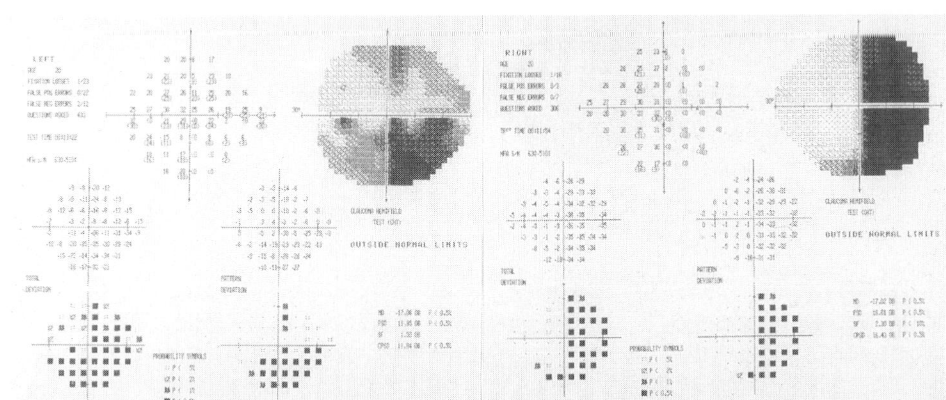

Figure 6.5B Automated perimetry of same patient showing right hemianopic field loss.

covered in Chapter 5. Traumatic chiasmal syndromes may follow severe head injury especially when complicated by sphenoid fracture and disruption of chiasmal branches of the internal carotid artery. However, not all patients have a history of severe injury and a history of relative minor closed trauma should always be sought in patients presenting with complete bitemporal field loss as such a pattern of field defect is most unusual in compressive chiasmal syndromes (Savino *et al.*, 1980; Tang *et al.*, 1994).

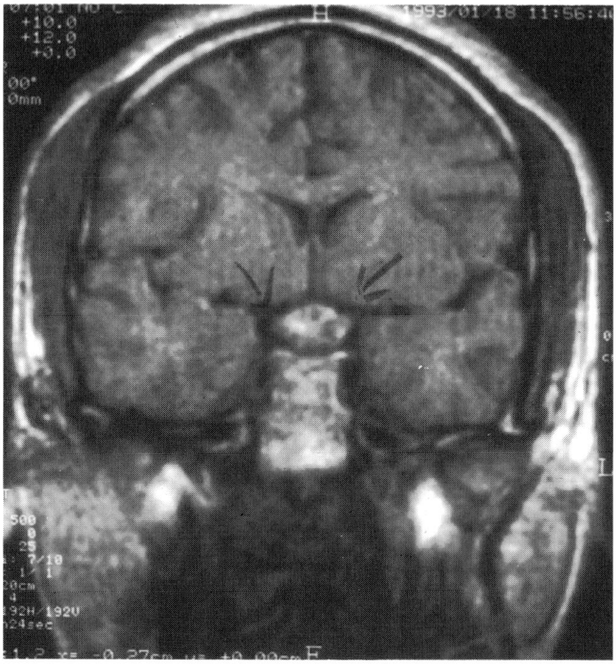

Figure 6.6A Coronal view MRI scan showing intrinsic expansion of the optic chiasm due to a pilocytic astrocytoma.

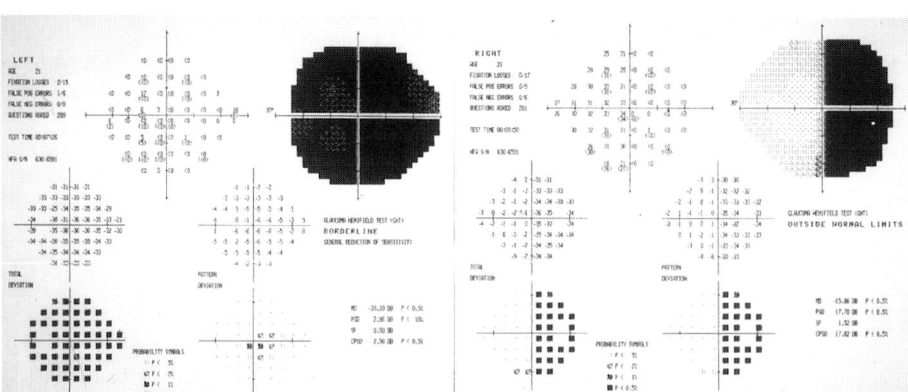

Figure 6.6B Automated perimetry of same patient showing right hemianopic field loss and complete loss of left central field.

RADIONECROSIS OF THE ANTERIOR VISUAL PATHWAYS

Radionecrosis of the chaism and intracranial optic nerves is a rare late complication of radiation therapy for sellar, parasellar and skull base tumours. Visual loss occurs 6 months to 3 years after completion of therapy with a peak incidence between 12 and 18 months. There is no correlation between patient age and the onset of visual loss which is typically rapid and relentless. Chiasmal, optic tract or unilateral and bilateral optic nerve patterns of loss may be seen. It has been suggested that in the case of patients with pituitary adenomas receiving radiotherapy, those with acromegaly are somehow more vulnerable. However, this may reflect the use of yttrium implants or external beam radiotherapy as sole treatment in selected cases of growth hormone secreting tumours during the 1970s. Pathological studies indicate a microvasculopathy and occlusive endarteritis similar to radiation retinopathy which is seen following radiation therapy of orbital and nasopharyngeal tumours.

The risk is greatest when the total dose is greater than 600 cGy or if fractional doses are greater than 200 cGy, and the topic is of great current interest because of the development of interstitial stereotactic delivery techniques which offer greater precision in targeting tissues for maximal dosage (Hammer, 1983; Kline *et al.*, 1985). With these techniques, radiotherapy may be offered in some centres even to patients with slowly growing chiasmal gliomas when previously this would have been thought to be too hazardous. When the study is performed shortly after the onset of visual loss MRI shows tissue swelling with normal signal on unenhanced sequences and focal enhancement on gadolinium injection within the posterior optic nerves and chiasm (Zimmerman *et al.*, 1990). This pattern of signal change is consistent with pathological reports of microvascular disease suggesting blood–brain barrier breakdown. Therefore, MRI is useful in discriminating visual loss due to radionecrosis from that due to recurrent tumour. Early use of anticoagulation with i.v. heparin followed by full warfarin treatment may be helpful in arresting visual loss, as may hyperbaric oxygen therapy (Borruat *et al.*, 1993; Guy and Schatz, 1986).

REFERENCES

Anderson D, Faber P, Marcovitz S *et al.* (1983). Pituitary tumors and the ophthalmologist. *Ophthalmology* **90**: 1265–1270.

Borruat FX, Schatz NJ, Glaser JS *et al.* (1993). Visual recovery from radiation-induced optic neuropathy: the role of hyperbaric oxygen therapy. *J Clin Neuro-Ophthalmol* **13**: 98–101.

Brodsky MC, Hoyt WF, Barnwell SL and Wilson CB (1988). Intrachiasmatic craniopharygioma: a rare cause of chiasmal thickening. *J Neurosurg* **68**: 300–302.

Cosman F, Post KD, Holub DA and Wardlaw SL (1989). Lymphocytic adenohypophysitis: report of 3 cases and review of the literature. *Medicine (Baltimore)* **68**: 240–256.

Davis PC, Hoffman JC, Spencer T *et al.* (1987). MR imaging of pituitary adenoma: CT, clinical, and surgical correlation *Am J Roentgenol* **148**: 797–802.

Freeman MP, Kessler RM, Allen JH *et al.* (1987). Craniopharyngioma: CT and MR imaging in nine cases. *J Comput Assist Tomogr* **11**: 810–814.

Gutman I, Melamed S, Ashkenazi I and Blumenthal M (1993). Optic nerve compression by carotid arteries in low tension glaucoma. *Graefe's Arch Clin Exp Ophthalmol* **231**: 711–717.

Guy J and Schatz NJ (1986). Hyperbaric oxygen in the treatment of radiation-induced optic neuropathy. *Ophthalmology* 93: 1083–1088.

Hammer HM (1983). Optic chiasmal radionecrosis. *Trans Ophthalmol Soc UK* 103: 208.

Horton JC (1992). The central visual pathways. In: *Adler's physiology of the Eye* 9th edn. (WM Hart ed.) St Louis: Mosby Year Book, Ch 23, p. 732.

Hoyt WH and Beeston D (1966). *The ocular fundus in neuro-ophthalmic diagnosis.* St Louis: CV Mosby.

Isayama Y, Takahashi T and Inove M (1980). Ocular findings of suprasellar germinoma: Long-term follow-up after radiotherapy. *Neuro-Ophthalmology* **1**: 53–61.

Kaufman LM, Tomask RL, Kaufman BA *et al.* (1989). Herniation of the suprasellar visual system and third ventricle into empty sellae: morphological and clinical considerations. *Am J Neurol Res* **10**: 65–76.

Kline LB, Kim JV and Ceballos R (1985). Radiation optic neuropathy. *Ophthalmology* **92**: 1118–1126.

McDonald WI (1982). The symptomatology of tumours of the anterior visual pathways. *Can J Sci Neurol* **9**: 381–390.

Marcus M, Vitale S, Calvert PC and Miller NR (1991). Visual parameters in patients with pituitary adenoma before and after transsphenoidal surgery. *Austral N Z J Ophthalmol* **19**: 111–118.

Miller N (ed.) (1982–1994); *Walsh and Hoyt's Clinical Neuro-Ophthalmology* 4th edn. Baltimore: Williams and Wilkins, pp. 62–63.

Moster ML, Savino PJ, Schatz NJ *et al.* (1985). Visual function in prolactinoma patients treated with bromocriptine. *Ophthalmology* **92**: 1332.

Norwood EG, Kline LB, Chandra Sekar B *et al.* (1986). Aneurysmal compression of the anterior visual pathways. *Neurology* **36**: 1035–1041.

Petty AM, Kun LE and Meyer GA. (1985). Radiation therapy for incompletely resected meningiomas. *J Neurosurg* **62**: 502–507.

Polyak S (1957). *The Vertibrate Visual System.* Chicago: Chicago University Press.

Regli I, de Triboulet N, Regli F and Bogousslavsky J (1989). Chiasmal apoplexy: haemorrhage from a cavernous malformation in the optic chiasm. *J Neurol Neurosurg Psychiat* **52**: 1095–1099.

Reid RL, Quigley ME and Yen SSC (1985) Pituitary apoplexy: A review. *Arch Neurol* **42**: 712–719.

Reynolds WD, Smith JL and McCrary JA (1982). Chiasmal optic neuritis. *J Clin Neuro-Ophthalmol* **2**: 93–101.

Rhoton AL, Harris FS and Renn WH (1977). *Neuro-Ophthalmology Symposium of the University of Miami; and the Bascom Palmer Eye Institute.* JS Glaser (ed.) SE Louis: CV Mosby, pp. 75–105.

Savino PJ, Glaser JS and Schatz NJ (1980). Traumatic chiasmal syndrome. *Neurology* **30**: 963–970.

Slavin ML, Lam BL, Decker RE *et al.* (1993). Chiasmal compression from fat packing after transsphenoidal resection of intrasellar tumour in two patients. *Am J Ophthalmol* **115**: 368–371.

Spector RH, Glaser JS and Schatz NJ (1980). Demyelinative chiasmal lesions. *Arch Neurol* 37: 757–762.

Spark RF, Bader R, Bienfang DC *et al.* (1982). Bromocriptine reduces pituitary tumor size and hypersecretion. *J Am Med Assoc* **247**: 311.

Tang RA, Grotta JC, Lee KF *et al.* (1983). Chiasmal syndrome in sarcoidosis. *Arch Ophthalmol* **101**: 1069–1073.

Tang RA, Kramer LA, Shiffman *et al.* (1994). Chiasmal trauma: clinical and imaging considerations. *Surv Ophthalmol* **38**: 381–383.

Teng MMH Huang CI and Chang T (1988). The pituitary mass after transsphenoidal hypophysectomy. *AM J Neuroradiol* **9**: 23–26.

Wass Jah, Williams J, Charlesworth M *et al.* (1982). Bromocriptine in management of large pituitary tumours. *Br Med J* **284**: 1908–1911.

Watnick RL and Trobe JP (1989). Bilateral optic nerve compression as a mechanism for the Foster Kennedy syndrome. *Ophthalmology* **96**: 1793–1798.

Yeakley JW, Kulkarni MV, McArdle DB *et al.* (1988). High-resolution MR imaging of juxtasellar meningiomas with CT and angiographic correlation. *Am J Neuroradiol* **9**: 279–285.

Zimmerman CF, Schatz NJ and Glaser GS (1990). Magnetic resonance imaging of radiation optic neuropathy. *Am J Ophthalmol* **110**: 389–394.

7

The posterior (retrochiasmal) visual pathways

OPTIC TRACT AND LATERAL GENICULATE GANGLION

A total interruption of the optic tract results in a complete fixation splitting homonymous hemianopia on the contralateral side – a pattern typical of any retrochiasmal lesion. However, because the retinotopic organization of fibres in the tracts is less complete than in the radiations, non-congruous defects are usually seen. The nerve fibres involved are those deriving from the retinal ganglion cells before their synapse at the lateral geniculate ganglion, and optic tract lesions result in optic atrophy most obvious in the contralateral eye, which typically is of a characteristic pattern. This is the 'bow-tie' (also referred to as band atrophy) pattern of atrophy where fibres from the crossing temporal hemifield entering the disc at the 3 o'clock and 9 o'clock positions are lost with preservation of normal disc colour at the upper and lower poles. Because the temporal hemifield served by the nasal hemiretina carries a greater number of cells which drive the pupillary light reflex then the nasal hemifield, lesions of the optic tract typically show a contralateral relative afferent pupil defect. This is in distinction to retrogeniculate causes of a homonymous hemianopia where the reflex arc for the pupillary light reflex is usually undisturbed (Newman and Miller, 1983; Bell and Thompson, 1978; Cibis *et al.*, 1975).

Pure optic tract syndromes are uncommon and almost always there are visual system abnormalities as a result of impairment of adjacent brain stem or chiasm. Tract lesions are typically seen in space-occupying suprasellar lesions (pituitary tumours, craniopharyngioma, aneurysms, optochiasmal gliomas) which extend posteriorly, especially when there is a prefixed chiasm. Demyelination and vascular occlusion are much less important causes of clinical deficits although are frequently present at autopsy (Savino *et al.*, 1978).

A pure lesion at the lateral geniculate ganglion is even less frequent, and is more often associated with a contralateral hemiparesis from involvement of the adjacent posterior limb of the internal capsule or contralateral hemisensory loss from thalamic involvement. Occlusive vascular disease (hypertension, emboli, vasculitis) of the deep perforating branches of the posterior cerebral (thalamogeniculate and lateral posterior choroidal) artery or anterior choroidal (from the internal carotid) are usually responsible. Horizontal bands of the ganglion may be destroyed resulting in a specific hemianopic wedge field defect (referred to as a geniculate hemianopia) but more often there is a congruous or non-congruous hemianopia. Because the afferent fibres serving the pupillary light reflex exit the tract proximally to the ganglion, a relative afferent pupil defect is not present (Gunderson and Hoyt, 1971).

THE VISUAL RADIATIONS

Ventral fibres in the geniculostriate pathway initially pass anteriorly and downwards in the temporal lobe forming Meyer's loop. Lesions in this area usually result in a congruous hemianopia primarily affecting the superior quadrant and with preserved normal visual acuity and pupillary light reflexes. Often there is a wedge-shaped extension into the inferior quadrant with a sloping margin. Field defects from lesions in this area arise as a result of intrinsic tumours (gliomas), metastases and demyelinating plaques more frequently than from vascular occlusion (Plant *et al.*, 1992; Trobe *et al.*, 1973). Temporal lobe surgery for epilepsy will normally spare the geniculostriate pathways if the resection is confined to the anteromost 4–5 cm only.

More dorsal fibres pass directly through the parietal lobe and result in a homonymous hemianopia which primarily involves the inferior quadrant, but because the entire geniculostriate tract passes through the parietal lobe more extensive lesions will cause a total homonymous hemianopia with macular splitting, acuity preservation and normal pupillary light reflexes. As with all acquired retrogeniculate lesions, the fundi are normal: this is in distinction to congenital and developmental lesions of the posterior visual pathways where retrograde transsynaptic degeneration results in anomalies of the optic nerve heads (homonymous hemioptic hypoplasia) (Beatty *et al.*, 1982; Hoyt *et al.*, 1972). In extensive parietal lesions patients frequently exhibit hemineglect of all sensory modalities together with abnormalities of spatial awareness (apraxia). Ocular motor abnormalities may also arise due to abnormal visual pursuit functions (Morrow and Sharpe, 1993): this is manifested clinically by showing asymmetric responses to the rotating optokinetic drum.

PRIMARY VISUAL CORTEX (STRIATE CORTEX, OR AREA V1)

Damage to the visual cortex causes a range of visual disturbances. Classically, attention has focused on various specific patterns of acquired field defect to derive a primary retinotopic map in the striate cortex which is also known as calcarine cortex, primary visual cortex, Brodmann area 17 and area V1 (see Chapter 1). However, many cortical visual deficits (Table 7.1) cannot simply be understood in terms of field loss and an awareness of the relationships between striate and extrastriate cortex is required for an adequate description. Area V1 connects reciprocally with V2, V3 and surrounding areas of visual association cortex. It also connects directly and reciprocally with areas V5 (middle temporal visual area, MT) and at least part of V4. V4 receives both M and P inputs, projects ventrally towards the intertemporal cortex and contains neurons which may contribute to colour and pattern processing. V5 (MT) receives mainly M inputs, projects dorsally towards the occipitoparietal regions and is concerned with processing of motion, attention and related visuospatial functions.

FIELD DEFECTS IN LESIONS OF AREA V1

Occipital lobe lesions may cause a full congruous homonymous hemianopia or more limited quadrantanopias (Holmes, 1918). If the occipital pole is selectively involved then the macular representation only is affected, causing a hemianopic scotoma. More anterior occipital cortical lesions may produce a monocular defect of the unpaired fibres serving the peripheral temporal hemifield: this is the only exception to the rule that all retrochiasmal lesions result in bilateral field defects. A temporal crescenteric scotoma lies 60 degrees from fixation and will be missed if field testing is confined to the central field

Table 7.1 Selected causes of cortical visual disturbances

Vascular
Posterior cerebral artery occlusion
Middle cerebral artery occlusion (posterior temporal and parietal branches)
Watershed zone infarction
Intracerebral haemorrhage (arteriovenous malformation, hypertension, amyloid angiopathy, vasculitis)
Migraine
Demyelinating disorders
Multiple sclerosis
Acute disseminated encephalomyelitis
Degenerative diseases
Alzheimer's disease
Infections
Bacterial or fungal abscess
Viral encephalitis
Progressive multifocal leukoencephalopathy
HIV
Creutzfeldt-Jakob disease
Tumours
Primary and metastatic
Trauma
Coup and contracoup
Drugs effects
Epilepsy

only. It is important to emphasize that such a uniocular peripheral scotoma is much more commonly the result of a peripheral retinal lesion. The reverse syndrome is also seen where the extreme anterior occipital cortex is preserved resulting in a complete homonymous hemianopia except for a temporal crescent of spared vision 60–100 degrees from fixation in one of the otherwise blind hemifields (Benton *et al.*, 1980). This temporal crescent will lie either inferiorly or superiorly depending on whether the lesion lies above or below the calcarine fissure.

Because the occipital pole is served by a dual blood supply deriving from both posterior and middle cerebral artery circulations in some individuals, macular vision may also be preserved in what is otherwise a complete homonymous hemianopia (Smith and Richardson, 1966). The precise explanation of 'macular sparing' is somewhat controversial (setting aside artifactual cases arising from poor patient fixation which account for the majority), as sparing extends only 10 degrees into the blind hemifield but modern anatomical accounts give at least 60% of the primary visual cortex to this part of the visual field (Horton and Hoyt, 1991b). This extensive portion of cortically magnified visual field in the primary visual cortex probably does not carry a dual blood supply. Earlier theories explaining macular sparing on the basis of bilateral representation of the central vision at both occipital poles have not been substantiated. An overlap of ganglion cell projections from either side of the vertical meridian at the fovea would explain only 1 degree at the most of macular sparing.

BLINDSIGHT

'Blindsight', or residual vision in the apparently blind hemifield – a V1 scotoma – continues to generate controversy. Using careful test techniques, a reflex perceptual facility for stimulus presence, location, orientation, direction of movement and colour can generate appropriate reflex motor responses in spite of deficient conscious awareness.

Subcortical pathways from optic tracts to superior colliculi and to the pulvinar of the thalamus have been implicated, as have extrageniculostriate pathways which project to areas of pre-striate cortex (avoiding area V1). Callosal connections accessing the functional capabilities of the intact hemisphere may also play a role. Great care is needed in the assessment of apparent residual vision which may simply be due to the normal functioning of the monocular temporal crescent of V1 serving the contralateral eye (Celesia *et al.*, 1991; Cowey and Stoerig, 1991; Sanders *et al.*, 1974; Barbur *et al.*, 1993).

A related effect is the Riddoch phenomenom of statokinetic dissociation and is demonstrated on Goldmann perimetry when a stimulus is perceived on movement in the periphery of a homonymous hemianopia despite failure to see colour or static forms (Riddoch, 1917). The explanation for this probably lies in the functional separation of neuronal channels into those primarily concerned with movement and those primarily concerned with form – for example the intrahemispheric pathways from V1 to V5 (MT), or the extrageniculostriate tectal pathways. In certain test paradigms the same effect can be shown in lesions of the anterior visual system as well (Safran and Glaser, 1980).

Bilateral occipital cortex lesions arise quite frequently because the two posterior cerebral arteries are terminal branches of the single basilar artery and therefore basilar occlusions give rise to cortical blindness. A variety of bilateral homonymous lesions ranging from bilateral homonymous hemianopias, bilateral macular sparing homonymous hemianopias (one cause of tunnel vision), quadrantanopias and scotomas may be seen. When bilateral homonymous hemianopic scotomas arise, a characteristic notch at the vertical meridian betrays the retrochiasmal location of the pathology (Newman *et al.*, 1984). The pupillary light reflexes are normal and the visual acuity is usually markedly reduced. Curiously, many patients with cortical blindness may appear to be unaware of their visual loss and use confabulation when asked to perform visual identification tasks. This is known as Anton's syndrome. Careful assessment is mandatory, as patients with functional (non-organic) visual loss may present with very similar symptoms and signs. Neuroimaging and electrophysiology are required to confirm the diagnosis of organic visual loss in these cases (Forstl *et al.*, 1993).

Vascular disease accounts for most acquired lesions of the occipital cortex – usually thromboembolism of vertebrobasilar or cardiac origin but all other possible causes of stroke may apply. Because the two occipital lobes together only account for less than 10% of the total cortical volume, tumours are rarely confined to this territory and meningiomas, gliomas and metastases usually extend into the ipsilateral parietal lobe with associated non-visual symptoms. Bilateral occipital cortex disease also arises in metabolic disease hypoglycaemia and heavy metal poisoning), neurodegenerative disease (the leukodystrophies, mitochondrial cytopathies) and inflammatory central nervous system (CNS) disease (Creutzfeldt-Jakob disease, encephalitis, meningitis, demyelination) (Table 7.2).

THE VISUAL ASSOCIATION AREAS (EXTRASTRIATE CORTEX AREAS V2–V6)

AREA V2/V3

Lesions affecting human area V1 often extend into underlying white matter, into the pre-striate areas (Brodmann 18 and 19) and adjacent parietal and temporal regions. Areas V2/V3 share a common border with V1 which they surround concentrically. Recently, it has been proposed that inferior quadrantic field defects which respect the horizontal as well as the vertical meridian are typical of dorsal V2/V3 lesions (Horton and Hoyt, 1991a).

Table 7.2 Visual disturbances caused by cortical damage

Disorders of colour processing
Central achromatopsia
Colour anomia
Disorders of visuospatial processing (localization, orientation, attention)
Reduced static visual acuity or contrast sensitivity
Balint's syndrome
• simultanagnosia (visual disorientation)
• optic ataxia
• optic apraxia
Metamorphopsia
Monocular diplopia or polyopia
Micropsia and macropsia
Disorders of pattern processing and recognition
Visual agnosia
Prosopagnosia
Pure alexia without agraphia
Disorders of temporal processing
Central akinetopsia (defective motion perception)
Reduced dynamic visual acuity
Palinopsia (visual perseveration)
Disorders of stereopsis
Astereopsis (static or dynamic)
Disorders of visual imagery
Visual hallucinations

(From Rizzo and Nawrot, 1993.)

AREAS V4–V6

It is helpful to conceptualize the pre-striate pathways, or visual association areas as two separate systems: a ventromesial pathway which occupies the occipital lobe below the calcarine fissure and the adjacent temporal lobe – these areas contain the human homologues of areas V4 in the simian model and IT in the primate model, and a dorsolateral area which is located in the occipital lobe above the calcarine fissures and in the adjacent parietal and temporoparietaloccipital regions – the human homologues of areas V5 and MT. The clinical significance of this is that there may be functional partitioning of the pre-striate cortex in such a way that focal lesions may result in selective impairment of aspects of higher visual function (Zeki, 1992). These regional localizations of function are supported by new cerebral activation study techniques using positron emission tomography (PET) and magnetic resonance imaging (MRI) techniques, although current methods do not show the superior colliculus or the lateral geniculate nucleus, nor allow discrimination of P and M pathways (Lueck *et al.*, 1989; Zeki *et al.*, 1991; Rizzo *et al.*, 1992; Rademacher *et al.*, 1992).

VENTROMESIAL PATHWAY – CEREBRAL DYSCHROMATOPSIA AND PROSOPAGNOSIA

Lesions of the ventromesial pathway may result in defects of object recognition, colour vision and reading. Acquired defects of colour vision are generally the result of lesions of the anterior visual pathways but sometimes cerebral lesions can cause generalized or hemianopic dyschromatopsia. The human equivalent of area V4 or its white matter connections has been implicated, although the exclusive significance of this territory is disputed. It has been shown that lesions which give rise to loss of colour vision in the contralateral hemifield in humans are located in the ventral occipitotemporal cortex, similar to that activated in normal subjects in PET studies (Green and Lessell, 1977). Pure alexia is frequently associated, as is an impairment of the ability to recognize familiar faces or to learn new faces (prosopagnosia), and typically patients may at the same time have normal acuity, spatial contrast sensitivity and motion perception. Hemianopic field defects are commonly found, often bilateral inferior quadrantanopias, as a result of damage to the adjacent ventral portions of the optic radiations (Meadows, 1974a,b; Zeki, 1990; Rizzo *et al.*, 1992; Damasio *et al.*, 1982).

DORSOLATERAL PATHWAY – BALINT'S SYNDROME VISUAL AGNOSIA AND CEREBRAL AKINETOPSIA

A further range of selective visual disabilities have been ascribed to lesions of the dorsolateral pathway, usually when damage is bilateral. These include the visual agnosias where patients have normal visual acuty but cannot identify objects by sight. In Balint's syndrome there is an inability to accurately reach out and grasp objects within the field of view (optic ataxia), an inability to voluntarily reposition gaze to fix on an object of interest (psychic paralysis of gaze) and an unawareness of objects lying to one side of the object of regard in spite of adequate acuity and field (simultanagnosia). Finally, cases of cerebral motion blindness (akinetopsia) have also been reported, in keeping with the model of localization of the processing of movement functions (magnocellular stream) to the dorsolateral pathways superior to the calcarine fissure in the occiptal cortex and ending in the human homologue of area V5 (MT). Unilateral lesions causing cerebral hemiakinetopsia are apparently possible (Rizzo, 1993; Plant and Nakayama, 1993; Plant *et al.*, 1993; Zeki, 1991; Watson *et al.*, 1993).

POSITIVE VISUAL PHENOMENA, HALLUCINATIONS AND MISCELLANEOUS DISORDERS

Visual hallucinations occur when the patient reports seeing an image which is not present to any other observer. They are only rarely associated with psychiatric disease, in contrast to auditory hallucinations.

Visual hallucinations may be classified as formed and unformed. Unformed flashes and streaks of light (phosphenes) may be a symptom of vitreous traction, retinal tear or retinal detachment. Phosphenes may also be stimulated by sudden eye movement or by loud noises in optic neuritis. Unformed visual hallucinations arising from the posterior visual pathways are a feature of classic migraine, in focal seizures involving the occipital cortex, and as release phenomena when there is a deficit of field or acuity in the visual pathways, especially after a vascular accident. By contrast, formed hallucinations arise in normal individuals on falling asleep or awakening (hypnagogic and hypnopombic), and in instances of use, abuse or withdrawal of a wide range of medicinal and recreational drugs. Of special interest is the Charles Bonnet syndrome (Brown and Murphy, 1992; Ulbrich, 1987) comprising well-formed visual hallucinations occuring in the elderly with visual loss. Strictly speaking, these are not hallucinations in the neuropsychiatric sense as the subject's insight and mental state is preserved. The patient experiences in vivid detail scenes of faces or complex objects such as fabric patterns or brickwork which are not recognized from previous experience. These tableaux impose themselves on the normally perceived world, usually for only a few minutes at a time, and seem to be related to visual sensory deprivation (Cogan, 1973).

PALINOPSIA AND CEREBRAL DIPLOPIA

Palinopsia or visual perseveration causes the patient to continue to perceive an object after it is no longer in view. Usually pallinopsia arises as a part of a generalized occipitoparietal syndrome, but is occasionally seen in isolation. The perseverated images may be perceived only in the blind hemifield of a patient with a homonymous hemianopia. A related phenomenon is cerebral diplopia where the patient experiences either monocular diplopia or polyopia in the absence of any abnormality of ocular motility or the intraocular structures (such as astigmatism or lens opacities). The mechanism remains obscure, but probably relates to lesions of V1 – the primary visual cortex (Bender *et al.*, 1968; Meadows, 1973).

REFERENCES

Barbur JL, Watson JDG, Frackowiak RSJ and Zeki S (1993). Conscious visual perception without V1. *Brain* **116**: 1293–1302.

Beatty B, Sadun A, Smith L *et al.* (1982). Direct demonstration of transsynaptic degeneration in the human visual system: A comparison of retrograde and anterograde changes. *J Neurol Neurosurg Psychiat* **45**: 143–146.

Bell RA and Thompson HS (1978). Relative afferent pupillary defect in optic tract hemianopias. *Am J Ophthalmol* **85**: 538–540.

Bender MB (1945). Polyopia and monocular diplopia of cerebral origin. *Arch Neurol Psychiat* **54**: 323.

Bender MB, Feldman M and Sobin AJ (1968). Palinopsia. *Brain* **91**: 321–328.

Benton S, Levy I and Swash M (1980). Vision in the temporal crescent in occipital infarction. *Brain* **103**: 83–97.

Brown GC and Murphy RP (1992). Visual symptoms associated with choroidal neovascularisation. Photopsias and the Charles Bonnet syndrome. *Arch Ophthalmol* **110**: 1251–1256.

Celesia GG, Bushnell MD *et al.* (1991). Cortical blindness and residual vision: is the "second" visual system capable of more than rudimentary visual perception? *Neurology* **41**: 862–869.

Cibis GW, Campos EC and Aulhorn E (1975). Pupillary hemiakinesia in suprageniculate lesions. *Arch Ophthalmol* **93**: 1322.

Cogan DG (1973). Visual hallucinations as release phenomena. *Graefe's Arch Clin Exp Ophthalmol* **1818**: 139–150.

Cowey A and Stoerig P (1991). The neurobiology of blindsight. *Trends Neurosci* **14**: 140–145.

Damasio AR, Damasio H and Van Hoesen GW (1982). Prosopagnosia: Anatomic basis and behavioural mechanisms. *Neurology* **32**: 331–341.

Dutton GN (1994). Cognitive visual dysfunction. *Br J Ophthalmol* **78**: 723–726.

Forstl H, Owen AM and David AS (1993). Gabriel Anton and 'Anton's syndrome'. On focal diseases of the brain which are not perceived by the patients (1898). *Neuropsychiat Neuropsychol Behav Neurol* **6**: 1–8.

Green GL and Lessell S (1977). Acquired cerebral dyschomatopsia. *Arch Ophthalmol* **95**: 121.

Gunderson CH and Hoyt WF (1971). Geniculate hemianopia: Incongruous homonymous field defects in two patients with partial lesions of the lateral geniculate nucleus. *J Neurol Neurosurg Psychiat* **24**: 1–6.

Holmes G (1918). Disturbances of vision caused by cerebral lesions. *Br J Ophthalmol* **2**: 353–384.

Horton JC and Hoyt WF (1991a). Quadrantic field defects: a hallmark of lesions in extrastriate (V2/3) cortex). *Brain* a **114**: 1703–1718.

Horton JC and Hoyt WF (1991b). The representation of the visual field in human striate cortex: a revision of the classic Holmes map. *Arch Ophthalmol* **109**: 816–824.

Horton JC, Dalgi LR, McCrane EP and Demonasterio FM (1990). Arrangement of ocular dominance columns in human visual cortex. *Arch Ophthalmol* **108**: 1025–1031.

Hoyt WF, Rios-Montenegro EN, Behrens MM *et al.* (1972). Homonymous hemioptic hypoplasia: Fundoscopic features in standard and red-free illumination in three patients with congenital hemiplegia. *Br J Ophthalmol* **56**: 537–545.

Lueck CJ, Zeki S, Friston KJ *et al.* (1989). The colour centre in the cerebral cortex of man. *Nature* **340**: 386–389.

Meadows JC (1973). Observations of a case of monocular diplopia of cerebral origin. *J Neurol Sci* **18**: 249–253.

Meadows JC (1974a). The anatomical basis of prosopagnosia. *J Neurol Neurosurg Psychiat* **37**: 489–501.

Meadows JC (1974b). Disturbed perception of colors associated with localized cerebral lesions. *Brain* **97**: 615–632.

Morrow MJ and Sharpe JA (1993). Retinotopic and directional deficits of smooth pursuit initiation after posterior and cerebral hemispheric lesions. *Neurology* **43**: 595–603.

Newman RP, Kinkel WR and Jacobs L (1984). Altitudinal hemianopia caused by occipital infarcts. Clinical and computerized tomographic correlations. *Arch Neurol* **41**: 413–418.

Newman SA and Miller NR (1983). Optic tract syndrome: Neuro-Ophthalmic considerations. *Arch Ophthalmol* **101**: 1241–1250.

Olbrch HM, Engelmeier MP, Pauleikhoff D and Wanbke T (1987). Visual hallucinations in ophthalmology. *Graefe's Arch Exp Clin Ophthalmol* **225**: 217–220.

Plant GT and Nakayama K (1993). The characteristics of residual motion perception in the hemifield contralateral to lateral occipital lesions in humans. *Brain* **116**: 1337–1353.

Plant GT, Kermode AG, Turano G *et al.* (1992). McDonald WI. Symptomatic retrochiasmal lesions in multiple sclerosis: clinical features, visual evoked potentials and magnetic resonance imaging. *Neurology* **42**: 68–76.

Plant GT, Laxer KD, Barbaro NM *et al.* (1993). Impaired visual motion perception in the contralateral hemifield following unilateral posterior cerebral lesions in humans. *Brain* **116**: 1303–1335.

Rademacher J, Galaburda AM, Kennedy DN *et al.* (1992). Human cerebral cortex: localisation, parcellation and morphometry with magnetic resonance imaging. *J Cogn Neurosci* **5**: 263–287.

Riddoch G (1917). Dissociation of visual perceptions due to occipital injuries, with especial reference to appreciation of movement. *Brain* **40**: 15–57.

Rizzo M (1993). Ballint's syndrome and associated visuospatial disorders. In *Visual Perceptual Defects: Ballière's Clinical Neurology* (ed C Kennard), pp. 415–437. London: Ballière Tindal.

Rizzo M and Nawrot M (1993). Human visual cortex and its disorders. *Curr Opin Ophthalmol* **4**: 38–47.

Rizzo M, Nawrot M, Blake R and Damasio AR (1992). A human disorder resembling area V4 dysfunction in the monkey. *Neurology* **42**: 1175–1180.

Safran AB and Glaser JS (1980). Statokinetic dissociation in lesions of the anterior visual pathways. *Arch Ophthalmol* **98**: 291.

Sanders MD, Warrington EK, Marshall J *et al.* (1974). 'Blindsight'. Vision in a field defect. *Lancet* **ii** 707–708.

Savino PJ, Paris M, Schatz NJ *et al.* (1978). Optic tract syndrome: A review of 21 patients. *Arch Ophthalmol* **96**: 656–663.

Smith CG and Richardson WFG (1966). The course and distribution of the arteries supplying the visual (striate) cortex. *Am J Ophthalmol* **61**: 1391–1396.

Trobe JD, Lorber ML and Schlezinger NS (1973). Isolated homonymous hemianopias: a review of 104 cases. *Arch Ophthalmol* **89**: 377–381.

Watson JDG, Myers R, Frackowiak RSJ *et al.* (1993). Area V5 of the human brain: evidence from a combined study using positron emission tomography and magnetic resonance imaging. *Cerebral Cortex* **3**: 79–94.

Zeki S (1990). A century of cerebral achromatopsia. *Brain* **113**: 1727–1777.

Zeki S (1991). Cerebral akinetopsia (visual motion blindness). A review. *Brain* **114**: 811–824.

Zeki S (1992). The visual image in mind and brain. *Scient Am* Sept 69–76.

Zeki S, Watson JD, Lueck CJ *et al.* (1991). A direct demonstration of functional specialization in human visual cortex. *J Neurosci* **11**: 641–649.

8

Eye movement abnormalities

1 Central control of eye movements: basic principles

THE ORGANIZATION OF EYE MOVEMENTS

The complex sensorimotor act of normal vision requires two essential components: one is the ability to shift gaze rapidly (a saccade) to bring the image of an object of interest on to the regions of the retina containing the highest density of photoreceptors, the fovea, and the other is to stabilize the new image on this area despite movement of the object (smooth pursuit and vergence), or of the head and body (vestibulo ocular and optokinetic reflexes). To serve these movements, viscous drag and elastic restoring forces of the orbital tissues must be overcome by powerful contractions of the extraocular muscles (Leigh and Zee, 1991).

THE NEURAL SUBSTRATE OF CONJUGATE EYE MOVEMENTS: SYNOPSIS OF ANATOMY AND PHYSIOLOGY AND METHODS OF CLINICAL ASSESSMENT

The vestibulo-ocular and optokinetic systems: anatomy and physiology
The vestibulo-ocular system (the vestibulo-oculo reflex or VOR) serves to stabilize gaze and ensure clear vision during rotational head movements, particularly those that occur during locomotion. For example, a rotational movement of the head to the right produces a compensatory eye movement in the orbit to the left so that the angle of gaze, or eye position in space does not change and the image of the world remains fairly stationary upon the retina. The VOR is a brain stem reflex involving the semicircular canals, the vestibular ganglion, central vestibular nuclei and the oculomotor nuclei in specific pathways reflecting the plane of head movement and the direction of the compensatory eye movement in question. For example, from the right horizontal labyrinthine canal, excitatory projections will drive the horizontally acting ipsilateral medial rectus muscle and the contralateral lateral rectus muscle, while inhibitory projections will act on the ipsilateral lateral rectus and contralateral medial rectus. The ratio of amplitudes of output and input is referred to as the VOR gain. In addition to the simple VOR, mechanisms also exist which are driven by the otoliths, to provide ocular compensation for non-rotational movements such as body tilt or impulsion (e.g lateropulsion, levitation). During combined, smooth eye-head tracking, the VOR is cancelled, probably at the level of the ocular motor neurons by an internal

neural signal. During sustained rotation, vesibulo-ocular compensation declines and visual images of the seen world increasingly slip across the retina. This is a stimulus for both the optokinetic and smooth pursuit systems.

Optokinetic stimulation therefore occurs naturally during sustained self-rotation in the light. In the laboratory and in clinical practice the optokinetic system is stimulated by a large patterned drum around the stationary subject. Even though there is no peripheral vestibular stimulation, the subject experiences a powerful sensation of self-rotation and nystagmus is generated with the slow phase in the direction of the rotation of the patterns. The nystagmus continues for a few moments after the stimulus is withdrawn. Retinal projections reach the vestibular nuclei via a subcortical pathway incorporating the nucleus of the optic tract and the accessory optic system of the thalamus, and also via inputs from the visual cortex (Büttner and Büttner–Ennever, 1987).

Clinical assessment of the vestibular system

Patients with vestibular disease complain of disequilibrium, unsteadiness, vertigo, inappropriate tilting and oscillopsia. Formal laboratory based neuro-otological testing is required for a full assessment. This includes quantitative eye movement recording, caloric testing, rotational tests and, in special instances, the use of elaborate equipment to assess otolith–ocular function. In the ophthalmology clinic some simple qualititative tests remain useful. Static vestibular imbalance is indicated by the presence of nystagmus which characteristically is accentuated when fixation is removed by Frenzel goggles or + 20 dioptre lenses.

Ophthalmoscopy is a good way of detecting more subtle nystagmus, although it should be noted that because the retina is behind the centre of rotation of the eye, the direction of movement is in the opposite direction to that occurring at the front of the eye. Dynamic tests of vestibular balance include positional testing and noting the effects of rapid head shaking. Abnormalities of VOR gain can be qualitatively noted by simply measuring visual acuity on a card during head rotation: if vestibular gain is abnormal, the visual acuity will drop by several lines compared with the level achieved with the head still.

Acute unilateral vestibular disease causes central imbalance of vestibular tone because there is a difference between the neural activity of left and right vestibular nuclei. This causes spontaneous nystagmus with the slow phases directed towards the side of the lesion. Disease confined to a single canal or its immediate projections causes nystagmus in the plane of that canal. With time, adaptation of central vestibular tone leads to loss of nystagmus, at least in the light. Lesions of central vestibular structures result in nystagmus that is usually present in the primary position and may be horizontal, vertical or torsional. In addition VOR gain abnormalities are prominent. Unilateral lesions of the central otolithic connections cause disturbances of head posture and skew deviation.

In the unconscious patient, bedside testing of the VOR (doll's eye movements) is very important. This is elicited either by head rolling or by caloric testing. If the VOR is absent there are either bilateral peripheral vestibular lesions, or severe brain stem dysfunction. If the VOR is present but asymmetrical or monocular, there is either a localized nuclear or an infranuclear ocular motor nerve lesion.

In the conscious patient with stable fixation, the VOR can also be utilized in the assessment of ophthalmoplegias: in supranuclear defects of voluntary eye movement, the VOR will drive the eyes fully in the opposite direction to the direction of rotation because of independent input to the ocular motor nuclei (Zee, 1991; Rosenberg, *et al.*, 1975).

The saccadic system: anatomy and physiology (Fig. 8.1)

Table 8.1 Classification of saccades

I. Intentional saccades	Volitional saccades made to a predetermined visual target (visually guided saccades) or generated when the goal for the saccade is known but there is no visible target (non-visually guided saccade).
A. Visually guided saccades	
B. Non-visually guided saccades	
1. Predictive saccades	Saccades generated before the target is stepped to a predictable location
2. Target searching	Saccades stepped into a homonymous hemianopia
3. Remembered target	Saccades stepped to a location at which a target has previously been presented
4. Anti-saccade	The subject generates a saccade to the mirror location of a target in the opposite direction
II. Reflexive saccades:	Saccades that draw the eyes to novel stimuli suddenly occurring in the environment
III. Spontaneous saccades	Random saccades generated when the subject is in the dark and not required to perform any behavioural task
IV. Quick phases of nystagmus	

This classification indicates a hierarchy of function from the most rudimentary of all saccades — the quick phases of vestibular nystagmus during rotation in the dark, through the reflexive saccades to the sudden appearance of a novel stimulus, to higher level volitional function such as saccades toward the remembered location of a visual target. In the clinic, if voluntary saccades cannot be generated, the examiner must move down through the saccade hierarchy and evaluate progressively more reflexive types including the quick phases of nystagmus.

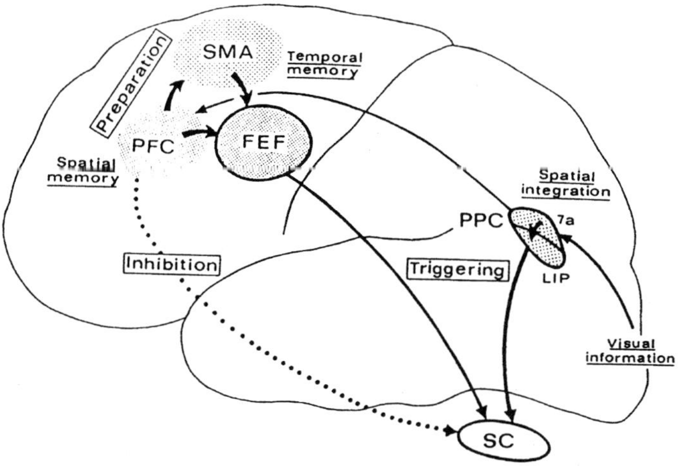

Figure 8.1 Main actions of the different ocular motor cortical areas in saccade initiation. FEF: frontal eye field; LIP: lateral intraparietal area; PFC: prefrontal cortex; PPC: posterior parietal cortex; SC: superior colliculus; SMA: supplementary motor area; 7a: area 7a. (From Pierrot–Deseilligny, 1991.)

The final common pathway for horizontal saccades is the pontine paramedian reticular formation (PPRF), and for vertical saccades it is the rostral interstitial nucleus of the medial longitudinal fasciculus (riMLF) in the mesencephalon (Büttner-Ennever *et al.*, 1989a). In the pons, the abducens nucleus contains motor neurons innervating the ipsilateral lateral rectus muscle, intermingled with internuclear neurons which, after decussating in the lower pons, project via the medical longitudinal fasciculus to the contralateral medical rectus subnucleus of the oculomotor nucleus. The abducens nucleus receives projections from the various cells of the PPRF. These include the excitatory burst neurons which discharge at high frequency just before and during saccades, providing the eye velocity commands known as the 'pulse', or 'burst'. Another type of neuron, the omnipause neuron, discharges tonically except just before and during saccades ('pause'). These neurons appear to exert an inhibitory influence on the 'burst' neurons during fixation. Finally, maintainance of the eccentric position of the eye requires a third set of integrator neurons to produce a tonic 'step' (Hanson *et al.*, 1986).

Higher level control of saccades

(i) Superior colliculus. The superior colliculus contains a retinotopic afferent projection of the visual field and descending efferents which project to structures in the brain stem concerned with the generation of premotor saccadic movement commands. Afferent fibres are also received from the frontal and parietal cortex. Patients with striate cortex lesions who make saccades presented in the blind hemifield even though they cannot consciously perceive the target's location may be relying on superior collicular function (Schiller et al., 1987; Pierrot-Deseilligny, 1991).

(ii) Frontal lobe. Stimulation of the frontal eye fields in premotor cortical area 8 generates a contralateral saccade. Other frontal areas which contribute to saccadic eye movement control lie in the supplementary eye fields and in the dorsolateral prefrontal cortex. Reflexive and anticipatory saccades, antisaccades and memory guided saccades may all be slow and hypometric in unilateral frontal lobe lesions. Projections from the frontal eye fields pass directly to the brain stem, and also indirectly via the caudate nucleus, substantia nigra and superior colliculus (Pierrot-Deseilligny et al., 1991a,b c; Duhamel *et al.*, 1992).

(iii) Parietal lobe. A posterior pathway arising in the posterior parietal cortex projects to the superior colliculus and then to the immediate premotor regions of the PPRF and riMLF. Patients with bilateral parietal lesions show an acquired form of ocular-motor apraxia and abnormal patterns of visual scanning (visually guided saccades) (Braun et al., 1992).

(iv) Thalamus, basal ganglia and cerebellum. The intramedullary lamina and the pulvinar within the thalamus appear to assist with spatial localization and informing higher structures of the occurrence of an eye movement, and for mediating changes of attention. The substantia nigra pars reticulata and caudate nucleus within the basal ganglia appear to gate, selectively, reflexive or voluntary saccades generated via the superior colliculus thereby preventing unwanted reflexive saccades to stimuli which might at any particular moment be disruptive. The cerebellum is important in the control of saccadic accuracy (Leigh and Zee, 1991).

The saccadic system: clinical examination and common abnormalities

Examination

Saccadic eye movements are best examined by instructing the patient to fixate alternately on two targets: saccades in each direction can be examined in each field of gaze in both horizontal and vertical planes. The examiner notes whether the saccades are of normal velocity, promptly initiated, accurate and correctly yoked.

Table 8.2 Saccadic abnormalities

Saccadic slowing with restricted amplitude	Internuclear ophthalmoplegia, gaze palsy, ocular myopathy, ocular motor palsy
Saccadic slowing with full amplitude	Central brain stem or hemisphere lesions drug intoxication, drowsiness
Saccadic hypermetria (overshoot)	Cerebellar vermis lesions, peripheral ocular motor disorders, ipsilateral hemianopia and cerebral hemisphere lesions
Saccadic hypometria (undershoot)	Cerebellar system disorders, parkinsonism, progressive supranuclear palsy, anticonvulsant medication
Increased saccadic latency	Voluntary saccades – Parkinson's and Huntington's disease, Congenital ocular motor apraxia
Inappropriate saccades (saccadic intrusions)	(see below)

Saccadic slowing, such as the lag of the adducting eye in internuclear ophthalmoplegia, is best seen when the subject is asked to rapidly refixate between two widely spaced targets. Slow adduction can also be demonstrated using the hand-held optokinetic drum or tape, where quick phases made by the affected eye are smaller and slower. Saccadic latency can be inferred from the time it takes the patient to initiate the saccade. Saccadic dysmetria can be appreciated by noting the direction and size of corrective saccades made to acquire the fixation target.

After noting an abnormality the examiner localizes the disturbance within the hierarchy of saccadic organization by testing nystagmus quick phases with the rotating optokinetic drum, then reflex movements to a suddenly appearing visual target, then volitional saccades and so on. If there is an abnormality of saccadic initiation, an accompanying head movement may help the patient in ocular motor apraxia. During steady fixation, extraneous saccadic eye movements (saccadic intrusions) may be noted.

Clinical abnormalities of saccades

More precise assessments are achieved using formal eye movement recording systems. Common abnormalities are given in Table 8.2.

Unilateral hemisphere lesions resulting in eye movement abnormalities can be termed 'paralytic' and 'irritative'. Following an acute right hemisphere lesion in a sufficiently alert subject, there may be a failure to generate saccades towards the side of the lesion with ipsilaterally directed conjugate gaze and preservation of smooth pursuit movements (Sharpe *et al.*, 1985). When the opposite hemisphere is intact the palsy is transient: this is thought to reflect the bilateral saccadic control of the frontal eye fields. Irritative lesions (epileptiform) of the frontal lobe may generate contralaterally directed saccades. Lesions of the posterior cortical saccadic pathway from the posterior parietal lobe result in increased latencies of visually guided saccades and decreased accuracy of memory guided saccades. The effects are more marked in right parietal lesions than left. In the brain stem, discrete lesions of the PPRF produce loss of saccades and quick phases of nystagmus to the side ipsilateral to the lesion, whereas a lesion of the abducens nucleus results in a complete ipsilateral gaze-palsy involving all types of eye movement. Slowed saccades may result from omnipause neuron lesions, while defects in the integrator (step cells) produce an exponential drift towards the primary postion which is corrected by a saccade to produce the pattern of gaze-paretic nystagmus. The cerebellum maintains additional influence on the saccadic integrator and is involved in calibrating the size of the saccadic pulse. In saccadic hypometria, an attempt to make a 20 degrees refixation will actually comprise two or three fragmented steps of 10 or 5 degrees each. Hypometric saccades are seen in cerebellar system disorders, Parkinsonism and progressive supranuclear palsy, and also as a side-effect of anticonvulsant medications. Abnormally large saccades (hypermetria) are typically a feature of lesions of the dorsal vermis (Bains *et al.*, 1992; Duhamel *et al.*, 1992; Lueck *et al.*, 1992a, b).

Saccadic intrusions

Saccadic intrusions (sporadic) and oscillations (sustained) take the fovea off target. In contrast to nystagmus, there is no smooth pursuit element.

The commonest saccadic intrusions are square wave jerks which occur during fixation when there is a conjugate displacement of the eyes followed by a refixational saccade. Square wave jerks are seen in cerebellar disease, progressive supranuclear palsy and multiple sclerosis. High amplitude (macro) jerks are seen in Alzheimer's and Huntingdon's diseases.

Saccadic oscillations can be analysed according to the presence or absence of an intersaccadic interval — usually formal eye movement recording is required to note this. Macrosaccadic oscillations comprise horizontal salvoes of saccades straddling the fixation point with a distinct intersaccadic interval of some 200ms are associated with cerebellar lesions. In opsoclonus and ocular flutter there is no intersaccadic interval — leading to the term 'back-to-back saccades'. Opsoclonus is a multidirectional sequence of conjugate saccadic eye movements which persist during sleep and may be a presenting, paraneoplastic phenomenom in children (neuroblastoma) and adults (carcinoma) in addition to associations with postinfective states and drug intoxication. In contrast, ocular flutter is milder, inconstant and always in the horizontal plane so it may be regarded as a form of the same instability of pause or burst neuronal activity (Ashe *et al.*, 1991).

The smooth pursuit system: anatomy and physiology (Fig. 8.2)

Smooth pursuit eye movements are used by foveate animals in tracking slow-moving objects to maintain their images at or near the fovea. The initial stimulus for smooth pursuit is movement of an image upon the retina, especially in the foveal and parafoveal regions. In the maintainance of normal smooth pursuit tracking, the gain (eye velocity/target velocity) is normally 1.0 and the eye does not lag behind the target (the phase shift is small). The pursuit pathway continues to the magnocellular portion of the lateral geniculate nucleus and then to the primary visual cortex. Unilateral lesions of the striate cortex abolish smooth pursuit for targets lying in the blind hemifield, but pursuit remains intact for targets presented in the normal hemifield. The striate cortex projects to the middle temporal visual area (MT), via a direct pathway and an indirect pathway which passes initially to other prestriate areas. Lesions in area MT cause a scotoma for motion within the affected portion of the visual field. In rhesus monkeys the middle temporal area lies in the superior temporal sulcus — the human homologue probably lies posterior to the superior temporal sulcus at the junction of areas 19, 37 and 39 — the junction of the occipital, temporal and parietal lobes. An adjacent area, the medial superior temporal area (MST) receives input related to eye velocity and combines this with the motion signal from MT. The areas MT and MST have been shown in experimental animals to project to the dorsolateral pontine nucleus, considered to be the next step in the pursuit pathway. Some projections pass via the posterior parietal cortex and frontal eye fields which are important in programming predictive pursuit movements. From the dorsal pontine nucleus, connections pass to the cerebellar flocculus and vermis. The flocculus is important in maintaining pursuit during steady-state tracking while the vermis is more important when target velocity changes. The cerebellar flocculus projects to the ipsilateral medial vestibular nucleus and nucleus propositus hypoglossi (NPH) before reaching the ocular motor nuclei (Sharpe and Morrow 1991; Komatsu and Wurtz, 1989).

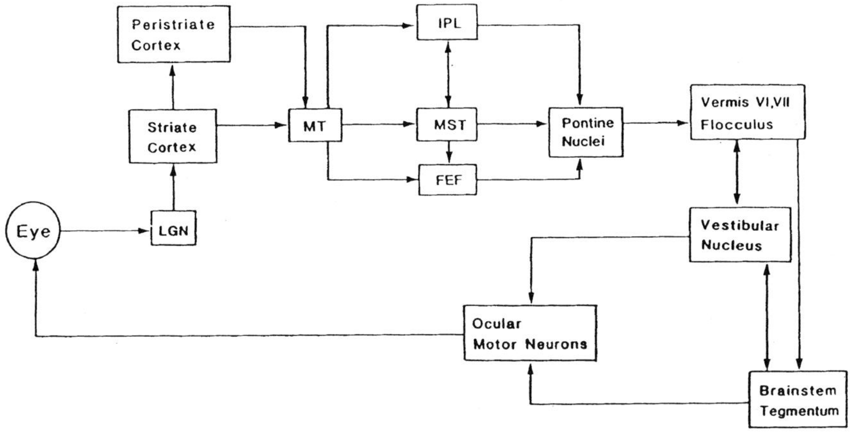

Figure 8.2 Schematic circuit of projections that process visual motion information and generate smooth ocular tracking. Homologous areas for MT and MST of monkey brain are areas 19 and 39 of the human brain, located in the angular gyrus. LGN, lateral geniculate nucleus; MT, middle temporal area; MST, middle superior temporal area; IPL, inferior parietal lobule; FEF, frontal eyefield, VI, VII, lobules VI and VII of the vermis in the cerebellum. (From Sharpe and Morrow, 1991.)

The smooth pursuit system — clinical examination and common abnormalities

The clinical examination of the smooth pursuit system starts with checking steady fixation, both under binocular viewing conditions and then with first one eye and then the other occluded to detect latent nystagmus. Examining the optic nerve head with the ophthalmoscope is a sensitive way of detecting drifts, nystagmus or saccadic intrusions while the other eye fixates.

The simplest method for testing tracking is to ask the patient to follow a small target such as a pencil tip moving at a low uniform speed about 1 metre in front of the eyes. Pursuit movements that do not match the target velocity require catch-up saccades if the gain is too low, and back-up saccades if the gain is too high. It is always important to ensure that the patient's concentration and visual attention are adequate to the task. When co-operation or attention is lacking a large hand-held mirror or hand-held optokinetic drums and tapes are useful. A mirror large enough to fill the visual field is a very powerful stimulus for visual tracking when rotated in front of the eyes and may be used to confirm non-organic visual loss. Hand-held optokinetic drums or tapes do not adequately test the optokinetic system, but do stimulate smooth pursuit and are very good for demonstrating pursuit asymmetries. The nature of the slow phases of nystagmus should be analysed. For example, a patient with a right posterior cortical lesion may show fewer quick phases when the drum is rotated to the right. This is mainly due to the fact that pursuit gain is lower to the right and since the eyes deviate more slowly from the primary position, fewer quick phases are needed.

In humans, bilateral occipital lobe lesions abolish or prevent the development of smooth pursuit, and it is also possible to identify specific abnormalities of ocular tracking arising as a result of lesions of the secondary visual areas. A patient may note difficulties in seeing moving but not stationary objects in the affected hemifield when routine (static) perimetry is normal. Other patients may show deficient tracking towards the side of the lesion. Asymmetry of horizontal smooth pursuit is seen in lesions at other parts of the pursuit pathways: large frontal lobe lesions, thalamus, dorsolateral pontine regions and cerebellum. Symmetrical low gain pursuit is also a common abnormality in old age, Parkinson's disease, progressive supranuclear palsy, Alzheimer's disease and schizophrenia (Morrow and Sharpe, 1990; Johnston *et al.*, 1992; Daniel *et al.*, 1995).

Steele–Richardson–Olszewski syndrome

The Steele–Richardson–Olszewski syndrome is a late onset progressive neurodegenerative disease characterized by supranuclear gaze palsy, pseudobulbar palsy, dysarthria, dystonic rigidity and dementia. Not all patients have a typical supranuclear gaze palsy but those who do may present with visual symptoms including diplopia, blurred vision and a 'staring gaze'. Some patients may complain of symptoms relating to blepharospasm and abnormal levator inhibition. This group may benefit symptomatically from treatment with local botulinum injections to the orbicularis muscle (see Chapter 9) (Daniel *et al.*, 1995).

The neural integrator — mechanisms for gaze holding

Both velocity and position components of the discharges of the ocular motor neurons are required to hold the eyes steady in a eccentric position of gaze. A neural network — the neural integrator — integrates these signals: for horizontal conjugate movements, the nucleus propositus hypoglossi and medial vestibular nucleus are of prime importance. For vertical movements, midbrain structures including the interstitial nucleus of Cajal contribute to neural integration.

Inadequate integration causes a rapid decay in eye position and consequent drift of the eyes back from an eccentric to a neutral position. Clinically this is seen as gaze-evoked nystagmus, where corrective saccades are required to carry the eye back into a desired eccentric position in the orbit. Impaired integration ('leaky integrator') is a common side-effect of anticonvulsant medications and is caused by focal disease of the brain stem and cerebellum.

Following complete cerebellar removal in monkeys, animals are unable to maintain an eccentric eye position: ocular postion is corrected with a saccadic fast phase toward the intended direction of gaze (gaze-paretic nystagmus). In unilateral cerebellar lobectomy studies, the same pattern is followed on the side of the lesion. In clinical practice lesions restricted to the cerebellum are unusual and the brain stem is often also involved.

Abnormalities of eye — head movements — clinical features

When smooth tracking takes place as a combination of eye and head movements the VOR must be suppressed (Land, 1992). Abnormalities of eye–head movements can be assessed by first noticing any spontaneous head tilt, turn or tremor. Eye-head pursuit is tested by rotating the patient's head during fixation on a head-fixed target. If there is impaired cancellation of the VOR the eyes will be continually taken off target by slow phases of the

Table 8.3 Typical clinically detectable abnormalities of eye movement in lesions of the cerebellum or its brain stem connections

Cogwheel (saccadic) pursuit
Hypometric and hypermetric saccades
Horizontal gaze palsy or paresis
Saccadic intrusions and oscillations
Skew deviation
Nystagmus
Failure to suppress VOR

VOR and corrective saccades will be made. Cerebellar disease and common diseases such as multiple sclerosis, Parkinson's disease and progressive supranuclear palsy frequently impair VOR suppression. Abnormalities of head posture and gaze are commonly caused by disturbance of vestibular function and patients frequently complain of disturbed vision and oscillopsia (illusory movement of the visual world). Loss of otolithic inputs is most evident clinically when it occurs unilaterally and acutely. The result is an ipsilateral head tilt together with a skew deviation and torsion (hypodeviation and excyclotorsion of the ipsilateral eye). Lesions involving the central otolithic pathways — the vestibular nuclei, medial longitudinal fasciculus, or interstitial nucleus of Cajal may cause a combination of skew deviation and head tilt — the ocular tilt reaction (Zee, 1991; Leigh, 1989; Galleta *et al.*, 1994).

Instability of head posture also arises in a variety of central disturbances. In benign familial tremor, head tremor rarely interferes with steady gaze because the VOR is adequate. However, in acquired cerebellar disease with titubation, it causes unstable fixation and reduced acuity (Barratt *et al.*, 1985). Congenital abnormalities also give rise to head tremor and gaze disturbances. In spasmus nutans there is a triad of head nodding, nystagmus and anomalous head positions. The nystagmus is typically intermittent, high frequency, variable and asymmetric, in distinction to congenital nystagmus and there is no visual sensory deficit. Usually there are no associated neurological abnormalities, although some patients do have strabismus and amblyopia. Spontaneous remission after 1–2 years is usual.

Patients with congenital nystagmus often have associated head oscillations. This is thought to represent a common neural mechanism for both forms of oscillation, possibly involving the eye–neck reticulospinal neurones in the pons. Head turns in congenital nystagmus bring the eyes close to the null position in the orbit where the nystagmus is minimal. In the nystagmus blockage syndrome, voluntary convergence suppresses the nystagmus and the patient acquires a head turn to direct the adducted viewing eye to the object of interest (Abadi and Dickinson, 1986; Tusa *et al.*, 1992; Troost, 1992).

Ocular motor apraxia

Ocular motor apraxia refers to a failure to generate saccades to command (Fielder *et al.*, 1986). Strictly speaking, as an apraxia, reflex and nystagmus quick phases should be intact, but the term is often used when reflex saccades are also abnormal. Children with congenital ocular motor apraxia present with abnormal visual fixation behaviour and the appearance of being blind. Within a few months characteristic head thrusts develop as the child attempts to change fixation. By performing this manoeuvre, the intact VOR drives the eyes into an extreme contraversive position in the orbit. As the head moves past the target, the eyes are dragged along in space until they become aligned to the target. Then the head rotates backward and the eyes maintain fixation as they are brought back to the primary postion in the orbit by the VOR. Vertical eye movements are normal in the congenital form of the disorder. The cause is unknown and usually the movement abnormalities improve with age. Associated intracranial anomalies including cerebellar hypoplasia and agenesis of the corpus callosum (Joubert's syndrome) have been described.

Patients with Louis-Bar syndrome (ataxia telangectasia), cerebral Whipple's disease and variants of Gaucher's have a horizontal saccadic palsy whereas patients with Niemann-Pick disease type C have a saccadic palsy which initially only involves vertical eye movements (Knox *et al.*, 1995). Blinking may be used to shift vertical gaze. Acquired ocular motor apraxia has been associated with bilateral lesions of the frontoparietal cortex. In Balint's syndrome there is additional peripheral visual inattention and optic ataxia (inaccurate visually guided hand movements).

Vergence eye movements

Stereoscopic vision is essential for the accurate perception of depth, especially in the space around which we use our hands. At greater distances, depth may be appreciated by monocular cues such as motion parallax and contour overlay. Thus, unless objects are viewed at optical infinity, the vergence system of dysjunctive eye movements must be used. For single vision to be derived from the inputs of two eyes, the images of an object of interest must fall on corresponding retinal points so that fusion (the perception of an object seen by both eyes as single) may take place. Corresponding retinal elements allow a subjective sense of visual direction based on the imaginary third cylcopean eye. If two images of an object fall on non-corresponding retinal areas in each eye, the object is simultaneously localized in two different directions resulting in diplopia. At the same time, two different objects are localized to the same positions in space resulting in visual confusion.

The vergence system operates to avoid diplopia and visual confusion and is driven by two primary stimuli: image disparity which produces diplopia, and retinal blur which leads to loss of sharpness of the perceived images. Disparity-induced vergence results in precise correspondence of images on the retina and blur-induced accommodative vergence ensures that they remain in focus. A residual disparity or steady-state vergence error is known as fixation disparity. Images within this residual disparity fall within Panum's area of single binocular vision. Because of the horizontal separation of the eyes in the orbits, each eye receives a slightly different image of an object. These dissimilar retinal images can be fused to allow the creation of a solid three-dimensional percept.

The combination of vergence, accommodation and pupillary constriction is known as the near triad: the degree of pupillary constriction is a useful clinical sign. There is a synkinetic relationship between the accommodation of the lens (A) and accommodative linked convergence (AC) expressed as the AC/A ratio. The AC/A ratio is usually smaller than that required for binocular fixation at all viewing distances and disparity-induced vergence must also be used. The sense of nearness provided by image size, texture and pattern provides an additional vergence stimulus. The relationship between vergence amplitude and disparity amplitude is under adaptive control which may have therapeutic applications in some cases.

The cells of the medial rectus motor neurons in the oculomotor nucleus do not lie in one discrete location, and three separate subgroups can be identified. Subgroup C appears to innervate the outer orbital portion of the medial rectus muscle which contain smaller muscle fibres and may be involved in the generation of slower vergence eye movements. However, the existence of a subpopulation of medial rectus neurons exclusively concerned with vergence as opposed to versional eye movements remains to be demonstrated. Premotor vergence velocity and tonic vergence position cells may be located dorsal and lateral to the oculomotor nucleus. Cortical control of voluntary vergence is thought to lie in the frontal eye fields, and for reflex movements in the posterior cortex, in the same manner as the organization of saccades.

Congenital abnormalities of vergence mechanisms are common. Abnormalities of the AC/A ratio are accompanied by concomitant strabismus in the forms of convergence excess, convergence insufficiency, divergence excess and divergence insufficiency. Sometimes these abnormalities present with intermittent diplopia in adulthood. Acquired neurological disorders cause vergence disturbances which may take the form of either impaired or absent convergence. In tumours of the pineal region and rostral midbrain and thalamus, excessive disconjugate eye movements appear together with convergence retraction nystagmus and spasm of the near reflex (Parinaud's syndrome).

In convergence retraction nystagmus there is a disorder of saccades in which attempted upgaze elicits rapid, bilateral simultaneous phasic adducting eye movements which also retract the globe. When the optokinetic drum is used, there are normal slow downward phases, but the quick moving upward phases are replaced by convergence movements.

Patients with acquired concomitant estropia may have either organic or non-organic disease. Organic disease includes a wide range of intra-axial upper brain stem lesions including Wernicke-Korsakoff syndrome and 'thalamic esotropia', as well as posterior fossa mass lesions. Non-organic causes, however, occur more commonly: in distinction to bilateral VIth nerve palsy the deviation is greater for near than for distance, there is a full range of eye movements and less pupillary constriction when one eye is viewing. Binocular viewing is associated with a strong pupillary miosis and horizontal doll's eye movements are full. In functional spasm of the near reflex there is considerable associated discomfort and the patient cannot sustain the abnormality for more than a brief period, during which time they may complain of blurred vision, 'eye strain', and diplopia. Convergence substitution may help a patient with a horizontal-gaze palsy to drive the adducting eye into the desired direction (Beigi, 1995).

Weakness of divergence may simulate bilateral VIth nerve palsies, and in this condition the esotropic deviation is greater for distance than for near, increasing the diagnostic difficulties. Sometimes formal eye movement recordings are required to make the distinction as abducting saccadic velocities and amplitudes are normal in divergence paralysis. Raised intracranial pressure, craniocervical junction lesions and drug intoxication are underlying causes. Divergence nystagmus may also arise (Zee and Levi, 1989).

2 Central disorders of eye movements — clinical applications

NYSTAGMUS

Nystagmus is a rhythmic to-and-fro oscillation of the eyes and is a common finding in patients with disease affecting the brain stem and cerebellum. It reflects any disorder of mechanisms which normally function to hold steady gaze — the vestibular system, the gaze-holding mechanism, the visual stabilization system and the smooth pursuit system. The evaluation of a patient's nystagmus requires the systematic examination of each of these classes of eye movement. In addition, it is important to note the direction of nystagmus in different angles of gaze and head positions and note the effects of binocular and monocular fixation. Measurement of the nystagmus waveform can be very helpful in achieving these goals, especially in the task of distinguishing acquired nystagmus from congenital forms of nystagmus and from saccadic disorders that lead to instability of gaze (Troost, 1989).

CLINICAL TERMS

Nystagmus is divided into two types according to the predominant waveform: pendular when the oscillation of the eyes is sinusoidal and jerk when the movement is a slow drift alternating with a corrective fast phase. Jerk nystagmus is characteristically exaggerated when gaze is into the direction of the fast phase (Alexander's law). As a general rule, the slow phase reflects the underlying abnormality. The observer should try to characterize nystagmus not simply according to its pendular or jerk wave form, but also in terms of frequency, direction of the fast phase, and amplitude.

When nystagmus is unidirectional, it is helpful to classify the degree of abnormality: *first* degree nystagmus is present only when looking in the direction of the fast phase, *second* degree is present when in the primary position and *third* degree is present when in all fields of gaze.

EYE MOVEMENT RECORDING TECHNIQUES

Eye movement recording is useful not only as a research tool, but also for the accurate documentation of clinical problems. A modern video camera can be used to record the eye movements, and by means of TV monitors provide a magnified picture of the subject's eyes for the purposes of clinical demonstrations and for quantitative videooculography. Electronystagmography is a method which depends on the standing potential of the eye (the electro-oculogram or EOG): the electric field that surrounds the eye as a result of metabolic activity in the retina moves as the eye moves and can be recorded using skin electrodes. Horizontal movements can be recorded more satisfactorily than vertical, and quantitative measurements are technically difficult to achieve. Electromagnetic search coils provide greater precision; a wire coil is embedded into a contact lens which is fitted to one or both eyes, the subject is placed in an alternating magnetic field and the eye position is recorded from the voltage induced in the coil. Contact lens fitting makes this an invasive technique and in some units satisfactory high resolution data can be gained using infrared differential reflection recordings. In this method, periorbital sensors are placed adjacent to the eye in spectacle-type frames and movement recordings are made, derived from corneal infrared reflections.

PHYSIOLOGICAL FORMS OF JERK NYSTAGMUS

Quantitative eye movement recording allows biomathematical modelling of nystagmus, and it is useful to define certain terms. Eye movements are classified as versions (conjugate) and vergence (disconjugate). Versions are subdivided into fast eye movements and slow eye movements. Fast eye movements include saccades and the fast phase of jerk nystagmus. Slow eye movements include smooth pursuit movements and the slow phase of jerk nystagmus. Nystagmus can be seen as one of a number of functional defects in the slow eye movement system.

1) High gain instability — there is a runaway, increasing velocity movement or a pendular oscillation. Horizontal jerk nystagmus with increasing velocity slow phases is characteristic of congenital nystagmus.
2) Vestibular tone imbalance — vestibular dysfunction results in asymmetric vestibular input to an otherwise normal horizontal eye movement system. This can result from abnormalities in labyrinths, vestibular nerve or brain stem nuclei and the consequence is a slow drift of the eyes towards the side with the damage. This type of nystagmus is enhanced by high plus (Frenzel) lenses and darkness.
3) Leaky integrator. Integrator leak nystagmus is evoked only in eccentric gaze positions (gaze evoked). The eyes are unable to maintain an eccentric position and drift back to the primary position reflecting the elastic forces within the orbital tissues. Nystagmus due to brain stem dysfunction of the neural integrator is called gaze paretic nystagmus.

It will be appreciated that each of the above forms of nystagmus can arise as a result of dysfunction in the brain stem, cerebellum and peripheral vestibular system, but there are certain specific nystagmus types in which neuroanatomic correlation is possible.

CONGENITAL NYSTAGMUS

The recognition of congenital nystagmus (CN) is of great importance in adult patients because they may be protected from unnecessary investigations (Abadi and Dickinson, 1986). It is more properly termed 'infantile' or 'early onset' nystagmus because the onset is at about 2–3 months of age and is not present at birth. The term is used to describe idiopathic nystagmus and does not include cases arising secondary to sensory deprivation as a result of ocular disease. Congenital nystagmus may be pendular or jerk, or a combination of both. A number of features are typical: the nystagmus is binocular, is usually horizontal in all directions of gaze, is accentuated by attempted fixation, is diminished on convergence and is not associated

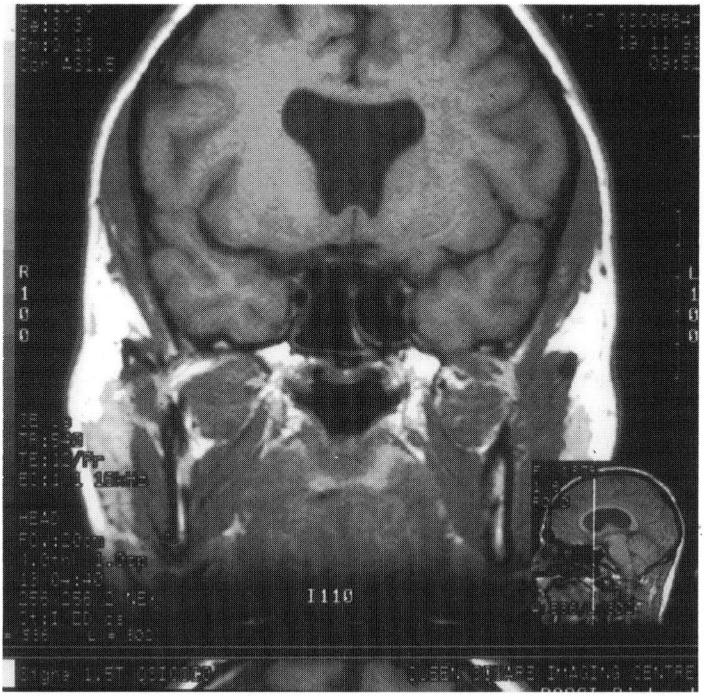

Figure 8.3 Coronal view MRI scan of the same patient with chiasmal dysplasia and a single ventricle.

with oscillopsia. Frequently the eyes are quieter when moved into a particular position in the orbit — the null position — and patients often adopt an abnormal head posture to facillitate this. About 15% of congenital nystagmus patients also have strabismus. Paradoxically, when the patient views a rotating optokinetic drum, the quick phases are directed in same direction as the drum rotates — 'inverted pursuit', or 'inverted OKN' (Halmagyi *et al.*, 1980). On formal eye movement recording sometimes a pure pendular waveform is seen. More typically however, a distinctive 'CN' waveform is seen where the velocity increases exponentially to the point of reversal (high gain instability).

The cause of congenital nystagmus is unknown: the suggestion that pendular forms are due to defects of vision (e.g. albinism, aniridia, retinal dytrophies, optic nerve colobomata) and that jerk forms are due to primary motor mechanisms is not always the case.

LATENT AND MANIFEST-LATENT NYSTAGMUS

Latent nystagmus is a congenital jerk nystagmus that is absent or minimal when both eyes are viewing, and appears or is enhanced when one eye is covered. Under uniocular cover, both eyes develop a conjugate jerk nystagmus in which the quick phases are directed towards the fixating eye. The opposite physical sign is easier to observe: the observed eye drifts towards and beats away from the covered eye. Latent nystagmus is invariably associated with strabismus, usually infantile esotropia, and often patients show upward deviation of the covered eye — termed 'dissociated vertical deviation'. Because of the presence of strabismus, sometimes latent nystagmus is apparent without occluding one eye as the patient is only fixing monocularly. This is termed 'manifest-latent nystagmus'. Latent nystagmus is common and must be correctly recognized if the adult patient is to avoid unnecessary investigation for a progressive neurological condition (Dell'Osso *et al.*, 1979).

ACQUIRED HORIZONTAL JERK NYSTAGMUS — VESTIBULAR NYSTAGMUS (VESTIBULAR TONE IMBALANCE) AND GAZE-EVOKED (GAZE-PARETIC) NYSTAGMUS

Vestibular nystagmus arises as a result of lesions of the vestibular end-organ (labyrinth), vestibular nerve, nucleus or cerebellar flocculus (vestibulocerebellum). In peripheral lesions, the nystagmus is unilateral with combined horizontal and torsional elements and with the fast phase directed away from the side of the lesion. The nystagmus is reduced by visual fixational efforts and is intensified in the dark and on wearing glasses which fog out vision (Freznel + 20 dioptre spectacles). Head shaking or a change in head position also intensifies the nystagmus. Tinnitus, vertigo and deafness are commonly present. Smooth pursuit and saccades are normal. In contrast, central vestibular nystagmus may be bidirectional and be purely vertical or torsional. Fixation does not suppress the amplitude, nor are the oscillations intensified by wearing Freznel spectacles or reducing the illumination.

Gaze-evoked nystagmus is elicited in attempting to maintain an eccentric eye position. The eyes drift slowly back towards the primary position followed by a corrective saccade. Formal recording shows a decreasing-velocity exponential slow phase. As referred to above, this is 'leaky integrator' nystagmus with a defect in step neuron function, specifically in the vestibulocerebellum — the flocculonodular lobe and nucleus propositus hypoglossi. Frequently, smooth pursuit eye movements are also abnormal and there may also be evidence of a horizontal gaze paresis as a result of cerebral hemisphere or brainstem disease. Patients with cerebellar–pontine angle lesions may show both a gaze-paretic nystagmus to the side of the lesion as a result of horizontal gaze paresis together with faster beating nystagmus when looking to the opposite side due to vestibular damage (Brun–Cushing nystagmus).

SOME SPECIAL TYPES OF NYSTAGMUS

Induced and physiological nystagmus

Nystagmus may be seen spontaneously or in special conditions without any implications of a pathological process. Spontaneous fatigue nystagmus is seen after maximal horizontal gaze sustained for more than 30 seconds, and a few beats of end-point nystagmus may normally be seen after a much shorter time especially at more than 30 degrees from fixation.

Nystagmus can be induced in a number of ways — which can be of great diagnostic value. Caloric-induced vestibular nystagmus is a valuable test for peripheral vestibular disease. The patient is positioned supine with his head 30 degrees from the horizontal and water is irrigated into the ear after checking that the tympanic membranes are intact. Cold water normally produces a slow eye movement to the side irrigated with corrective rapid eye movement (saccades) to the opposite side. Warm water produces nystagmus in the opposite direction. The direction of the induced nystagmus can be remembered by the acronym COWS — 'cold: opposite; warm: same'. When assessing brain stem function in the unconscious patient caloric testing produces no corrective saccade and no nystagmus. Instead intact vestibular pathways are indicated by a tonic deviation of the eyes to the irrigated side when cold water is used, and to the opposite side when warm water is used.

Nystagmus may also be induced with the optokinetic drum which is of value in the topical diagnosis of both supranuclear and infranuclear eye movement disorders and in the identification of congenital nystagmus (Table 8.4).

Nystagmus induced by certain postures is a characteristic of position-dependent vertigo requiring formal neuro-otological assessment. Finally nystagmus may be induced in virtually any form as a side-effect of barbiturate, phenothiazine, anticonvulsant and tranquillizer therapy.

Table 8.4 Some clinical applications of testing nystagmus induced with the optokinetic drum

Pursuit deficits (slow phase) towards the side of the field defect in homonymous hemianopia due to deep parietal lesions
Asymmetric saccades (fast phase) in internuclear ophthalmoplegia
Asymmetric pursuit (nasotemporal asymmetry) in congenital esotropia
Normal nystagmus pattern in functional visual loss (can be voluntarily inhibited by some individuals)

See-saw nystagmus

In see-saw nystagmus, which may be either pendular or jerk, one eye intorts and rises while the opposite eye extorts and falls in a rapidly alternating sequence. The pendular form is most frequent and is associated with a bitemporal hemianopia due to large parasellar masses expanding upwards to the third ventricle and to distort structures in the mesencephalic-diencephalic region. Because of abnormalities of both the afferent and efferent visual system it is not always possible to separate their respective contributions in acquired forms which are also seen in association with craniocervical junction abnormalities. It is interesting to note that half of the see-saw movement is in fact an ocular tilt reaction (see below) and it is reasonable to attribute most cases to dysfunction of the rostral mesencephalon in the region of the intestitial nucleus of Cajal (Halmagyi, 1994). However, congenital forms have also been recorded in association with apparently isolated anterior afferent visual pathway dysplasia (Apkarian *et al.*, 1995).

Convergence-retraction nystagmus

Convergence-retraction nystagmus forms part of the Sylvian aquaduct syndrome or Parinaud's syndrome. Best elicited with a downward moving optokinetic drum, typically there are slow downward pursuit movements but the expected saccadic upward movement is replaced by rapid convergent movements which also retract the globe due to co-firing of the extraocular muscles. This constellation of physical signs should be distinguished from convergence-induced nystagmus which is usually voluntary and associated with spasm of the near reflex.

Periodic alternating

In periodic alternating nystagmus (PAN) there is a persisting horizontal jerk nystagmus which changes direction approximately every 90–120 seconds. Usually the direction change is marked by an interval, or neutral phase, lasting about 10 seconds. A complete cycle therefore takes over 3–4 minutes and may easily be missed in shorter clinical examination time. Acquired PAN is associated with posterior fossa lesions, in particular with structural abnormalities at the craniocervical junction and is also seen in instances of marked bilateral visual loss. The γ-aminobutyric acid (GABA)-ergic agent Baclofen frequently abolishes acquired PAN.

Downbeat and upbeat

Disturbance of central vestibular tone results in vertical nystagmus (downbeat or upbeat). Less commonly, torsional or horizontal nystagmus results. Downbeating nystagmus is associated with a number of clinical diseases, but is most commonly seen with lesions in the posterior fossa near the craniocervical junction including the Arnold–Chiari malformations and basilar invagination (Halmagyi *et al.*, 1983; Hirose *et al.*, 1991; Fisher *et al.*, 1983). Spinocerebellar degenerations, intra-axial brain stem lesions and drug toxicity may also be implicated.

Downbeating nystagmus often presents an exception to Alexander's law by showing an increased intensity not when gaze is directed downwards in the direction of the fast phase, but when the eyes are in lateral gaze. Upbeating nystagmus is sometimes seen in patients with intrinsic brain stem or cerebellar disease of any cause.

Nystagmus and instability of gaze caused by afferent visual pathway disease
In binocular visual loss, nystagmus arises which has both horizontal and vertical components and which changes direction over the course of seconds and minutes. Monocular visual loss may lead to instability of gaze, most frequently taking the form of low frequency bi-directional drifts. Monocular oscillations in children may take the form of vertical pendular movements and raise the possibility of optochiasmal glioma for which imaging studies are indicated. If present in infancy, monocular visual loss also leads to horizontal nystagmus with features of latent nystagmus (see above). In retrochiasmal afferent visual disease asymmetry of smooth pursuit may result in a constant-velocity drift toward the intact hemisphere (Weiss and Biersdorf, 1989).

Muscle paresis
A weak extraocular muscle will fatigue quickly during contraction and muscle-paretic nystagmus will result. Myasthenic patients may appear to have a gaze-evoked nystagmus which is asymmetrical. Sometimes the nystagmus appears only in the abducting eye mimicking an internuclear ophthalmoplegia with an adduction deficit. Ocular myasthenia may mimic central nervous disorders including gaze palsies, one-and-a-half syndrome and internuclear ophthalmoplegia.

Acquired pendular nystagmus
Several features help to distinguish acquired pendular nystagmus from the pendular form of congenital nystagmus: in the congenital form movements are conjugate, horizontal and tend to convert to jerk forms in lateral gaze, whereas in acquired pendular nystagmus there usually are vertical and torsional components. Oscillopsia is a common symptom and visual acuity is usually impaired (Gresty *et al.*, 1982, 1991). Tremors in other parts of the body may coexist such as in the palate, head or limbs in which the movements occur at roughly the same frequency as the nystagmus. In these cases the term ocular myoclonus is used. In particular, patients develop oculopalatal myoclonus following brain stem strokes, the ocular oscillations are vertical, difficult to treat and the syndrome is characterized pathologically by hypertrophy of the inferior olivary nucleus (Nakada and Kwee, 1986). Patients with multiple sclerosis may also have acquired pendular nystagmus. Although optic atrophy may also occur in these patients, the cause of poor vision is the ocular oscillations.

Eyelid nystagmus
Eyelid nystagmus normally simply consists of a rhythmic upward jerking movement of the upper lids in co-ordination with ocular nystagmus. However, in some patients lid nystagmus has a distinct clinical appearance. The amplitude of the lid movement may be greater than that of the eyes, or may be evoked by lateral gaze, or ocular convergence (Pick's sign). Intrinsic brain stem disease is usually present such as the lateral medullary syndrome, but the mechanism for abnormal synkinesia between the lids and the eye movements is unexplained (Sanders *et al.*, 1968).

Epileptic
Nystagmus associated with epileptic activity includes retraction, pendular, torsional and divergent–convergent forms. The pupils may also dilate and constrict. If the patient is conscious during the seizure then diagnostic confusion with nystagmus due to anticonvulsant medication may result.

OPHTHALMIC ASPECTS OF THE MANAGEMENT OF NYSTAGMUS

Numerous methods have been sought in attempts to find treatment for nystagmus and its visual consequences which are blurred vision and oscillopsia (Leigh 1994).

Only a few reliably improve symptoms. Baclofen is usually effective in treating periodic alternating nystagmus, and acetazolamide is effective in treating some patients with familial periodic ataxia and nystagmus. Biofeedback may be of use in congenital nystagmus, as may a number of optical devices (Tusa *et al.*, 1992). These include base-out prisms to stimulate convergence together with low myopic lenses to stimulate accommodation and the near triad. A combination of prisms may be used which both encourages convergence and deviates the eyes towards the null point. The null point in congenital nystagmus can be shifted towards the primary position by moving the muscle attachments of the extraocular muscles (Kestenbaum's procedure). In most cases of acquired nystagmus, treatment of the underlying disease is the only option, where possible. For example, foramen magnum decompression for the Arnold–Chiari malformation with cerebellar herniation may occasionally improve downbeat nystagmus and prevent the progression of other neurological deficits. Attempts to control oscillopsia by weakening or detaching the rectus muscle or by using retrobulbar botulinum toxin may help in extreme cases but the results are frequently disappointing (Ruben *et al.*, 1994; Repka *et al.*, 1994; Tomsak *et al.*, 1995).

SKEW DEVIATION AND THE OCULAR TILT REACTION

Skew deviation comprises any vertical deviation of ocular alignment as a result of acquired supranuclear or vestibulo-ocular dysfunction (Lueck *et al.*, 1991; Hedges and Hoyt, 1982). The hypertropia may be the same (concomitant) in all positions of gaze, or may vary and alternate in left and right gaze (Moser *et al.*, 1988). Non-comitant skew deviation can mimic a single extraocular muscle paresis, but usually there are are accompanying signs suggesting a brain stem lesion. Acquired monocular elevation palsy (also termed the double elevator palsy because of the apparent underaction of both elevators of one eye — the inferior oblique and the superior rectus) is an unusual variant of skew deviation in which the eyes are straight in the primary position of gaze but the affected eye will not elevate (Jampel and Fells, 1968). Full elevation on eyelid closure (Bell's phenomenon) confirms the supranuclear origin of the defect which is most probably located immediately rostral to the oculomotor nucleus to explain the paradox that the superior rectus muscle is innervated from the contralateral oculomotor nucleus complex whilst the inferior oblique supply is ipsilateral.

In some patients, the skew deviation is associated with ocular torsion which may be sustained (tonic) or paroxysmal and gives rise to a compensatory head tilt. The head tilt reflects a response to subjective changes in the perception of the vertical meridian (the visual vertical) rather than to observed degrees of cyclodeviation. The pathologic head tilt (ear to shoulder) is contralateral to the hypertropic eye and may represent a compensatory response to the perceived tilt of the visual vertical. When observed, the torsion is conjugate in the direction of the lower eye.

Skew deviations are seen in peripheral and central vestibular disease, with intrinsic brain stem lesions, commonly in association with unilateral internuclear ophthalmoplegia, and with pure cerebellar lesions such as paraneoplastic degeneration (Brandt and Dietrich, 1991).

PERIPHERAL VESTIBULAR DISEASES

Diseases of the semicircular canals and otoliths cause vertigo and tilt, and also nystagmus and skew deviation (Brandt, 1990). Vertigo is the illusory sensation of motion either in oneself or in the environment. Unlike oscillopsia, vertigo persists when the eyes are closed. Vertigo can be described as acute, recurrent or posturally induced.

Acute vertigo may be due to viral vestibular neuronitis or neurolabyrinthitis, although in most cases a definite aetiology is never proved. Herpes zoster (Ramsay Hunt syndrome) and in children bacterial middle ear disease may also be the underlying cause. In such cases functional recovery within a few weeks is the norm. Other causes include head trauma, ethanol and aminoglycoside ingestion, vertebrobasilar insufficiency and brain stem strokes.

Recurrent vertigo is seen in Menière's disease where hearing loss and tinnitus are prominent. Other causes include, migraine, benign paroxysmal vertigo of childhood, Cogan's syndrome of interstitial keratitis, hearing loss and recurrent vertigo. Specific treatment of the underlying cause is indicated.

In benign paroxysmal positional vertigo, symptoms are provoked by changes in head posture such as looking up at a ceiling, or reversing the car. In clinical examination, vertigo, nausea and nystagmus will be precipitated by lying the patient down, turning the head to one side, and moving the head and neck, together into a head hanging position. Vestibular exercises or specific surgical measures to the vestibular apparatus may be helpful (Baloh *et al.* 1987).

OSCILLOPSIA

Oscillopsia is an illusion of movement of the seen world, usually as a result of excessive motion of images of stationary objects on the retina. The relationship between the retinal image velocity and the development of oscillopsia is indirect and varies between subjects as a result of central adaptive processes: patients with congenital nystagmus rarely complain of oscillopsia. Acquired disease results in oscillopsia for three reasons:

1) VOR inadequacy
2) extraocular muscle weakness
3) ocular oscillations.

An abnormal VOR produces oscillopsia because of abnormal gain or because of a mismatch between the vectors of eye movement and head rotation. This is the result of peripheral or central vestibular disease. Extraocular muscle paresis may lead to oscillopsia during head movements because the VOR is prevented from working in the paretic field of gaze. In nystagmus and in other ocular oscillations such as superior oblique myokymia, oscillopsia occurs even when the head is still (Kommerell and Schaubele, 1980).

DISEASES OF THE MEDULLA

The vestibular nuclei, perihypoglossal nuclei, and inferior olive are important structures for the control of eye movements which lie in the medulla oblongata. The vestibular and perihypoglossal nuclei are frequently involved in Wernecke's disease, and also in tumours and paramedian infarction. Vertical nystagmus and horizontal gaze-paretic nystagmus may be seen in lesions of these structures. In palatal and oculopalatal myoclonus, the inferior olivary nucleus hypertrophies. This condition develops several months following brain stem or cerebellar infarction.

In Wallenberg's syndrome of posterior inferior cerebellar artery occlusion (the lateral medullary syndrome), the typical findings are ipsilateral loss of pain and temperature sensation in the face, Horner's syndrome, and bulbar palsy, together with contralateral pain and temperature sensory loss over the trunk and limbs. Symptoms include vertigo, and sensations of environmental tilt and of the body being pulled laterally (lateropulsion). Spontaneous nystagmus, skew deviation and deviation of the eyes toward the side of the lesion on blinking may also be observed (Daroff *et al.*, 1968; Kommerell and Hoyt 1973; Brazis, 1992).

CEREBELLAR DISORDERS

Cerebellar disorders frequently coincide with brain stem problems, so that the pure effects of cerebellar disease are only rarely seen. Saccadic dysmetria is seen in lesions of the dorsal vermis, whilst lesions of the flocculus and paraflocculus have abnormalities of VOR cancellation (Waterson *et al.*, 1992).

DISEASES OF THE PONS

The PPRF contains the pause and burst neurons which are important in the generation of saccades. Unilateral destructive lesions of the PPRF as a result of infarction or haemorrhage therefore cause an ipsilateral conjugate horizontal gaze palsy (Bronstein *et al.*, 1990; Meienberg, 1981). Because the abducens nucleus contains interneurons which innervate the contralateral medial rectus muscle via the medial longitudinal fasciculus (MLF) in addition to neurons innervating the ipsilateral lateral rectus, nuclear lesions also cause a horizontal gaze palsy.

The MLF carries fibres serving conjugate horizontal eye movements from the abducens internuclear neurons to the medial rectus subnucleus and also fibres concerned with vertical eye movements from the vestibular nuclei. Lesions of the MLF characteristically produce an internuclear ophthalmoplegia (INO), but the precise features also depend on the size and location of the lesion in the pathway. Rostral lesions which also involve the oculomotor subnuclei may impair convergence, but more caudal lesions do not. The finding of exotropia with bilateral internuclear ophthalmoplegia ('wall-eyed bilateral internuclear ophthalmoplegia — WEBINO') indicates a rostral lesion.

Unilateral lesions of the MLF produce weakness of the ipsilateral medial rectus and dissociated ('ataxic') nystagmus of the abducting eye. The adduction weakness may range from complete absence of movement to an adduction lag on making larger horizontal saccades. This can be demonstrated readily by observing the quick phases of nystagmus produced by the optokinetic drum. Nystagmus in the abducting eye may be rapid (gaze evoked), slow (gaze paretic) or irregular and associated with convergence abnormalities. Skew deviation frequently accompanies INO as a result of disrupted otolithic–ocular motor connections: the higher eyed is usually on the side of the lesion. In bilateral lesions impaired vertical VOR movements can be seen.

Combined lesions of the abducens nuceus or PPRF and the adjacent MLF on one side of the brain produce an ipsilateral horizontal-gaze palsy and INO, so that the only horizontal eye movement which is preserved is abduction of the contralateral eye. This is known as the 'one-and-a-half syndrome' (Wall and Wray, 1983). Such patients show an exotropia when attempting to look straight ahead, with the eye opposite the side of the lesion deviated outwards — a paralytic pontine exotropia (Sharpe *et al.*, 1974). Bilateral pontine lesions will abolish all horizontal eye movements, although in chronic lesions such as tumour infiltration, reflexive movements may be spared. The Wernicke–Korsakoff syndrome is a treatable cause of central abnormalities of horizontal eye movements which include internuclear ophthalmoplegia, abduction weakness and horizontal gaze palsies which may progress to total ophthalmoplegia. Administration of thiamine usually causes a rapid improvement in the eye signs. Similar abnormalities may be seen in Leigh's disease — an untreatable subacute necrotizing encephalopathy of infancy and childhood.

In a variety of metabolic, toxic and degenerative conditions, selective disorders of ocular motility arise, suggesting predominant loss of one population of brain stem neurons. This may explain both slow saccades and saccadic oscillations. For example, horizontal saccades may be slowed in spinocerebellar and olivopontocerebellar degeneration with sparing of vertical saccades. In progressive supranuclear palsy vertical saccades are the first to slow. Loss of burst cells in the PPRF may be responsible for the horizontal slowing, while loss of pause cells may cause saccadic oscillations which lack an intersaccadic interval (opsoclonus and ocular flutter). Diseases causing opsoclonus and ocular flutter include viral encephalitis, the paraneoplastic syndromes in particular due to neuroblastoma, metabolic diseases and drug intoxication (Ridley *et al.*, 1987).

DISEASES OF THE MIDBRAIN

Midbrain disorders result in disturbances of vertical eye movements which can be related to involvement of three structures: the rostral interstitial nucleus of the MLF, the posterior commissure and the interstitial nucleus of Cajal (iC). Lesions of the posterior commissure cause loss of upgaze and the characteristic clinical constellation of associated features is referred to as Parinaud's syndrome, the Sylvian aqueduct syndrome, the dorsal midbrain syndrome or the pretectal syndrome. These features include lid retraction (Collier's sign) and occasionally ptosis, downward gaze preference (setting sun sign), disturbances of vergence eye movements including convergence-retraction nystagmus, skew deviation and pupillary light-near dissociation. Normally all types of vertical eye movements are involved, although in some cases the VOR and Bell's phenomenom is spared. In most cases there is a bilateral lesion, but unilateral abnormalities may cause the dorsal midbrain syndrome by interrupting the afferent and efferent connections of the posterior commissure (Hommel and Bogousslavsky, 1991; Mehler, 1988, Bogousslavsky *et al.*, 1990; Büttner-Ennever *et al.*, 1989a, b).

The dorsal midbrain syndrome may be produced by tumours (pinealoma, glioma, metastasis), by obstructive hydrocephalus, and by vascular occlusion (perforating branches of the posterior cerebral artery). Bilateral defects of the riMLF are much less common and result either in paralysis of downward eye movements or of all vertical saccades depending on the extent of the lesion. Rarely, both elevator muscles of one eye may be selectively impaired with midbrain lesions ('double elevator palsy'). This is a supranuclear palsy of monocular elevation in which the eyes are straight in the primary position and only become disconjugate on attempted upgaze: the VOR is variably affected. A focal lesion of the prenuclear inputs to the ipsilateral inferior oblique and contralateral superior rectus has been implicated (Lepore *et al.*, 1985).

Selective vulnerability of vertical saccades is seen in a number of degenerative and metabolic storage diseases, including progressive supranuclear palsy and Niemann-Pick disease type C, also known as the DAF syndrome of *D*own-gaze paralysis, *A*taxia/*A*thetosis, and *F*oam ('sea-blue histiocytes') cells in the bone marrow (Palmer *et al.*, 1985; Cogan *et al.*, 1981). Other metabolic conditions which may be associated with supranuclear vertical gaze abnormalities include Wilson's disease, Whipple's disease, kernicterus and barbiturate overdose.

THALAMUS AND BASAL GANGLIA

Thalamic lesions cause abnormalities of both horizontal and vertical gaze. Conjugate deviation of the eye s away from the side of the lesion is typical. An esotropia occurs in caudal thalamic lesions which may not be associated with any abnormality of vertical movements. Thalamic esotropia may reflect disturbance of vergence inputs to the oculomotor nuclei (Williams and Hoyt, 1989; Gomez *et al.*, 1988).

Patients with Parkinson's disease show a number of eye movement abnormalities including square wave saccadic jerks, hypometric voluntary saccades, and catch-up saccades on horizontal smooth pursuit due to loss of gain (Gibson *et al.*, 1987). In an oculogyric crisis, seen in postencephalitic Parkinson's and as a side-effect of neuroleptic medication, the eyes show conjugate upward deviation, and downgaze can only be achieved by a combination of a blink and a downward saccade. Huntington's disease produces abnormalities of saccadic initiation and an obligatory blink or head turn may be required to start a horizontal eye movement.

EYE MOVEMENT ABNORMALITIES IN STATES OF ALTERED CONSCIOUSNESS

EPILEPSY

During epileptic seizures horizontal conjugate gaze abormalities may be seen, which appear to reflect focal seizure activity in cortical areas which are concerned with the generation of saccades and pursuit. Seizures emanating from the superior temporal lobes may cause a variety of vestibular sensations, and occipital lobe seizures have been reported to produce oscillopsia. There are reports of the precipitation of seizures by eye movements — either convergence or lateral deviation.

COMA

The ocular motor examination is very useful in evaluating the unconscious patient because both the level of consciousness and the control of eye movements are controlled from the brain stem. Tonic conjugate horizontal deviations due to lesions above the ocular motor decussation are usually towards the side of the lesions and away from the side of the hemiparesis, whilst those due to lesions below the decussation tend to be away from the side of the lesion and towards the hemiparesis. Deviations of the visual axes are due to peripheral cranial nerve or orbital injury. The presence of spontaneous roving eye movements indicates that the brain stem gaze mechanisms are intact. Conjugate vertical ocular bobbing is a classic sign of intrinsic pontine haemorrhage but can be seen in cerebellar stroke as well as in metabolic and toxic encephalopathies (Susac *et al.*, 1970). 'Ping-pong' gaze consists of slow horizontal conjugate deviations alternating every few seconds, usually in association with bilateral cerebral hemisphere infarction. Patients with the locked-in, de-efferent syndrome are conscious but quadriplegic as a result of pontine lesions. Voluntary vertical eye movements are preserved unless midbrain structures are also involved.

Reflex eye movements may be elicited in the unconscious patient either by head rotation ('doll's head' or oculocephalic manoeuvre) or by caloric testing (the oculovestibular test). Often both tests are performed, noting whether the ocular deviation which results is conjugate and whether any nystagmus is induced. Patients with a persistent vegetative state leaving severe cerebral hemisphere damage and preserving the brain stem will have normal brain stem ocular reflexes. In the acute phase, quick phases of nystagmus on caloric testing are lost, but may be regained without evidence of cortical recovery (Büttner and Zee, 1989).

3 Peripheral disorders: basic principles

THE ANATOMY AND ACTIONS OF THE EXTRAOCULAR MUSCLES

The eye is suspended in the orbit by fascia and by the rectus muscles, supported by retro-ocular fat. Fibrous bands connect the rectus muscle sheaths to the lower surface of the levator palpebrae superioris and the inferior oblique muscle superiorly and inferiorly, and to the adjacent orbital wall in the horizontal plane. Each eye is rotated by six muscles: four rectus and two oblique which pull the eye in the transverse, parasagittal and vertical axes depending on the starting position of the eye. The primary action of a muscle refers to the axis about which the eye principally rotates when that muscle contracts; the secondary and tertiary actions refer to the axes about which there are lesser rotations (see Table 8.5).

The four recti and the superior oblique arise from the apex of the orbit and the inferior oblique arises from the anterior, inferior nasal aspect. The tendons of the four rectus muscles insert into the sclera anterior to the equator of the globe; the superior and inferior oblique muscle tendons approach the globe from its anterior and medial aspect and insert posterior to the equator. The superior oblique achieves this position after passing through the trochlea — a fibrous cartilagenous ring lying just inside the superior medial orbital rim.

The pulling actions of the vertically acting muscles depend upon the horizontal position of the eye. The superior and inferior rectus muscles act as a pure elevator and depressor when the eye is abducted by 23 degrees. In an adducted position, the superior rectus starts to rotate the eye in (incyclotorsion) and the inferior rectus to rotate the eye out (excyclotorsion). The superior oblique only acts as a pure depressor of the eye when the eye is adducted by 51 degrees. The more the eye is abducted, the more the superior oblique acts so as to intort the globe, rather than as a depressor.

Extraocular muscle fibres are smaller and more richly innervated than skeletal muscle fibres and are amongst the fastest contracting in the body as well as being relatively fatigue resistant (Table 8.6). Twitch fibres with a single end-plate per fibre generate all-or-nothing propogation responses, while non-twitch (tonic) fibres have multiple nerve terminals per fibre and are capable of smoothly modulated muscle contraction. In standard accounts, two populations of fibres are defined within each muscle — one lying centrally and extending to the globe known as the global fibre layer, and the other lying peripherally and referred to as the orbital fibre layer. The orbital layer is predominantly made up of non-twitch, tonic fibres, and the global layer includes the twitch fibres. However, recent work indicates that all fibre groups participate in all types of eye movement (Porter *et al.*, 1995)

Table 8.5 Actions of extraocular muscles with the eye in the primary position

Muscle action	Primary action	Secondary action	Tertiary
Medial rectus	Adduction	—	—
Lateral rectus	Abduction	—	—
Superior rectus	Elevation	Intorsion	Adduction
Inferior rectus	Depression	Extorsion	Adduction
Superior oblique	Abduction	Intorsion	Depression
Inferior oblique	Extorsion	Elevation	Abduction

Table 8.6 Classification of mammalian extraocular muscles fibres

Type A	Type B	Type C
Large diameter Single end-plate Fast twitch Required for saccadic movements	Intermediate diameter Multiple end-plates Slow twitch Needed for smooth pursuit movements	Small diameter Small *en grappe* plates Tonic contractions Function to align both visual axes, i.e. fine local contractions

BINOCULAR VISUAL FUNCTION

The two eyes are separated horizontally in the skull and each eye has a slightly different horizontal view of the world. Fusional reflexes in the cortex result in a single panoramic ('cyclopean') view in which the image disparity contributes to the appreciation of depth. The neural substrate for fusion consists of both sensory and oculomotor elements: sensory fusion being the process whereby a stimulus projecting onto corresponding points on each retina are perceived as one, and motor fusion where saccadic and vergence eye movements are used to maintain the stimulus onto the corresponding retinal points at different viewing distances.

In most individuals, the correct alignment of the eyes depends on powerful motor fusion keeping in check a greater or lesser tendency of ocular muscle balance to drift. When normal binocular viewing conditions are interrupted by alternately occluding one eye and then the other (alternate cover test), a latent deviation or phoria can be unmasked. When one eye is misaligned under binocular viewing conditions there is a manifest deviation or a tropia. An individual with a latent esophoria may temporarily develop a frank convergent squint — esotropia, and an individual with a latent exophoria may similarly develop a frank divergent squint — an exotropia. Vertical slippage is much less common and the terms used are 'hyperphoria' and 'hypertropia', hyper referring to the higher eye. Deviations arising from fusional disruption are usually constant in all directions and are called concomitant. By contrast, deviations which change according to the angle of gaze are non-comitant and are due to extraocular muscle weakness or mechanical hindrance.

CONJUGATE EYE MOVEMENTS AND CLINICAL TESTING IN DIPLOPIA

The physiological mechanisms co-ordinating conjugate eye movements are summarized by the laws of reciprocal innervation and of motor correspondence.

1) The law of reciprocal innervation (Sherrington's law) determines that the extraocular muscles do not co-contract because as one muscle — the agonist, for example the lateral rectus — receives an impulse to contract, an equivalent inhibitory impulse is sent to the antagonist, the ipsilateral medial rectus.
2) The law of motor correspondence (Hering's law) determines that the muscles of a yoked pair of extraocular muscles (e.g the right lateral rectus and left medial rectus which both serve right horizontal gaze) receive equal innervation.

Misalignment of the visual axes — strabismus — causes the two images of a seen object to fall on non-corresponding areas of the two retinas. This is diplopia. In addition, the two fovea are simultaneously presented with different images, causing visual confusion. The first point to establish is whether diplopia is truly binocular or is monocular by covering one eye. Monocular diplopia is commonly due to uncorrected refractive error, early cataract or corneal distortion. Very rarely it is due to cerebral disorders (cerebral diplopia). Patients who have an obvious ocular misalignment but no diplopia usually have a concomitant developmental strabismus, although exceptions are seen in supranuclear and internuclear disorders. The patient should be asked whether the diplopia is horizontal, vertical or torsional and in which direction of gaze the images are most widely separated. This provides important clues to the muscle or cranial nerve responsible.

The physical examination must be conducted in a logical sequence. Preliminaries include the measurement of best corrected visual acuity in each eye, tests for binocularity, confrontation assessment of visual fields and when required objective refraction. These are followed by four steps:

1) examination of the range of eye movements
2) subjective diplopia testing
3) cover testing
4) the head-tilt test.

The range of eye movements is assessed first with one eye covered and the other fixating (ductions) and then with both eyes together (versions) in the nine cardinal or diagnostic positions of gaze. When the range of movement is limited a forced duction test is helpful in determining whether the cause is muscle weakness or mechanical restriction. A Tensilon® test may be useful to confirm the suspicion of myasthenia gravis although a negative result does not necessarily exclude the diagnosis.

Subjective tests for diplopia are useful in the co-operative patient. The patient must have binocular vision for the test to work. The two images of diplopia are maximally separated when the patient looks in the direction of action of the paretic muscle and the target seen by the paretic eye is projected more peripherally, particularly as the patient looks into the paretic field. More accurate versions of this technique rely on preventing fusional vergence eye movements by using red-green goggles or a Maddox rod. With red-green goggles (the Lancaster red-green test) the abnormalities of conjugate vision in the nine positions of gaze can be plotted on a chart.

Cover testing requires less patient co-operation. When the fixating eye is covered, the deviating eye makes a saccade to take up foveal fixation. This is repeated in the cardinal positions of gaze and the direction in which the corrective saccade is the largest indicates the field of action of the paretic muscle.

In assessing a vertical deviation, a series of steps are performed to correctly identify the paretic muscle (the Marshall Parks three step test) (Spector, 1993; Trobe, 1984):

1) determine the side of the hypertropia using the cover test.
2) determine whether the deviation is greater in left or right gaze.
3) determine the effect on the deviation of a head tilt to the right or left shoulder (the Bielschowsky test).

For example, in a patient with a left superior oblique palsy, there will be:

1) a left hypertropia
2) the hypertropia will increase on right gaze
3) tilting the patient's head to the left will generate a reflex torsional eye movement normally causing intorsion of the left eye; the tertiary action of the left superior oblique is intorsion — if this muscle is weak, the second intorter of eye will overact. This is the left superior rectus, causing the left hyperdeviation to increase.

SPECIFIC PHYSICAL SIGNS IN STRABISMUS

PRIMARY AND SECONDARY DEVIATION

Most patients with diplopia will fixate with the normal eye, and the eye with the paretic muscle deviates a certain amount from the line of sight. This is the primary deviation. If, however, the patient is forced to fixate with the paretic eye, either by covering the other eye during examination, or when an eye disease has caused reduced acuity in the non-paretic eye, the angle of deviation increases. This is the secondary deviation. The main reason for this is that when the paretic eye fixates, it holds a central orbital position, further into the field of action of the weak muscle.

ABNORMAL HEAD POSTURES

When patients with stabismus turn or tilt their heads to minimize diplopia, this suggests a paralytic deviation. Typically the head is turned toward the side of the weakness to minimize the action of the paretic muscle. A patient with a left lateral rectus palsy will turn his head to the left so that the eyes are deviated to the right in the primary position and diplopia is avoided. Head turns and tilts also are seen in congenital nystagmus in which the amplitude of nystagmus is least and acuity greatest in a null position of gaze which is often eccentric. Patients with horizontal deviations which increase in elevation or depression ('A' and 'V' patterns) may elevate or depress their chin.

CONCOMITANT STRABISMUS

A common diagnostic problem arises in the distinction between paralytic and concomitant strabismus. The history is important as strabismus since childhood will answer the question. Diplopia is typically absent because of suppression of the image from one eye, and lack of stereoacuity and the presence of latent nystagmus will confirm this conclusion.

In non-paralytic strabismus the deviations of the optical axes are the same in all positions of gaze (concomitant) and are the same whichever eye is fixating. Horizontal concomitant tropias (deviations which fusional mechanisms cannot correct) are frequently associated with refractive error — especially hypermetropia — abnormalities of vergence-accommodation synkinesis (AC/A ratio) and strabismic amblyopia. Sometimes non-paralytic strabismus has acute onset in adulthood. This is seen following head injury, upper brain stem and thalamic tumours and in the Arnold–Chiari malformation. These conditions are also associated with loss of fusional vergence eye movements.

4 Peripheral disorders: clinical features

CLASSIFICATION OF PARALYTIC STRABISMUS

1) Neurogenic
2) Myogenic
3) Mechanical

Infranuclear abnormalities of eye movements give rise to a paralytic squint, where the angle of deviation increases as the eyes are directed into the field of action of the muscle involved. The term paralysis is used when there is no movement in the affected muscle, and paresis for reduced movement.

Paralytic squint can be classified as neurogenic, myogenic or mechanical (Richards *et al.*, 1992). Neurogenic abnormalities relate to the functioning of the IIIrd, IVth and VIth cranial nerves which supply the extraocular muscles. Myogenic causes comprise disorders of the extraocular muscles themselves, and mechanical causes include developmental, inflammatory and mass lesions of the orbital structures which limit free movement of the globe.

ABDUCENS NERVE PALSIES

Abducens (VIth cranial nerve) nerve palsy is the most common ocular motor paralysis. In the assessment of patients with abduction deficits, the clinician must first exclude local explanations at the level of the lateral rectus muscle and the orbit, before diagnosing an abducens nerve palsy. These include dysthyroid eye disease (fibrotic medial rectus), myasthenia gravis, orbital inflammatory pseudotumour, orbital trauma (ethmoid blowout), congenital innervation defects (Mobius and Duane's syndromes) and convergence spasm. Causes of a true abducens nerve paralysis can be classified as follows:

Table 8.7 Aetiology of abducens nerve palsy

A. Nuclear (horizontal gaze palsy)	Congenital and hereditary gaze palsies Infarction Tumour Wernicke–Korsakoff syndrome
B. Fascicular	Infarction Demyelination Tumour
C. Subarachnoid space	Subarachnoid haemorrhage Trauma Meningitis Clivus tumour Cerebellopontine angle tumours Trigeminal and abducens nerve tumours
D. Petrous	Infection of petrous tip (Gradinego's syndrome) Inferior petrosal sinus thrombosis Trauma Raised intracranial pressure Post-CSF tap Aneurysm and vascular anomaly
E. Cavernous sinus and superior orbital fissure	Carotid aneurysm or dissection Cavernous sinus thrombosis Carotid–cavernous fistula: direct and indirect Granulomas Neoplasms Herpes zoster
F. Orbit	Neoplasms
G. Non-localizing	Microvascular disease (including diabetes, hypertension and vasculitis) Parainfectious Migraine

Abducens palsy arising in the brain stem (nuclear and fascicular lesions)

Applied anatomy

The abducens nerve nucleus is situated in the caudal portion of the paramedian pontine tegmentum beneath the floor of the fourth ventricle. Facial nerve fibres loop around the nucleus to form the facial colliculus before exiting in the cerebellopontine angle. The MLF passes medially. There are two populations of cells in the abducens nucleus: the first form the VIth nerve and pass ventrally to exit at the pontomedullary junction; the second form internuclear neurons passing in the MLF to the contralateral medial rectus subnucleus in the oculomotor complex. These arrangements explain how a nuclear lesion of the VIth nerve gives rise to both a horizontal gaze palsy and also, commonly, a lower motor neuron facial nerve palsy.

The abducens nerve has a long intrapontine course of about 10mm coming into close contact with brain stem structures such as the nucleus of the tractus solitarius, the central tegmental tract, the spinal tract of the trigeminal nerve and the superior olivary nucleus. Consequently, in the vast majority of cases, lesions of the fascicle are associated with other neurological signs. The aetiology is generally vascular, but tumours and inflammatory lesions may also be responsible.

The blood supply of the pons is clinically important in the understanding of the brain stem vascular syndromes. A paramedian/basal territory is supplied by short circumferential and direct branches of the basilar artery, and a dorsolateral territory supplied by the anterior inferior cerebellar artery, long circumferential arteries and the superior cerebellar artery.

Acquired nuclear and fascicular lesions

Among the pontine syndromes, Foville's syndrome of the anterior inferior cerebellar artery is the most common whereby a lesion of the pontine tegmentum causes an ipsilateral paralysis of abduction (or gaze palsy), lower motor neuron facial palsy, loss of taste in the anterior two-thirds of the tongue, Horner's syndrome, facial analgesia and peripheral deafness. Partial forms are more frequent than the full syndrome (Donaldson and Rosenberg, 1988; Johnson and Hepler, 1989; Mastrianni *et al.*, 1994). A lesion in the ventral paramedian pons may damage, in addition to the abducens nerve fascicle, the corticospinal tract and/or the ventral portion of the facial nerve fascicle resulting in an ipsilateral abducens palsy, and contralateral hemiplegia with additional facial palsy.

Congenital lesions

Isolated congenital paralysis of abduction is exceedingly rare and much more frequently

Table 8.8 Pontine syndromes involving the abducens nerve classified by vascular territory

Vascular territory	Structures involved	Ipsilateral signs	Contralateral signs
Paramedian/basal	VIth and VIIth fascicle; pyramidal tract	VIth and VIIth nerve paralysis	Hemiparesis or hemiplegia
Dorsolateral	VIth prenuclear fibres/nucleus/fascicle; VIIth nucleus and fascicle; spinal root of Vth/spinothalamic tract	Horizontal gaze palsy, VIIth nerve paralysis; hemianesthesia of face	Hemianaesthesia of limbs

congenital disorders of the abducens nerve are seen together with additional physical signs in the Möbius syndrome and Duane's syndrome.

Möbius syndrome

The Möbius syndrome includes facial diplegia and bilateral abducens palsy. Musculoskeletal dysplasias and cleft palate may be associated. According to Towfighi and others, the Möbius syndrome is due to heterogeneous neuropathological findings (Towfighi *et al.*, 1979). These include hypoplasia or atrophy of cranial nerve nuclei (group I), primary peripheral nerve involvement (group II), brain stem focal necrosis (group III) and myopathies (group IV). Hypoxic or ischaemic insult during pregnancy is implicated in groups I, II and III while group IV patients have facioscapulohumeral muscular dystrophy. Acquired Möbius syndrome resulting from hypoxic destruction of the internal genu of the facial nerve is described, as are familial patterns of the congenital form (Raroque *et al.*, 1988).

Duane's retraction syndrome

Duane's syndrome is characterized by limitation or absence of abduction and variable limitation of adduction, together with retraction of the globe and narrowing of the palpebral apperture on attempted adduction of the eye. Duane's syndrome is usually unilateral; the left eye is more commonly involved, but 15–20% of cases are bilateral. Usually the disorder is sporadic, but familial cases do occur. Numerous ocular, skeletal and neural abnormalities are associated, notably the Klippel-Fiel anomaly, Goldenhar's syndrome, deafness, urinary tract abnormalities and cardiac defects. These anomalies may be seen singly or in combination throughout certain families and may represent the pleiotrophic effects of the same gene (Hoyt and Nactigäller, 1965).

The clinical classification of Duane's syndrome is based on electromyographic recordings by Huber (Huber, 1974):

type I — is by far the commonest, consisting of limited abduction and relatively preserved adduction,
type II — limited adduction and relatively preserved abduction,
type III — a combination of types I and II.

Electromyographic evidence clearly points to paradoxical innervation underlying these patterns. Types I and II represent dual innervation of the lateral rectus by both the abducens and oculomotor nerves; type II represents innervation of both the lateral and medial rectus muscles by the oculomotor nerve. The consequence of these misrouting patterns is co-contraction of both agonist and antagonist muscles on attempted lateral eye movement with consequent retraction of the globe into the orbit. Frequently there are vertical deviations of the eye on attempted adduction, thought to be the result of the globe slipping around the tight leash of contracted horizontal recti (Metz, 1982; Saad and Lee, 1993).

In contrast to patients with acquired lateral rectus palsy, sensory adaptations are common in Duane's syndrome so that the patient usually does not experience diplopia. This is primarily because of suppression when the affected eye moves into the field of action of the relevant muscle. An abnormal head posture is common in order to maximize binocular function. Autopsy evidence has confirmed that the lateral rectus receives partial or complete innervation from branches of the inferior division of the oculomotor nerve in association with a hypoplastic abducens nucleus and nerve. In one case reported by Miller, the rostral part of the abducens nucleus was preserved, containing the interneurons to the contralateral medial rectus (Miller *et al.*, 1982). Duane's retraction syndrome is not the only cause of retraction of the globe on attempted lateral movements: this may also be seen following idiopathic orbital inflammatory disease (orbital pseudotumour), dysthyroid eye disease and following orbital trauma.

Abducens palsy due to peripheral lesions

Applied anatomy

The abducens nerve emerges from the brain stem ventrally and ascends the anterior face of the pons where it is crossed by the anterior inferior cerebellar artery to pierce the dura 2 cm below the posterior clinoids. The abducens nerve traverses or passes above the inferior petrosal sinus and runs beneath the pertroclinoid ligament to enter the cavernous sinus. Within the cavernous sinus it lies freely, unsupported by the dural wall. At this point some sympathetic fibres are briefly attached before passing onwards to the ophthalmic trigeminal. From the cavernous sinus, the nerve passes through the annular segment of the superior orbital fissure and innervates only the lateral rectus (Depper, 1993).

Acquired lesions

Within the subarachnoid space the abducens nerve may be damaged by meningeal inflammation and infiltration, fusiform basilar aneurysms, transtentorial herniation from supratentorial space occupying lesions, and raised intracranial pressure due to other causes. Lesions at the clivus are often bilateral as both abducens nerves are in close proximity at this point — tumours including meningioma, chordoma and naso-pharyngeal carcinoma (Volpe and Lessell, 1993) may be found. In the cavernous sinus, the abducens nerve is more vulnerable to compressive effects of mass lesions because it is not tethered to the dural wall, in contrast to the trochlear and oculomotor nerves (Striph and Burde, 1988). The aetiology is frequently an intracavernous vascular lesion e.g. aneurysm or carotid–cavernous fistula (Fig. 8.4), but skull base and parasellar tumours may also be responsible.

By comparison with unilateral palsies, bilateral abducens nerve palsies are more commonly due to tumours, demyelination, subarachnoid haemorrhage, meningitis, Wernicke's encephalopathy and raised intracranial pressure. Bilateral abducens palsy must be differentiated from convergence spasm and divergence paresis (Savino *et al.*, 1982). In practice, the greatest clinical difficulties arise in patients where the abducens

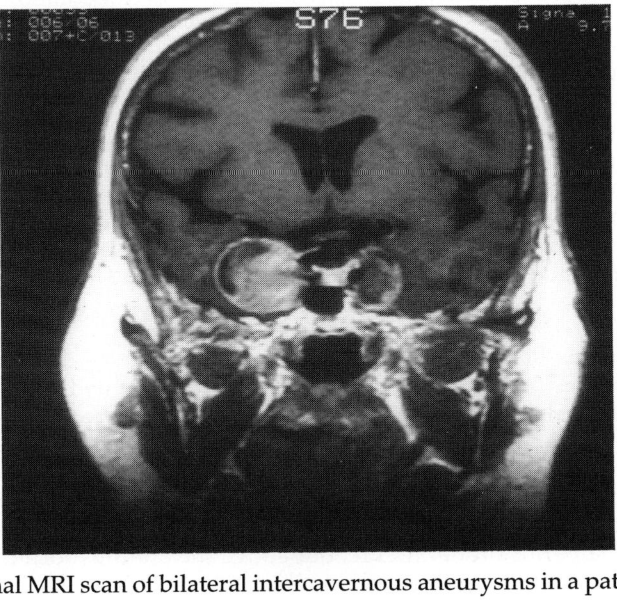

Figure 8.4 Coronal MRI scan of bilateral intercavernous aneurysms in a patient with bilateral VIth nerve palsey.

palsy apparently arises in isolation. The age of the patient may be a helpful guide to the likely aetiology. In infants, VIth nerve palsy must be differentiated from Duane's syndrome and infantile esotropia with cross fixation. In any child with a sudden ocular deviation efforts must be made to exclude a tumour arising in the retina or anterior visual pathways. Abduction weakness in children may be the first sign of a tumour in the posterior fossa. In these cases a coexistent gaze palsy suggests a pontine glioma, while coexistent cerebellar signs usually indicate astrocytoma, ependymoma or medulloblastoma. In adults aged between 16 and 50 years, vasculopathies, trauma, antral nervous system (CNS) inflammatory disease including demyelination and tumours are more likely; in the elderly degenerative vascular disease is a common cause. In most patients, even when inital investigations including imaging and cerebrospinal fluid (CSF) studies are negative, the cause becomes apparent on careful follow-up and repeat imaging.

Ophthalmic aspects of the management of unrecovered lateral rectus palsy
Several measures are available for the relief of diplopia, abnormal head turns and eccentric fields of binocular single vision. Prisms fitted to spectacle lenses are useful in the acute phase. Extraocular muscle surgery using adjunctive botulinum toxin chemodenervation of the antagonist medial rectus can be very effective in chronic cases (King *et al.*, 1995; Murray, 1989; Lee *et al.*, 1994; Repka *et al.*, 1994b).

TROCHLEAR PALSIES

Clinical features
Trochlear nerve palsy accounts for the majority of cases with acquired vertical strabismus (Brazis, 1993; Richards *et al.*, 1992). Most patients complain of vertical and torsional diplopia that is worse looking down. A head tilt away from the side of the lesion with the chin down is usual. Trochlear nerve palsy causes a hypertropia of the affected eye. On performing the head tilt test, the hypertropia is maximized on tilting the head towards the side of the lesion and minimized on tilting to the other side. The superior oblique acts as an intorter of the globe and weakness may result in excyclodeviation. The patient will typically tilt his or her head away from the side of the weak muscle to compensate for this by rolling the excyclodeviated eye inwards. Not all patients follow this pattern, however, and some may tilt their head the other way so as to achieve greater separation of images which may be easier to adapt to. A further valuable test is the assessment of torsional diplopia in downgaze. The false image is tilted outwards. Large degrees of torsion (greater than 10 degress) may suggest a bilateral weakness of the superior obliques, as does a V pattern esotropia.

The differential diagnosis of trochlear palsy includes skew deviation, thyroid ophthalmopathy and other restrictive ocular myopathies, and childhood strabismus syndromes which include inferior oblique overaction and superior oblique underaction.

Anatomy
The trochlear nucleus lies in midbrain at the caudal aspect of the oculomotor nuclear complex. The trochlear fascicles pass dorsally, lateral to the aqueduct to exit the midbrain and crosses the contralateral IVth nerve in the anterior medullary velum, just caudal to the inferior colliculi. The trochlear nerve is the only cranial nerve to decussate and to exit the brain stem dorsally. The nerve continues laterally around the midbrain tectum, crosses the superior cerebellar artery, and reaches the free edge of the tentorium, where it enters the dura and runs forward into the cavernous sinus. The trochlear nerve enters the orbit through the superior orbital fissure, but above the annulus formed by the origin of the rectus muscles, innervating the superior oblique only.

Table 8.9 Causes of trochlear nerve palsies

A. Nuclear and fascicular	Congenital aplasia Infarction and arteriovenous malformation Tumour and other mass lesions
B. Subarachnoid space	Trauma Meningitis Tumour Raised intracranial pressure Post-CSF tap
C. Cavernous sinus and superior orbital fissure	Carotid aneurysm Tolosa-Hunt syndrome Herpes zoster Tumours
D. Orbit	Neoplasms and inflammatory infiltration
E. Non-localizing	Microvascular disease (including diabetes, hypertension and vasculitis) Idiopathic

Congenital lesions

Congenital trochlear nerve palsies are relatively common in contrast to those of the oculomotor and abducens nerves. Often, the cause is a developmental anomaly of the superior oblique tendon in the orbit, but cases of congenital aplasia of the trochlear nucleus have been described. Patients who grow up with a superior oblique deficit undergo a number of sensory adaptations including the development of large vertical fusional amplitudes which may break down in later adulthood giving rise to symptomatic diplopia. Old photographs will reveal a very longstanding characteristic head tilt. The decompensation is apparently precipitated by age or minor injury.

Brown's superior oblique tendon syndrome and the familial fibrosis syndromes

Brown's syndrome presents as an apparent selective weakness of the inferior oblique muscle, so that the eye will not elevate in adduction. However, there is a positive forced duction test in which the eye cannot be actively rotated upwards indicating that the globe is impeded from movement by failure of the antagonist superior oblique tendon to relax as the inferior oblique contracts. In most cases there is a congenital abnormality at the trochlear limiting free movement of the superior oblique tendon (Sevel, 1981). Occasionally, inflammatory, neoplastic and traumatic orbital lesions can result in an acquired Brown's syndrome. Rarely, entire extraocular muscles are replaced with fibrous tissue. This congenital fibrosis is usually familial and bilateral with the eyes deviated downwards and inwards and with associated ptosis.

Nuclear and fascicular lesions

It is virtually impossible to distinguish clinically between nuclear and fascicular lesions of the trochlear nerve with the exception of the combination of unilateral trochlear nerve palsy with a contralateral Horner's syndrome indicating dorsolateral midbrain damage to the fascicle together with the central sympathetic pathways (Guy *et al.*, 1989; Mansour and Reinecke, 1986). The trochlear nerve is rarely involved (only 3%) in intrinsic brain stem lesions because of its short intrapontine course. However, the following aetiologies have been reported: mesencephalic haemorrhage or infarction, trauma, tumours, demyelination and decompensated hydrocephalus. Bilateral trochlear nerve palsies in the absence of a history of trauma may indicate a single lesion of the superior medullary velum.

Superior oblique myokymia
The syndrome of monocular torsional nystagmus causing intermittent vertical diplopia and oscillopsia is referred to as superior oblique myokymia, although strictly speaking the term microtremor is more appropriate. Slit lamp biomicroscopy may be helpful to see the oscillations clearly. The pathophysiology is obscure but an intermittent failure of supranuclear inhibition following a nuclear IVth nerve lesion with subsequent recovery has been postulated. Medical treatment includes the membrane stabilizing drugs carbamazepine and phenytoin while surgical weakening of the superior oblique tendon and inferior oblique muscle has been reported to help in some refractory cases (Kommerell and Schaubele, 1980; Lee, 1984; Brazis, 1994).

Peripheral lesions
Trauma accounts for at least 50% of cases. This is said to reflect the susceptibility of the trochlear nerves because of their proximity to the tentorial free margin in the posterior fossa — the tectum of the midbrain suffers a contracoup injury against the tentorial notch and the IVth nerves are damaged either as they sweep laterally around the midbrain, or dorsally in the substance of the superior medullary vellum. In this situation, bilateral IVth nerve injury is common (Lee and Flynn, 1985).

Of the remaining causes of IVth nerve palsy, causes may be localizing (lesions of the posterior fossa course in the subarachnoid space, cavernous sinus, superior orbital fissure and orbit) or non-localizing. Microvascular ischaemic disease is probably the commonest overall cause after trauma. As in apparent lateral rectus weakness, when a patient presents with a non-comitant vertical strabismus, the possibilities of myasthenia and dysthyroid eye disease must be considered.

Ophthalmic aspects of the management of unrecovered trochlear palsy
Prisms may correct a small vertical deviation in the primary position, but will not correct torsion or increasing diplopia in downgaze. With quantitative measurement of vertical deviations, torsional elements and fusion it is possible to select patients who may be suitable for extraocular muscle surgery.

OCULOMOTOR NERVE PALSIES

Clinical features
The oculomotor nerve supplies the medial rectus, inferior oblique, inferior rectus and superior rectus muscles, in addition to the lid levator and the parasympathetic innervation of the pupillary sphincter and ciliary body. A complete IIIrd nerve palsy is easily recognized by the features of ptosis, a fixed dilated pupil and an eye deviated 'down and out' with residual function only in abduction (lateral rectus) and intorsion (superior oblique). Incomplete palsies are more common, and careful assessment is essential to avoid confusion with myopathies with selective involvement (myasthenia) or restrictive disease (dysthyroid eye disease and orbital inflammatory disease). Although exceptions are sometimes seen, it is helpful in an emergency to distinguish between 'surgical' oculomotor palsies with pupillary involvement and 'medical' palsies where the pupil is spared. In the subarachnoid space and cavernous sinus the pupillomotor fibres of the IIIrd nerve lie superficially and dorsally so that compression from an expanding aneurysm is likely to involve these fibres eventually. By contrast, these fibres are characteristically spared by microvascular disease of the vasa nervorum which tends to primarily affect the central fibres only. In cases of acute compression, as many aneurysms fail to involve the pupil, this distinction is less reliable (Richards *et al.*, 1992; Brazis, 1991).

Applied anatomy of the oculomotor nerve and fascicle

The nuclear complex of the third (oculomotor) nerve lies beneath the aqueductal grey matter of the rostral midbrain at the level of the superior colliculus. The MLF passes just lateral to the oculomotor nuclei, and the IVth (trochlear) cranial nerve nucleus is contiguous caudally. Within the complex both lid levators are served by a single dorsal–caudal midline nucleus as are the visceral efferent pupillomotor fibres. The superior rectus subnucleus sends fibres across to the contralateral oculomotor nerve, and subnuclei for the medial rectus, inferior rectus and inferior oblique send fibres to the ipsilateral nerve (Atsaver *et al.*, 1993; Bienfang, 1975; Büttner-Ennever *et al.*, 1981). From the oculomotor complex the fibres pass through the red nucleus to exit the brain stem ventrally passing through the medial aspect of the cerebral peduncles to emerge in the interpeduncular space as the paired oculomotor nerves.

Table 8.10 Classification of oculomotor palsy

A. Nuclear	Congenital aplasia Infarction and arteriovenous malformation Trauma Tumour and other mass lesions
B. Fascicular	Demyelination Haemorrhage Infarction
C. Subarachnoid space (interpeduncular)	Aneurysm — typically posterior communicating artery or basilar artery Meningitis Microvascular disease — infarction Primary nerve tumours Trauma
D. Tentorial edge	Uncal herniation Trauma
E. Cavernous sinus and superior orbital fissure	Cavernous sinus thrombosis Carotid aneurysm Granulomas Herpes zoster Tumours Microvascular disease — infarction
F. Orbit	Trauma Neoplasms and inflammatory infiltration
E. Non-localizing	Idiopathic Para-infectious Migraine

Nuclear and fascicular lesions: applied neurovascular anatomy

Because vascular occlusion is the most common cause, a brief overview of applied neurovascular anatomy is appropriate. The arterial territories of the upper and lower midbrain are schematized in Fig. 8.5. The upper midbrain and thalamomesencephalic junction are supplied by the posterior subthalamic paramedian branches of the P1 segment of the posterior cerebral artery. In the lower midbrain, three vascular territories can be identified: the paramedian territory (IIIrd nerve nucleus, part of the MLF), supplied by direct twigs coming off the basilar tip, the basal territory (IIIrd nerve fascicular fibres and brachium conjunctivum) supplied by short circumferential branches of the superior cerebellar artery (SCA) and P1; and dorsolateral branches supplied by the long circumferential branches of the SCA and P1.

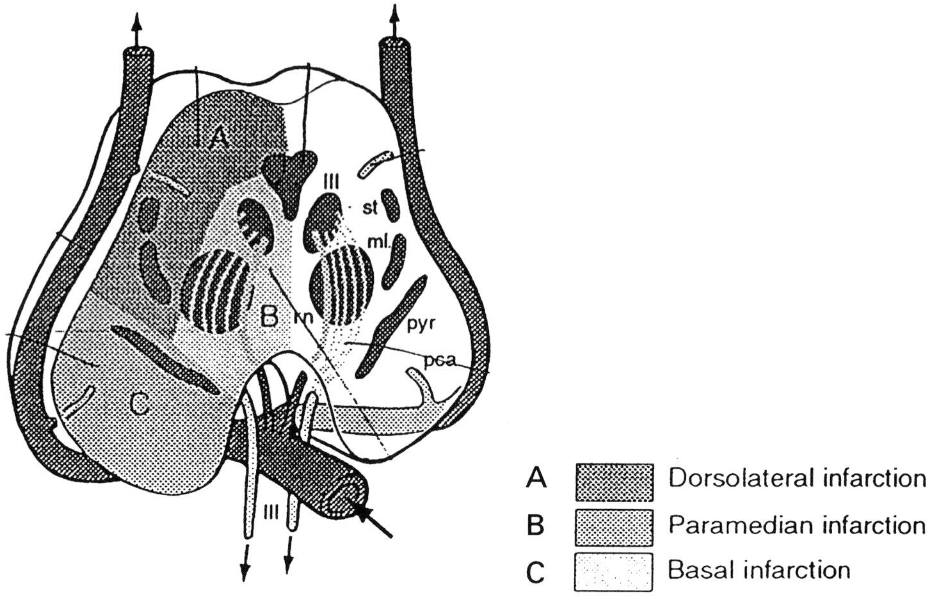

Figure 8.5 Schematic diagram of the neurovascular territories of the midbrain: III, oculomotor nucleus and nerve; pca, posterior cerebellar artery; pyr, pyramidal tract; ml, medial lemniscus; st, spinothalamic tract.

Acquired nuclear and fascicular lesions: clinical features

Two patterns of ocular motility abnormality are characteristic of lesions of the oculomotor complex:

1) An isolated complete bilateral ptosis. This arises from lesions exclusively affecting the caudal part of the oculomotor nerve complex, where the common cell group for both levator palpebrae superioris muscles lies. Cells for the various extraocular muscles lie rostrally and are not damaged in a purely caudal lesion.
2) A unilateral palsy of the medial rectus, inferior rectus and inferior oblique together with a contralateral superior rectus palsy. This is seen when half of the oculomotor complex is damaged: most axons from the subnucleus of the superior rectus decussate to innervate the contralateral muscle.

In Daroff's scheme (Daroff, 1970), a nuclear lesion in oculomotor palsy

is certain when there is:

1) unilateral oculomotor palsy with contralateral superior rectus weakness and bilateral ptosis
2) bilateral total oculomotor palsy with spared levator function

is impossible when there is:

1) a unilateral complete oculomotor palsy with normal contralateral superior rectus function
2) unilateral internal ophthalmoplegia
3) unilateral ptosis

and is possible when there is

1) bilateral ptosis
2) bilateral medial rectus palsy
3) bilateral internal ophthalmoplegia
4) bilateral total oculomotor palsy.

Nuclear oculomotor palsies are often associated with supranuclear eye movement disorders because of the close relationship to the supranuclear pathways and centres, especially when the cause is infiltrative or neoplastic (Bogousslavsky and Meienberg, 1987; Bogousslavsky *et al.*, 1994). Isolated nuclear IIIrd nerve palsies of vascular origin may be seen as a result of selective occlusion of paramedian branches of the basilar artery (Castro *et al.*, 1990). Other causes include trauma and infection.

Fascicular lesions
Fascicular lesions of the oculomotor nerve are usually associated with other abnormalities including contralateral hemiplegia, tremor and ataxia. There is evidence to suggest the following topographic organization within the oculomotor nerve fascicle: the most medial fibres are for the pupil, followed by fibres for the inferior rectus, levator, medial rectus, superior rectus and most laterally the inferior oblique. Isolated fascicular lesions are caused by infarction, haemorrhage or sometimes demyelination (Büttner and Brandt, 1992; Gauntt *et al.*, 1995; Hriso *et al.*, 1991; Ksiazek *et al.*, 1989, 1994).

Congenital lesions associated with the oculomotor nerve
Isolated congenital oculomotor palsy is usually due to perinatal trauma to the peripheral nerve, but absent or incomplete development has been demonstrated in some cases (Balkan and Hoyt, 1984; Victor, 1986). The pupil is often miotic rather than dilated because of aberrant sphincter innervation. Other misdirection syndromes arise including:

1) congenital adduction palsy with synergistic divergence
2) atypical vertical retraction syndrome
3) cyclic oculomotor paresis with cyclic spasm
4) Marcus–Gunn jaw-winking synkinesis.

In congenital adduction palsy with synergistic divergence ('the splits') there is a bilateral paralysis of adduction together with bilateral simultaneous abduction on attempted gaze into the field of action of the paretic medial rectus (Thomas *et al.*, 1993). In the atypical vertical retraction syndrome, co-contraction of superior and inferior rectus muscle results in retraction of the eye into the orbit with narrowing of the palpebral aperture. In cyclic oculomotor paresis with cyclic spasm there is transient oculomotor nerve palsy with ptosis, mydriasis and ophthalmoplegia together with involuntary spastic movements in which the eyelid elevates, the pupil constricts and the eye moves towards the midline, occurring every 2 minutes and lasting for between 10 and 30 seconds. The exact pathogenesis is obscure, but primary (developmental) aberant regeneration of nuclear and supranuclear fibres is a likely explanation (Hoyt and Nactigäller, 1965).

Jaw-winking synkinesis (trigemino-oculomotor synkinesis, or Marcus–Gunn phenomenon)

Jaw-winking synkinesis presents as a unilateral ptosis in infancy associated with rhythmic jerking of the upper lid, often as the infant suckles. Some 5% of cases of congenital ptosis are associated with jaw-winking. Two major groups are described: external pterygoid-levator synkinesis with lid elevation when the jaw is moved to the opposite side, and internal pterygoid-levator synkinesis with lid elevation on clenching the jaw closed. The first group is the most common.

Table 8.11 Classification of oculomotor palsies arising in the brain stem

Vascular territory(syndrome)	Structures involved	Ipsilateral signs	Contralateral signs
Basal territory (Weber)	IIIrd fascicle, anterior to red nucleus; pyramidal tract	IIIrd nerve paralysis (may be pupil sparing)	Hemiparesis or hemiplegia (hemiparaesthesia)
Paramedian territory (Benedict, Nothnagel, Claude)	IIIrd fascicle, red nucleus, medial lemniscus, substantia nigra	IIIrd nerve paralysis	Extrapyramidal movement disorders (hemianaesthesia)
Dorsolateral territory Interpeduncular syndrome	Both IIIrd fascicles Both pyramidal tracts	IIIrd nerve paralysis Hemiplegia/paresis	IIIrd nerve paralysis Hemiplegia/paresis

Brain stem syndromes involving oculomotor nerve
The eponymous syndromes with defining various combinations of neurological signs due to brain stem lesions remain of value in modern clinical practice insofar as the localization of small or early lesions is still based on clinical observation rather than neuroimaging. However, the syndromes are only rarely observed in their pure forms and several variations and combinations are possible. Confusingly, different texts tend to give slightly different details and an appreciation of the vascular territories involved is helpful.

Weber's syndrome, or the syndrome of the cerebral peduncle is the most frequently observed. It consists of an ipsilateral fascicular oculomotor nerve palsy and a contralateral hemiplegia due to a lesion at the crus cerebri in the ventral part of the mesencephalon. A supranuclear facial palsy may also be present. Partial forms of oculomotor palsy including pupillary sparing are possible, and laterally placed lesions are associated with additional contralateral hypoaesthesia. Infarction of the basal midbrain vascular territory is the usual cause. Benedict's syndrome is characterized by an ipsilateral fascicular oculomotor nerve palsy with a hemiparesis and involuntary movements (hemiballismus or choreoathetosis) contralateral to the lesion due to red nucleus or subthalamic damage. Variants include Nothnagel's syndrome in which there is ipsilateral cerebellar ataxia, and Claude's syndrome of the red nucleus (Gaymar *et al.*, 1991). Infarction of the paramedian vascular territory is the usual cause.

Acquired peripheral lesions of the oculomotor nerve

Applied anatomy
In the interpeduncular space the nerve passes beneath the origin of the posterior cerebral artery and lateral to the posterior communicating artery to run along the free edge of the tentorium and pierce the dura to enter the cavernous sinus lateral to the posterior clinoid. The oculomotor trunk occupies the superior aspect of the cavernous sinus and separates into superior and inferior divisions at about 5mm before the superior orbital fissure. The inferior branch supplies the medial and inferior recti, the inferior oblique and the ciliary ganglion; the superior branch innervates the superior rectus and levator muscle only.

Clinical features
Within the subarachnoid space the oculomotor nerve is vulnerable to meningeal processes such as infection and haemorrhage, and to compression by arterial aneurysm. The most common site for an aneurysm is the internal carotid — posterior

communicating artery junction. Usually the pupillomotor fibres are involved in such cases (the 'surgical IIIrd nerve palsy'), but especially in the first few days of symptoms the pupil may be spared (O'Connor *et al.*, 1983). Resolution of an oculomotor nerve palsy does not necessarily mean that an aneurysm is excluded, especially if there is a history of facial or orbital pain. Modern neuroimaging (MR angiography) is often adequate to exclude an aneurysm without needing to resort to formal angiography. Partial forms of oculomotor palsy may also be due to aneurysm at this site affecting the superior or inferior division of the nerve, and implying that functionally at least the separation may take place at a more proximal location than the superior orbital fissure (Bortolami *et al.*, 1993).

The oculomotor nerve may also be compressed against the tentorial edge, petrous ridge and clivus by the uncus of the temporal lobe during cerebral herniation. Classically the pupillomotor fibres are involved first in this medical emergency (Van Dalen and Van Mourek–Noordenbos, 1984). Within the cavernous sinus, the oculomotor nerve may be compressed by infraclinoid carotid aneurysm, when facial pain and trochlear and abducens involvement are common. Pituitary apoplexy and idiopathic inflammatory disease are other causes (Guy and Day, 1989).

Isolated oculomotor palsy may be due to infarction of the subarachnoid or intracavernous portions, usually in association with diabetes, hypertension or systemic vasculitis (Jacobson *et al.*, 1994). Typically the pupil is spared, reflecting involvement of the perforating vasa nervorum which supply the neurons innervating extraocular muscle fibres. In some cases, nerve infarction arises in the brain stem. Trauma may also be responsible — mechanisms include root avulsion at the brain stem origin, or damage at the point of dural perforation or in the supraorbital fissure (Cahill *et al.*, 1996).

Oculomotor synkinesis

The process whereby following neuronal damage, regenerating axons may come to innervate structures remote from their original destination is commonly seen following facial nerve injury. Typical examples include intrafacial dyskinesia, paradoxical gustatory sweating and gustatory tearing. A comparable syndrome arises following oculomotor nerve injury: observed patterns include co-contraction of the levator and medial rectus on attempted adduction or co-contraction of levator and inferior rectus on attempted depression, and pupillary constriction on medial or downward eye movement. Oculomotor synkinesia may be primary or secondary. Primary synkinesia is seen in slowly growing mass lesions of the cavernous sinus, such as a meningioma or infraclinoid aneurysm where there is no prior acute episode (Schatz *et al.*, 1977). Secondary synkinesia is seen following incomplete recovery from an oculomotor palsy of acute onset.

Ocular neuromyotonia

Ocular neuromyotonia is a rare disturbance of ocular motility resulting from powerful neuronal discharges from a radiation-injured ocular motor nerve causing episodic tonic contraction of the corresponding ocular muscle(s). Most commonly there is a history of radiotherapy for skull base or thalamic tumours. Patients experience intermittent diplopia and may show an intermittent abnormal head posture. The condition has been attributed to anomalous interaxonal connections forming a self-perpetuating reverberating neural circuit (Schultz, *et al.*, 1986; Lessell *et al.*, 1986; Barroso and Hoyt, 1993; Ezra *et al.*, 1996).

Ophthalmoplegic migraine and oculomotor palsy in childhood

The syndrome of vomiting, headache, photophobia and irritability together with variable pupillary involvement of an oculomotor nerve palsy in children always suggests the possibility of an intracranial aneurysm. However, presentation of berry aneuryms is

Table 8.12 Aetiology of multiple ocular motor nerve palsies

A. Brain stem	Encephalitis and AIDS Infarction and arteriovenous malformation Tumour and other mass lesions
B. Subarachnoid space	Aneurysm Meningitis Clivus tumours Trauma
C. Cavernous sinus and superior orbital fissure	Cavernous sinus thrombosis Carotid aneurysm Tolosa-Hunt syndrome Herpes zoster Tumours Microvascular disease — infarction
F. Orbit	Trauma Neoplasms and inflammatory infiltration
E. Non-localizing	Para-infectious (Guillain-Barré and Miller-Fisher syndromes)

exceptionally rare in children under 10 years of age, and where a family history of migraine can be elicited and there is rapid resolution of symptoms and signs following a period of sleep, the diagnosis of ophthalmoplegic migraine can be made. The availability of high resolution imaging (usually MRI) means that difficult clinical decisions with regard to angiography are seldom required. In teenagers, aneurysms enter the differential diagnosis as for adults. Other causes of oculomotor palsy in childhood include congenital / developmental anomalies, cranial and orbital trauma, and viral meningitis. In contrast to abducens palsies, neoplastic disease is a most uncommon cause of a clinically isolated oculomotor palsy (Fox, 1989; Gabianelli *et al.*, 1989; Kodski and Younge, 1992).

PAINFUL AND COMBINED OPHTHALMOPLEGIAS

Combined ocular cranial nerve palsies are most commonly unilateral as a result of lesions in the cavernous sinus or superior orbital fissure. In the case of abnormalities located at the superior orbital fissure, visual loss, proptosis and conjunctival venous congestion may also be seen. Confusion is sometimes caused by the minor degree of proptosis which may accompany loss of tone in multiple extraocular muscles, such as in a complete oculomotor nerve palsy. However, in distinction to true proptosis of orbital disease, resistance to retropulsion of the globe is not seen. Bilateral combined palsies are seen in a diverse range of conditions including postinfectious polyneuropathy (Miller–Fisher variant of Guillain–Barré syndrome), infiltrative brain stem lesions, inflammatory, infective and neoplastic disease of the basal meninges or cavernous sinus, pituitary apoplexy and carotid–cavernous fistulae and cavernous sinus thrombosis. The differential diagnosis rests of the history of the clinical course, associated signs and symptoms, CSF findings and neuroimaging (Hamed *et al.*, 1988; Hoogland *et al.*, 1993; Marsh *et al.*, 1977).

Painful combined ophthalmolplegias suggest a more specific set of diagnostic possibilities which can be summarized under the headings of inflammatory neoplastic and vascular disease.

Inflammatory disease

This may be infective or non-infective. In orbital cellulitis a characteristic picture of ophthalmoplegia together with fever, lid swelling and proptosis complicates local

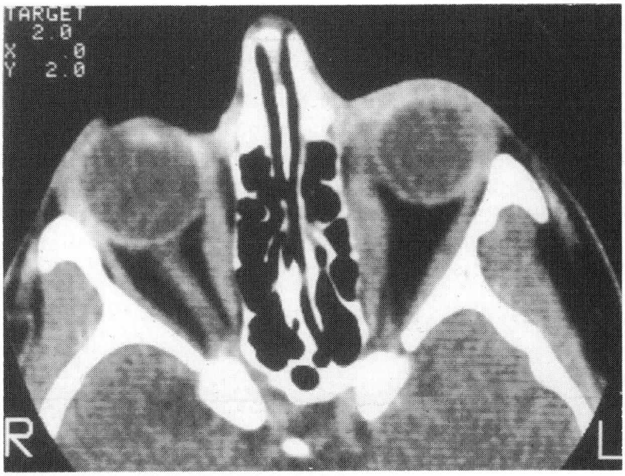

Figure 8.6 Axial CT scan of orbits showing bilateral medial rectus muscle enlargement in a patient with orbital myositis.

paranasal sinus or metastatic infection. In debilitated patients, orbitocerebral mucormycosis may present with a similar clinical picture but the disease progresses to ischaemic necrosis of orbital and intraocular structures. Commonly, however, the inflammatory process arises apparently without any infective aetiology. The terms 'orbital pseudotumour', 'idiopathic orbital inflammatory disease' and 'Tolosa–Hunt syndrome' are all used in this context. However, it is preferable to describe this group of conditions according to the anatomical location and physical signs encountered: thus orbital myositis (Fig. 8.6), non-infective dacryoadenitis, scleritis and granulomatous optic perineuritis may each or all be seen in orbital pseudotumour; proptosis, ophthalmoplegia, trigeminal sensory loss and Horners' syndrome form the superior orbital fissure syndrome; while ophthalmoplegia without proptosis is characteristic of inflammatory disease in the cavernous sinus (Rootman and Nugent, 1982; Stern *et al.*, 1985). Great care is required to exclude the possibility of infective granulomatous disease (tuberculosis), systemic vasculitis (Wegener's granulomatosis) (Power *et al.*, 1995) or unsuspected neoplasia (non-Hodgkin's lymphoma and metastases) and a tissue biopsy is obtained in order to plan definitive treatment in addition to standard imaging.

Neoplastic disease

Although often painless and insidious, primary and metastatic tumours in the cavernous sinus, superior orbital fissure and orbital apex may nevertheless occasionally present with painful ophthalmoplegia. Nasopharyngeal carcinoma most frequently affects men in late middle age and in some series accounts for 20% of all parasellar syndromes. Metastatic carcinomas and invasive squamous cell skin carcinoma are further candidates, the later arising sometimes many years after apparently adequate treatment to the original skin lesion.

Vascular disease

The constellation of multiple cranial nerve palsies, headache and variable visual disturbance is strongly suggestive of pituitary apoplexy: by contrast slowly progressive lateral extrasellar expansion of pituitary tumours into the cavernous sinus may be associated with sparing of the function of the oculomotor nerves until late in the disease process. The other vascular lesion of note in the context of painful ophthalmoplegia is infraclinoid (intracavernous) aneurysm. In this condition there is progressive diplopia with features of single followed by combined abducens and oculomotor nerve palsies, Horner's syndrome or combined sympathetic and parasympathetic pupillary paresis, trigeminal dysaesthesia together with periorbital pain which may be severe. Giant and infraclinoid carotid aneuryms are typically found in middle aged to elderly women. Intracavernous meningiomas may sometimes produce a very similar clinical picture, and high resolution imaging together with angiography are required to make the distinction.

MYOGENIC PARALYTIC STRABISMUS

Myogenic paralytic strabsimus includes disorders of eye movements due to abnormalities at the neuromuscular junction and disorders of the muscles themselves.

Myasthenia gravis

The clinical syndrome of myasthenia gravis comprises muscle weakness with intact tendon reflexes, normal pupillary reflexes, normal sensation, variability of muscle function (often worse after a day's activities), remissions and relapses and a tendency to primarily involve the extraocular, facial and oropharyngeal muscles. Myasthenia is seen at all ages, but as in other autoimmune disorders, women are more commonly affected especially in the under-40 age-group. Transplacental transmission of maternal auto-antibodies can cause a self-limiting neonatal myasthenia syndrome. Approximately 10% of myasthenia patients have a thymoma, and 5% have autoimmune thyroid disease (which may give rise to an additional ophthalmopathy). Myasthenia is an autoimmune disorder in which the number of post-synaptic acetyl choline receptor end-plates at the neuromuscular junction of skeletal muscle is reduced in association with the presence of a polyclonal humoral IgG response and anti-acetyl choline receptor antibodies. Antibodies are found in 80% of patients with generalized disease and 50% of those with disease limited to the extraocular muscles (Soliven *et al.*, 1988). The thymus gland is implicated in the pathogenesis, as hyperplasia and neoplastic change may arise.

Ocular involvement occurs eventually in over 90% of all myasthenic patients and is the presenting complaint in more than 75% (Kaminski *et al.*, 1990). In some patients who present with a limited ocular form of myasthenia, the disease remains confined to the extraocular muscles, levator palpebrae superioris and orbicularis oculi, whilst in other patients there is progression to generalized disease often within only 1 or 2 years (Oosterhuis, 1989). The extraocular muscle involvement of ocular myasthenia does not follow any set pattern and indeed can mimic a great range of other ocular motility disorders, especially single motor cranial nerve palsies and internuclear ophthalmoplegia. Nystagmus in the abducting eye of a myasthenic 'pseudo-internuclear ophthalmoplegia' may also be seen. Weakness of the orbicularis oculi is very commonly seen in ocular forms of myasthenia and is elicited by demonstrating a readiness of the examiners fingers to prise apart tightly closed eyelids. Some degree of ptosis is almost invariable, and may change from one eye to the other between examinations. The ptosis can also be accentuated by fatiguing movements in which the patient is required to sustain upgaze for a period of up to 30 seconds: this manouvre may also provoke an increased vertical squint due to fatigue of elevators of the globe.

Electromyography (EMG) is widely used to support the diagnosis of myasthenia. In ocular myasthenia positive abnormalities of limb muscle may be absent, and single fibre studies of the orbicularis or even the extraocular muscles may be useful (Milone *et al.*, 1993; Uyama *et al.*, 1993). The Tensilon (edrophonium) test is also useful: Tensilon transiently acts to block the action of the enzyme acetylcholinesterase, thereby making more acetyl choline available at the neuromuscular junction. A negative result does not rule the diagnosis out in the presence of strongly suggestive symptoms and signs but in a positive result 10mg of intravenous edrophonium will temporarily reverse the muscular weakness so that diplopia and ptosis may resolve. The changing diplopia and range of extraocular movements can be plotted on a Hess chart, but this refinement is difficult to apply in practice because of the variability of these measurement prior to Tensilon, and also because the test may take longer than the 3 minutes available before the effects of the diagnostic injection wear off. Injection of a bolus of edrophonium may be associated with powerful cholinergic cardiac effects and because of the risk of dysrhythmias a test dose of 1mg together with atropine 0.4mg are given initially in a setting where full resuscitation facilities are quickly available.

Thoracic imaging to detect a thymoma is routine, and thymectomy may benefit younger patients especially those with reactive hyperplasia. In addition to standard cholinergic agents such as pyridostigmine and prostigmine, immunosuppression with corticosteroids, azothiaprine, antithymocyte globulin and plasmapheresis all may be required. Close collaboration between the ophthalmologist and the neurologist is required in those patients with ocular forms of the disease who continue to require major immunosuppression (Rowland, 1980; Weinberg *et al.*, 1994). Occasionally, myasthenia may go into remission and leave the patient with a stable concomitant or paralytic squint which is amenable to surgical correction (Acheson, *et al.*, 1991).

Myasthenia-like syndromes

Occasionally chronic myasthenia may present as an end-stage ocular myopathy with severe ptosis, complete external ophthalmoplegia and lagophthalmos. A history of fatiguability is absent, the Tensilon is negative and the distinction between myasthenia and other myopathies (chronic progressive external ophthalmoplegia) can only be made after demonstrating fatigue on single fibre EMG and autoantibodies. Myasthenic syndromes of fatiguability may arise outside the context of autoimmune disease in:

Neoplasms: paraneoplastic Eaton–Lambert syndrome (extraocular muscle involvement very rare) (O'Neill *et al.*, 1988)

Drugs: penicillamine, aminoglycosides, vinca alkaloids, corticosteroids (corticosteroids may aggravate myasthenia gravis and hospital in-patient monitoring is required if this therapy is to be introduced in case the patient requires ventilatory support in the short term)

Neurotoxins: botulinum (effect used therpeutically for the treatment of strabismus and blepharospasm) (Burns *et al.*, 1986; Hedges *et al.*, 1983).

Dysthyroid eye disease

Dysthyroid eye disease (Graves' disease, thyroid eye disease, endocrine ophthalmopathy) presents as a constellation of orbital abnormalities, usually in association with biochemical and immunological evidence of thyroid gland dysfunction. Two phases are recognized: active and fibrotic (Sergott and Glaser 1981; Char, 1992; Sanders and Brown, 1986). In the active phase the patient develops lid changes (upper lid retraction and lid lag, puffiness), conjunctival congestion (chemosis), orbital congestion (proptosis) and extraocular muscle swelling (ophthalmoplegia) in association with water and glycosaminoglycan deposition in the orbital structures together with an inflammatory infiltrate. Vision may be compromised either by such severe proptosis as to cause corneal exposure, or by optic nerve compression at the orbital apex. In the fibrotic phase of the disease, evidence of inflammation resolves leaving the patient with variable degrees of proptosis, lid lag and ophthalmoplegia (Hudson *et al.*, 1991). The limitation of eye movements in the fibrotic phase is principally due to healing with fibrosis of the inflammatory infiltrate of the acute phase leaving a restrictive myopathy (Fells *et al.*, 1994). In some patients the acute phase is florid and readily diagnosed; in others it is limited and subclinical so that the patient presents with a restrictive myopathy. The disease may be highly asymmetric or unilateral and extraocular muscle involvement may be selective or generalized. The inferior and medial recti are the two most commonly involved muscles. The diagnosis is made from the history and typical physical signs.

Sometimes orbital and lid changes are minimal or absent so that the patient may present with diplopia, most commonly vertical. Imaging of the orbit by CT or MR reveals characteristic enlargement of the rectus muscles, and in the acute phase the increased water content of the recti is reflected in increased signal intensity on T1- and T2-weighted sequences on fat-suppressed MRI. The diagnosis is supported by the demonstration of thyroid associated autoantibodies and abnormal thyroid function. There is no single diagnostic test for dysthyroid eye disease and great care should always be exercised because of the possible co-existence of myasthenia or diagnostic confusion with orbital pseudotumour or true neoplasms.

In general terms, management is directed towards rendering the patient euthyroid and opting for conservative measures including ensuring adequate corneal protection during the acute phase of the orbital disease. In severe cases, immunosuppression or lens sparing orbital radiotherapy may be used (Ravin *et al.*, 1975; Kao *et al.*, 1993) — these measures are much more effective when used in the acute phase. The question of the influence on the natural history of the orbital disease by the choice of treatment used to control initial hyperthyroidism (carbimazole, radioiodine, thyroidectomy) is controversial (Bartalena *et al.*, 1989). In the fibrotic phase of the disease, ophthalmic surgery has much to offer towards functional and cosmetic rehabilitation in the form of orbital decompression for severe proptosis or optic nerve compression (Leone *et al.*, 1989), plastic procedures for retracted lids, and strabismus surgery to maximize the field of single binocular vision (Shorr and Seif, 1986).

Muscular dystrophies including chronic progressive external ophthalmoplegia

1. Chronic progressive external ophthalmoplegia (Kearns-Sayre syndrome)
2. Oculopharyngeal dystrophy
3. Myotonic dystrophy

Chronic progressive external ophthalmoplegia (CPEO) is characterized clinically by a slowly progressive symmetrical limitation of eye movements. Strabismus and diplopia are rarely seen. Reflecting the infranuclear origin of the ophthalmoplegia, oculocephalic and caloric stimulation do not increase the range of movement. There is usually a symmetrical ptosis and moderate orbicularis oculi weakness in addition. Familial occurrence and the absence of any spontaneous remission and relapse distinguish CPEO from chronic myasthenia. Many patients with CPEO have some degree of retinal pigment epithelial degeneration, ranging from clinically asymptomatic ERG changes, to a mild 'salt-and-pepper' retinopathy, through to a symptomatic field constriction with bone spicules and disc pallor typical of 'retinitis pigmentosa' (Eagle *et al.*, 1982; Mullie *et al.*, 1985). Cardiac conduction defects, cerebellar signs and raised CSF protein may also be present. These additional features have been designated 'ophthalmoplegia plus' or Kearns-Sayre syndrome (Kearns, 1965; Butler and Gadoth, 1976). Muscle biopsy specimens show the presence of 'ragged-red' muscle fibres within a population of relatively normal fibres on modified Gomori trichrome staining representing degenerate mitochondria. Electron microscopy of apparently normal fibres reveals further abnormal mitochondria. The disease is now characterized as a mitochondrial cytopathy in which a deletion from the circular strand of mitochondrial DNA may result in defects of intracellular respiratory chain and in morphological and functional changes in a range of tissues. (Bresolin *et al.*, 1990; Moraes *et al.*, 1989; Harding, 1991).

Oculopharyngeal dystrophy is a hereditary, usually autosomal dominant, muscular dystrophy in which the bulbar musculature is conspicuously involved in addition to external ophthalmoplegia, ptosis and orbicularis weakness. 'Ragged-red' fibres are not described in this condition.

Myotonic dystrophy is a further cause of external ophthalmoplegia. The myotonia may be apparent in the extraocular movements, when after sustained gaze in one particular direction, gaze in the reverse direction may then be abnormally slowed. Patients may suffer visual loss as a result of cataracts and less commonly from retinal pigment epithelial degeneration (Ter Bruggen *et al.*, 1993).

Other ocular myopathies

A variety of other diseases cause limited movements and muscle enlargement on imaging (Rootman and Nugent, 1982). These include:

1. orbital myositis (as the predominant feature of an orbital pseudotumour)
2. amyloidosis (Katz *et al.*, 1989)
3. parasitosis (trichinosis, echinococcosis)
4. neoplastic infiltration
5. giant cell arteritis
6. carotid-cavernous fistula.

ORBITAL DISEASES AND THE NEURO-OPHTHALMIC ASSESSMENT

Orbital disease is a common cause of double vision (most often due to dysthyroid eye disease) and it is appropriate to include a short section on the differential diagnosis and clinical features of orbital lesions (Wright, 1988; Kennerdell and Dresner, 1984; Rootman, 1988).

Table 8.13 Differential diagnosis of orbital mass lesions

The likelihood of different orbital disease can be considered on the basis of probability, based on Rootman's series of 1400 consecutive adult cases

Grave's disease	47%	
Neoplasms	22%	Primary • optic gliomas • perioptic meningiomas • sphenoid meningioma • mesenchymal / bone • lacrimal • lymphoproliferative • nerve sheath Contiguous • sinus • lids Metastatic
Vacular	7%	Lymphangioma / haemangioma A-V shunts and malformations
Miscellaneous	10%	Trauma Dermoid / epidermoid mucocoele

Eyelids

The lids are examined for abnormalities of position: ptosis or retraction, abnormalities of movement: lid lag, reduced levator function, and the presence of swelling or a mass. Although thyroid eye disease is a frequent cause of lid retraction, there are other possibilities. Ptosis in one eye, may result in lid retraction on the contralateral side because of the action of Hering's law of equal innervation to yoked muscles in each orbit: as the levator on the abnormal ptotic side receives additional innervation in an attempt to raise the lid, the contralateral levator overacts with consequent lid retraction. Other causes include aberrant regeneration of the oculomotor nerve and Parinaud's dorsal midbrain syndrome.

Lid swelling is a cardinal sign of orbital disease either in association with dysthyroid eye disease or with other inflammatory processes, especially cellulitis and non-infective pseudotumour. When the cardinal signs of inflammatory lid disease are present — calor, dolor and rubor, it is helpful to make the distinction between pre- and postseptal cellulitis. In preseptal cellulitis the inflammatory process is confined to the lid, usually complicating severe conjunctivitis or tarsal gland infection, whereas in postseptal cellulitis the disease process involves the orbital tissues including fat and the extraocular muscles. Not only are the lids inflamed, but there is proptosis, ophthalmoplegia and on occasion visual loss from optic nerve impairment as well (Jarrett and Gutman, 1969) (see Chapter 5).

Conjunctivae

The conjunctivae may show oedema (chemosis), dilated vessels or neoplastic infiltration. Chemosis is a non-specific sign of any orbital disease which may interfere with venous drainage. In the acute phase of dysthyroid eye disease localized conjunctival injection and oedema over the insertion of the rectus muscle tendons may be a more specific sign. Dilatation and arterialization of the larger conjunctival vessels is associated with diseases of increased orbital venous pressure: arteriovenous fistula and dural fistula. Diffuse hyperaemia of the episclera and sclera, with failure to blanche after instillation of vasoconstricting phenylephrine eye drops, together with pain indicate inflammation of deeper coats of the eye in association with pseudotumour.

Globe

The globe may show axial or non-axial proptosis with pulsation and resistance to retropulsion (Fig. 8.7). Proptosis may in practice be difficult to determine as there is considerable inter-individual and racial variation in the degree to which the globe extends anterior to the bony orbital margins. Up to 2mm of asymmetry is within normal limits, as measured by exophthalmometry. Subtle degrees of proptosis are best seen by viewing the position of the eyes and lids from above the brows. Apparent proptosis may be attributed to extraocular muscle paresis in the case of a IIIrd nerve pasy, but local causes should be excluded first. Resistance to retropulsion is a useful physical sign confirming the impression of an orbital mass. Pulsation is seen in congenital sphenoid dysplasia with partial orbital-cranial encephalocoele in neurofibromatosis, after orbital trauma, in carotid-cavernous and other arteriovenous fistulae.

Fundus

The fundus may show disc oedema, the presence of choroidal folds and exudative retinal detachment. Optic disc swelling does not necessarily indicate actual infiltration of the nerve or meninges but may simply reflect the presence of any orbital mass. Optociliary shunt vessels are seen in primary optic nerve tumours. Choroidal folds are seen when a mass deforms the shape of the globe from behind.

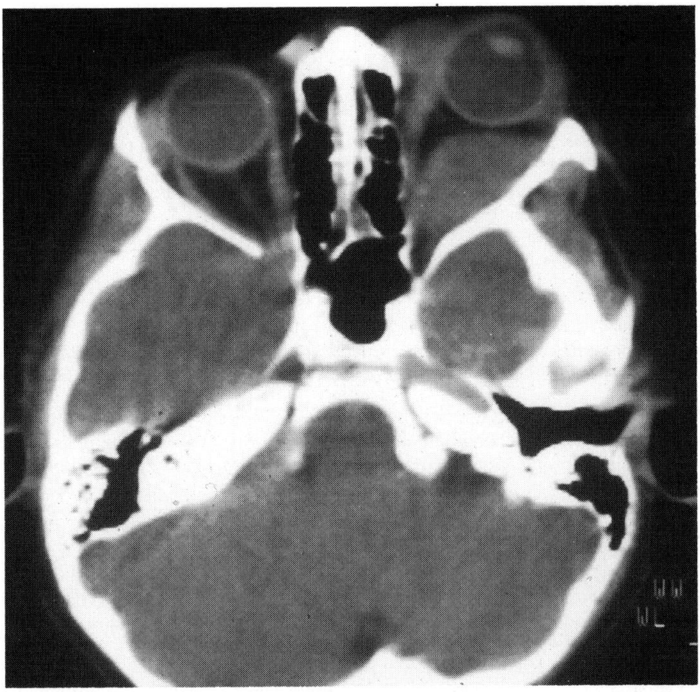

Figure 8.7 Axial CT scan of orbits showing righ proptosis due to a posterior-lateral mass: Biopsy showed a rhabdomyosarcoma.

Specific physical signs

A mass in the anterior orbit may be palpable at the boney margin of the orbit. Auscultation may reveal a bruit, the eye movements may be restricted at a positive forced duction test. Intraocular pressure may elevate when gaze is directed away from the field of action of a tethered muscle and in arteriovenous fistulas there may be an abnormally wide pulse pressure on applanation tonometry. Ausculatation may reveal vascular bruits due to congenital and acquired arteriovenous fistulae. The Valsalva manoeuvre may transiently increase proptosis in arteriovenous fistulae and venous varices.

REFERENCES

Abadi RV and Dickinson CM (1986). Waveform characteristics in congenital nystagmus. *Doc Ophthalmol* **64**: 153–167.

Acheson JF, Elston JS, Lee JP and Fells P (1991). Extraocular muscle surgery in myasthenia gravis. *Br J Ophthlamol* **75**: 232–235.

Apkarian P, Bour LJ, Barth PG *et al.* (1995). Non-decussating retino-fugal fibre syndrome. An inborn achiasmatic malformation associated with visuotopic misrouting, visual evoked potential ipsilateral asymmetry and nystagmus. *Brain* **118**: 1195–1216.

Ashe J, Hain TC, Zee DS and Schatz NJ (1991). Microsaccadic flutter. *Brain* **114**: 461–472.

Atlas SW, Grossman RI, Savino PJ *et al.* (1987). Surface-coil MR of orbital pseudotumor. *Am J Roentgenol* **148**: 803–808.

Atsaver A, Durgun B, Celik HH and Yilmaz E (1993). Somatotropic organisation of the axons innervating the superior rectus muscle in the oculomotor nerve of the rat. *Acta Anat* **146**: 251–254.

Bains RA, Crawford JD, Cadera W and Vilis T (1992). The conjugacy of human saccadic eye movements. *Vision Res* **32**: 1677–1684.

Balkan R and Hoyt CS (1984). Associated neurologic abnormalities in congenital third nerve palsies. *Am J Ophthalmol* **97**: 315–319.
Baloh RW, Honrubia V and Jacobson K (1987). Benign positional vertigo: Clinical and oculographic features in 240 cases. *Neurology* **37**: 371–378.
Barnes D and McDonald WI (1992). The ocular manifestations of multiple sclerosis: part 2. *J Neurol Neurosurg Psychiat* **55**: 863–868.
Barratt H, Gresty MA and Page NGR (1985). Neurological evidence for dissociation of pursuit and optokinetic systems. *Acta Otolaryngol (Stockh)* **100**: 89–97.
Barroso L and Hoyt WF (1993). Episodic exotropia from lateral rectus neuromyotonia: appearance and remission after radiation therapy for a thalamic glioma. *J Pediat Ophthalmol Strab* **30**: 56–57.
Bartalena L, Marcocci C, Bogazzi F *et al.* (1989). Use of corticosteroids to prevent progression of Grave's ophthalmopathy after radioiodine therapy for hyperthyroidism. *New Engl J Med* **321**: 1349–1352.
Beigi B, O'Keefe M, Logan P and Eustace P (1995). Convergence substitution for paralysed horizontal gaze. *Br J Ophthalmol* **79**: 229–232.
Bergin DJ and Wright JE (1986). Orbital cellulitis. *Br J Ophthalmol* **70**: 174–178.
Bienfang DC (1975). Crossing axons in the third nerve nucleus. *Invest Ophthalmol Vis Sci* **14**: 927–931.
Bogousslavsky J and Meienberg O (1987). Eye-movement disorders in brainstem and cerebellar stroke. *Arch Neurol* **44**: 141–148.
Bogousslavsky J, Miklossy J, Regli F and Janzer R (1990). Vertical gaze palsy and selective unilateral infarction of the rostral interstitial nucleus of the medial longitudinal fasciculus (riMLF). *J Neurol Neurosurg Psychiat* **53**: 67–71.
Bogousslavsky J, Maeder P, Regli F and Meuli R (1994). Pure midbrain infarction: clinical syndromes, MRI and etiologic patterns. *Neurology* **44**: 2032–2040.
Borruat FX, Bogousslavsky J, Uffer S *et al.* (1993). Orbital infarction syndrome. *Ophthalmology* **100**: 562–568.
Bortolami R, D'Alessandro R and Manni E (1993). The origin of pain in 'ischaemic-diabetic' third nerve palsy. *Arch Neurol* **50**: 795.
Brandt T (1990). Positional and positioning vertigo and nystagmus. *J Neurol Sci* **95**: 3–28.
Brandt T and Dieterich M (1991). Different types of skew deviation. *J Neurol Neurosurg Psychiat* **54**: 549–550.
Braun D, Weber H, Mergner T and Schulte-Mönting J (1992). Saccadic reaction times in patients with frontal and parietal lesions. *Brain* **115**: 1359–1386.
Brazis PW (1991). Localisation of lesions of the oculomotor nerve: recent concepts. *Mayo Clin Proc* **66**: 1029–1035.
Brazis PW (1992). Ocular motor abnormalities in Wallenberg's lateral medullary syndrome. *Mayo Clin Proc* **67**: 365–368.
Brazis PW (1993). Palsies of the trochlear nerve: diagnosis and localisation: recent concepts. *Mayo Clin Proc* **68**: 501–509.
Brazis PW, Miller NR, Henderer JD, Lee AG. The natural history and results of treatment of superior oblique myokymia. *Arch Ophthalmol* **112**: 1073–1077.
Bresolin N, Doriguzzi C, Ponzettto C *et al.* (1990). Ubidecarenone in the treatment of mitochondrial myopathies: A multi centre double-blind trial. *J Neurol Sci* **100**: 70–78.
Bronstein AM, Morris J, Du Boulay G *et al.* (1990). Abnormalities of horizontal gaze. Clinical, oculographic and magnetic resonance imaging findings. I: Abducens palsy. *J Neurol Neurosurg Psychiat* **53**: 194–199.
Burns CL, Gammon A and Gemmill MC (1986). Ptosis associated with botulinum toxin treatment of strabismus and blepharospasm. *Ophthalmology* **93**: 1621–1627.
Butler IJ and Gadoth N (1976). Kearnes-Sayre syndrome. A review of a multisystem disorder of children and young adults. *Arch Int Med* **136**: 1290–1293.
Büttner U and Brandt T (1992). Ocular motor disorders of the brainstem. *Clinical Neurology, International Practice and Research* Vol 1, No 2. London: Ballière Tindall.
Büttner U and Büttner-Ennever JA (1987). Pathophysiology of horizontal and vertical eye movement disorders. In *Eye Movement Disorders*. (eds EACM Sanders, RJW de Kaizer, DS Zee), pp. 37–46. Dordrecht: Junk.
Büttner UW and Zee DS (1989). Vestibular testing in comatose patients. *Arch Neurol* **46**: 561.
Büttner-Ennever JA and Akert K (1981). Medial rectus subgroups of the oculomotor nucleus and their abducens internuclear input in the monkey. *J Comp Neurol* **197**: 17–27.
Büttner-Ennever JA, Büttner U, Cohen B *et al.* (1982). Vertical paralysis and the rostral interstitial nucleus of the medial longitudinal fasciculus. *Brain* **102**: 125–149.
Büttner-Ennever JA, Acheson JF, Buttner U *et al.* (1989a). Ptosis and supranuclear downgaze palsy. *Neurology* **39**: 385–389.
Büttner-Ennever JA, Horn AKE and Schmidtke K (1989b). Cell groups of medial longitudinal fasciculus and paramedian tracts. *Rev Neurol* **145**: 533–539.
Cahill M, Bannigan J and Eustace P (1996). Anatomy of the extraneural supply to the intracranial oculomotor nerve. *Br J Ophthalmol* **80**: 177–181.
Castro O, Johnson LN and Mamourian AC (1990). Isolated inferior oblique paresis from brainstem infarction. Perspective on oculomotor fascicular organisation in the ventral midbrain tegmentum. *Arch Neurol* **47**: 235–237.
Char DH (1992). Advances in thyroid orbitopathy. *Neuro-Ophthalmology* **12**: 25–39.
Cogan DG, Dhu FC, Bachman DM *et al.* (1981). The DAF syndrome. *Neuro-Ophthalmology* **2**: 7.
Cowan WM, Fawcett JW, O'Leary DDN *et al.* (1984). Regressive events in neurogenesis. *Science* **225**: 1258–1265.
Daniel SE, de Bruin VMS and Lees AJ (1995). The clinical and pathological spectrum of Steele-Richardson-Olszewski syndrome (Progressive supranuclear palsy): a reappraisal. *Brain* **118**: 759–770.
Daroff RB (1970). Oculomotor manifestations of brainstem and cerebellar dysfunction. In *Neuro-Ophthalmology* (ed. JL Smith), Vol. 5, pp. 62–71. Florida: Huffman, Hallandale.

Daroff RB, Hoyt WF, Sanders MD and Nelson LR (1968). Gaze-evoked eyelid and ocular nystagmus inhibited by the near reflex. Unusual ocular motor phenomena in a lateral medullary syndrome. *J Neurol Neurosurg Psychiat* **31**: 362–367.
Davis GV and Shock JP (1975). Septo-optic dysplasia associated with see-saw nystagmus. *Arch Ophthalmol* **93**: 137–139.
Dehaene I and Van Zandijcke M (1984). See-saw jerk nystagmus. *Neuro-Ophthalmology* **4**: 261.
Dell'osso LF, Schmidt D and Daroff RB (1979). Latent, manifest latent and congenital nystagmus. *Arch Ophthalmol* **97**: 1877–1885.
Depper MH, Truwit CL, Dreisbah JN and Kelly WM (1993). Isolated abducens nerve palsy: MR imaging findings. *Am J Roentgenol* **160**, 837–841.
Donaldson D and Rosenberg EP Jr (1988). Infarction of abducens nerve fascicle as a cause of isolated sixth nerve palsy related to hypertension. *Neurology* **38**: 1654.
Downie JA, Francis IC, Arnold JJ *et al.* (1993). Sudden blindness and total ophthalmoplegia in mucormycosis: a clinicopathological correlation. *J Clin Neuro-Ophthalmol* **13**: 27–34.
Duhamel JR, Goldberg ME, Fitzgibbon EJ *et al.* (1992). Saccade dysmetria in a patient with a right fronto-parietal lesion. *Brain* **115**: 1387–1402.
Eagle RC, Barker PB, Phil D *et al.* (1982). The atypical pigmentary retinopathy of Kearnes-Sayre syndrome: a light and electron microscope study. *Ophthalmology* **89**: 1433–1440.
Ezra E, Spalton D, Sanders MD *et al.* (1996). Ocular neuromyotonia. *Br J Ophthalmol* **80**: 350–355.
Fells P, Kousoulides L, Pappa A *et al.* (1994). Extraocular muscle problems in thyroid eye disease. *Eye* **8**: 497–505.
Fielder AR, Gresty MA, Dodd KL *et al.* (1986). Congenital ocular motor apraxia. *Trans Ophthalmol Soc UK* **105**: 589–598.
Fisher A, Gresty MA, Chambers B and Rudge P (1983). Primary position upbeating nystagmus: A variety of central positional nystagmus. *Brain* **106**: 949–964.
Fox AJ (1989). Angiography for third nerve palsy in children (editorial). *J Clin Neuro-Ophthalmol* **9**: 37–38.
Gabianelli EB, Klingele TG and Burde RM (1989). Acute oculomotor nerve palsy in childhood: is arteriography necessary? *J Clin Neuro-Ophthalmol* **9**: 33–36.
Galetta SL, Liu GT, Raps EC *et al.* (1994). Cyclodeviation in skew deviation. *Am J Ophthalmol*, **118**: 509–514.
Gauntt CD, Kaskii S and Nagata I: Monocular elevation paresis caused by an oculomotor fascicular impairment. *J Neuro-Ophthlamol* **15**: 11–14.
Gaymar B, Saudeau D, de Toffol B *et al.* (1991). Two mesencephalic lacunar infarcts presenting as Claude's syndrome and pure motor hemiparesis. *Eur Neurol* **31**: 152–155.
Gibson JM, Pimlott R and Kennard C (1987). Ocular motor and manual tracking in Parkinson's disease and the effect of treatment. *J Neurol Neurosurg Psychiat* **50**: 853–860.
Gomez CR, Gomez SM and Selhorst JB (1988). Acute thalamic esotropia. *Neurology* **38**: 1759–1762.
Grafton ST, Mazziotta JC, Woods RP and Phelps ME (1992). Human functional anatomy of visually guided hand movements. *Brain* **115**: 565–587.
Gresty MA, Ell JJ and Findley LJ (1982). Acquired pendular nystagmus: Its characteristics, localising value and pathophysiology. *J Neurol Neurosurg Psychiat* **45**: 431–439.
Gresty MA, Bronstein AM, Page NG and Rudge P (1991). Congenital-type nystagmus emerging in later life. *Neurology* **41**: 653–656.
Guy J and Day AL (1989). Intracranial aneurysms with superior division paresis of the oculomotor nerve. *Ophthalmology* **96**: 1071–1076.
Guy J, Day AL, Mickle JP and Schatz N (1989). Contralateral trochlear nerve paresis and ipsilateral Horner's syndrome. *Am J Ophthalmol* **107**: 73–76.
Hamed LM, Schatz NJ and Galetta SL (1988). Brainstem ocular motility defects and AIDS. *Am J Ophthalmol* **106**: 437–442.
Hanson MR, Hamid MA, Tomsak RL *et al.* (1986). Selective saccadic palsy caused by pontine lesions: clinical, physiological and pathological correlations. *Ann Neurol* **20**: 209–217.
Harding AE (1991). Neurological disease and mitochondrial genes. *Trends Neurosci* **14**: 132.
Halmagyi GM, Gresty MA and Leech J (1980). Reversed optokinetic nystagmus (OKN): Mechanism and clinical significance. *Ann Neurol* **7**: 429–435.
Halmagyi GM, Rudge P, Gresty MA and Sanders MD (1983). Downbeating nystagmus: A review of 62 cases. *Arch Neurol* **40**: 777–784.
Halmagyi GM, Aw ST, Dehaene I *et al.* (1994). Jerk-wave from see-saw nystagmus due to unilateral meso-diencephalic lesion. *Brain* **117**: 789–803.
Hedges TR and Hoyt WF (1982). Ocular tilt reaction due to an upper brainstem lesion: Paroxysmal skew deviation, torsion, and oscillation of the eyes with head tilt. *Ann Neurol* **11**: 537–540.
Hedges TR, Jones A, Stark L and Hoyt WF (1983). Botulin ophthalmoplegia: Clinical and oculographic observations. *Arch Ophthalmol* **101**: 211–213.
Hirose G, Kawada J, Tsukada K *et al.* (1991). Upbeat nystagmus: clinico-pathological and pathophysiological considerations. *J Neurol Sci* **105**: 159–167.
Holt IJ, Harding AE, Cooper JM *et al.* (1989). Mitochondrial myopathies: clinical and biochemical features of 30 patients with major deletions of muscle mitochondrial DNA. *Ann Neurol* **26**: 699–708.
Hommel M and Bogousslavsky J (1991). The spectrum of vertical gaze palsy following unilateral brainstem stroke. *Neurology* **41**; 1229–1234.
Hoogland YT, Kattah JC and Cupps T (1993). Ophthalmoplegia: differential diagnostic considerations in sarcoidosis. *J Rheumatol* **20**: 1262–1263.
Hoyt WF and Nactigäller H (1965). Anomalies of ocular motor nerves. Neuro-anatomic correlates of paradoxical innervation in Duane's syndrome and related congenital ocular motor disorders. *Am J Ophthalmol* **60**: 443–448.

Hriso LA, Masdeu JC and Miller A (1991). Monocular elevation weakness and ptosis: an oculomotor fascicular syndrome? *J Clin Neuro-Ophthalmol* **11**: 111–113.
Huber A (1974). Electrophysiology of the retraction syndromes. *Br J Ophthalmol* **58**: 293–300.
Hudson HL, Levin L and Feldon SE (1991). Graves' exophthalmos unrelated to extraocular muscle enlargement: superior rectus muscle inflammation may induce venous obstruction. *Ophthalmology* **98**: 1495–1499.
Imes RK, Schatz H, Hoyt WF *et al.* (1985). Evolution of optociliary veins in optic nerve sheath meningioma. *Arch Ophthalmol* **103**: 59–60.
Jacobson DM, McCanna TD and Layde PM (1994). Risk factors for ischaemic ocular motor nerve palsies. *Arch Ophthalmol* **112**: 961–966.
Jampel RS and Fells P (1968). Monocular elevation paresis caused by a central nervous system lesion. *Arch Ophthalmol* **80**: 45–57.
Jarrett WH and Gutman FA (1969). Ocular complications of infection in the paranasal sinuses. *Arch Ophthalmol* **81**: 683.
Johnston JL, Sharpe JA and Morrow MJ (1992). Paresis of contralateral smooth pursuit and norma, vestibular smooth eye movements after unilateral brainstem lesion. *Ann Neurol* **31**: 495–502.
Johnson LN and Hepler RS (1989). Isolated abducens nerve paresis from intrapontine, fascicular aducens nerve injury. *Am J Ophthalmol* **108**: 459–460.
Kaminski HJ, Maas E, Spiegel P and Ruff RL (1990). Why are eye muscles frequently involved in myasthenia gravis? *Neurology* **40**: 1663–1669.
Kao SC, Kendler DL, Nugent RA *et al.* (1993). Radiotherapy in the management of thyroid orbitopathy, computed tomography and clinical outcomes. *Arch Ophthalmol* **111**: 819–823.
Katz B, Leja S, Melles BB and Press GA (1989). Amyloid ophthalmoplegia. Ophthalmoparesis secondary to primary systemic amyloidosis. *J Clin Neuro-Ophthalmol* **9**: 39–42.
Kearns TP (1965). External ophthalmoplegia, pigmentary degeneration of the retina, and cardiomyopathy. A newly recognised syndrome. *Trans Am Ophthalmol Soc* **63**: 559.
Kennerdell JS, Dresner SC (1984). The nonspecific orbital inflammatory syndromes. *Surv Ophthalmol* **29**: 93–103.
King AJ, Stacey E, Stephenson G and Trimble RB (1995). Spontaneous recovery rates for unilateral sixth nerve palsies. *Eye* **9**: 476–479.
Knox DL, Green WR, Troncoso JC *et al.* (1995). Cerebral ocular Whipple's disease: A 62 year odessey from death to diagnosis. *Neurology* **45**: 617–625.
Kodski SR and Younge BR (1992). Acquired oculomotor, trochlear and abducens cranial nerve palsies in pediatric patients. *Am J Ophthalmol* **114**: 568–574.
Komatsu H and Wurtz RH (1989). Modulation of pursuit eye movements by stimulation of cortical areas MT and MST. *J Neurophysiol* **62**: 31–47.
Kommerell G and Hoyt WF (1973). Lateropulsion of saccadic eye movements. *Arch Neurol* **28**: 313–318.
Kommerell G and Schaubele G (1980). Superior oblique myokymia. An electromyographical analysis. *Trans Ophthalmol Soc UK* **100**: 504–506.
Ksiazek SM, Repka MX, Maguire A *et al.* (1989). Divisional oculomotor nerve paresis caused by intrinsic brainstem disease. *Ann Neurol* **26**: 714–718
Ksiazek SM, Slamovitz TL, Rosen CE *et al.* (1994). Fascicular arrangement in partial oculomotor paresis. *Am J Ophthalmol* **118**: 97–103.
Land MF (1992). Predictable eye-head co-ordination during driving. *Nature* **359**: 318–320.
Lee J and Flynn JT (1985). Bilateral superior oblique palsies. *Br J Ophthalmol* **69**: 508–513.
Lee J, Harris S, Cohen J *et al.* (1994). Results of a prospective randomised trial of botulinum toxin therapy in acute unilateral sixth nerve palsy. *J Pediat Ophthalmol Strab* **31**: 283–286.
Lee JP (1984). Superior oblique myokymia. *Arch Ophthalmol* **102**: 1178–1179.
Leone CR Jr, Piest KL and Newman RJ (1989). Medial and lateral wall decompression for thyroid ophthalmopathy. *Am J Ophthalmol* **108**: 160–166.
Leigh RJ (1989). The cortical control of ocular pursuit movements. *Rev Neurol* **145**: 605–612.
Leigh RJ and Zee DS (1991). *The Neurology of Eye Movements* 2nd edn. Philadelphia: FA Davis.
Leigh RJ, Averbuch-Heller L, Tomsak RL *et al.* (1994). Treatment of abnormal eye movements that impair vision: Strategies based on current concepts of physiology and pharmacology. *Ann Neurol* **36**: 129–141.
Lepore FE, Gulli V and Miller DC (1985). Neuro-ophthalmological findings with neuropathological correlation in bilateral thalamic-mesencephalic infarction. *J Clin Neuro-Ophthalmol* **5**: 224–228.
Lessell S, Lessell IM and Rizzo JF (1986). Ocular neuromyotonia after radiation therapy. *Am J Ophthalmol* **102**: 766–770.
Lim L, Rosenbaum AL and Demer JL (1995). Saccadic velocity analysis in patients with divergence paralysis. *J Pediatr Strab* **32**: 76–81.
Lueck CJ, Hamlyn P, Crawford TJ *et al.* (1991). A case of ocular tilt reaction and torsional nystagmus due to direct stimulation of the midbrain in man. *Brain* **114**: 2069–2079.
Lueck CJ, Tanyeri S, Crawford TJ *et al.* (1992a). Saccadic eye movements in Parkinson's disease I: Delayed saccades. *Q J Exp Psychol (A)* **45**: 193–210.
Lueck CJ, Crawford TJ and Henderson L (1992b). Saccadic eye movements in Parkinson's disease II: Remembered saccades — Towards a unified hypothesis? *Q J Exp Psychol (A)*, **45**: 211–223.
Mansour AM and Reinecke RD (1986). Central trochlear palsy. *Surv Ophthalmol* **30**: 279–297.
Marsh RJ, Dulley B and Kelly V (1977). External ocular motor palsies in ophthalmic zoster: A review. *Br J Ophthalmol* **61**: 677–682.

Mastrianni JA, Galetta SL, Raps EC *et al.* (1994). Isolated fascicular abducens nerve palsy and Lyme disease. *J Neuro-Ophthalmol* **14**: 2–5.
Mehler MF (1988). The neuro-ophthalmologic spectrum of the rostral basilar artery syndrome. *Arch Neurol* **45**: 966–971.
Meienberg O, Büttner-Ennever JA and Kraus-Ruppert R (1981). Unilateral paralysis of conjugate gaze due to lesion of the abducens nucleus. Clinico-pathological case report. *Neuro-Ophthalmology* **2**: 47–52.
Metz HS (1982). Duane's retraction syndrome. *Arch Ophthalmol* **100**: 843–844.
Miller NR, Kiel SM, Green WR and Clark AW (1982). Unilateral Duane's retraction syndrome (type I). *Arch Ophthalmol* **100**: 1468–1472.
Milone M, Monaco ML, Evoli A *et al.* (1993). Ocular myasthenia: diagnostic value of single fibre EMG in the orbicularis oculi muscle. *J Neurol Neurosurg Psychiat* **56**: 720–721.
Moore AT and Morin JD (1985). Bilateral acquired inflammatory Brown's syndrome. *J Pediat Ophthalmol Strab* **22**: 26.
Moraes CT, Dimauro S, Zeviani M *et al.* (1989). Mitochondrial DNA deletions in progressive external ophthalmoplegia and Kearns-Sayre syndrome. *New Engl J Med* **20**: 1293–1299.
Morrow JM and Sharpe JA (1990). Cerebral hemispheric localisation of smooth pursuit asymmetry. *Neurology* **40**: 284–292.
Moser ML, Schatz NJ, Savino PJ *et al.* (1988). Alternating skew on lateral gaze (bilateral abducting hypertropia). *Ann Neurol* **23**: 190–192.
Mullie MA, Harding AE, Petty RKH *et al.* (1985). The retinal manifestations of mitochondrial myopathy. *Arch Ophthalmol* **103**: 1825–1830.
Murray AND (1989). Early and late botulinum toxin treatment of acute sixth nerve palsy. *Austral NZ J Ophthalmol* **17**: 239–245.
Nakada T and Kwee IL (1986). Oculopalatal myoclonus. *Brain* **109**: 431–441.
O'Connor PS, Tredici TJ and Green RP (1983). Pupil-sparing third nerve palsies caused by aneurysm. *Am J Ophthalmol* **95**: 395–397.
O'Neill JH, Murray NMF and Newsom-Davis J (1988). The Lambert-Eaton myasthenic syndrome. *Brain* **111**: 577–596.
Oosterhuis HJGH (1989). The natural course of myasthenia gravis: A long-term follow-up study. J *Neurol Neurosurg Psychiat* **52**: 1121.
Palmer M, Green WR, Maumenee IH *et al.* (1985). Niemann-Pick Disease-Type C. *Arch Ophthalmol* **103**: 817–822.
Pierrot-Deseilligny C (1991). Cortical control of saccades. *Neuro-Ophthalmology* **11**: 63–75.
Pierrot-Deseilligny C, Rivaud S, Gaymard B and Agid Y (1991a). Cortical control of reflexive visually-guided saccades. *Brain* **114**: 1473–1485.
Pierrot-Deseilligny C, Rivaud S, Gaymard B and Agid Y (1991b). Cortical control of memory-guided saccades in man. *Exp Brain Res* **83**: 607–617.
Pierrot-Deseilligny C, Roas A, Masmoudi K *et al.* (1991c). Saccade deficits after a unilateral lesion affecting the superior colliculus. *J Neurol Neurosurg Psychiat* **54**: 1106–1109.
Porter JD, Baker RS, Rugusa RJ and Bruekner JK (1995). Extraocular muscles: basic and clinical aspects of structure and function. *Surv Ophthalmol* **39**: 451–483.
Power WJ, Rodrigues A, Neves RA *et al.* (1995). Disease relapse in patients with ocular manifestations of Wegener granulomatosis. *Ophthalmology* **102**: 154–160.
Ranalli PJ and Sharpe JA (1988). Vertical vestibulo-ocular reflex, smooth pursuit and eye-head tracking dysfunction in internuclear ophthalmoplegia. *Brain* **111**: 1299–1317.
Raroque HG, Hershewe GL and Snyder RD (1988). Möbius syndrome and transposition of the great vessels. *Neurology* **38**: 1894–1895.
Ravin JG, Sisson JC and Knapp WT (1975). Orbital radiation for the ocular changes of Grave's disease. *Am J Ophthalmol* **79**: 285–288.
Repka MX, Savino PJ and Reinecke RD (1994a). Treatment of acquired nystagmus with botulinum neurotoxin A. *Arch Ophthalmol* **112**: 1320–1324.
Repka MX, Lam GC and Morrison NA (1994b). The efficacy of botulinum neurotoxin A for the treatment of complete and partially recovered chronic sixth nerve palsy. *J Pediat Ophthalmol Strab* **31**: 79–83.
Richards BW, Jones FR and Younge BR (1992). Causes and prognosis in 4278 cases of paralysis of the oculomotor, trochlear and abducnes cranial nerves. *Am J Ophthalmol* **113**: 489–496.
Ridley A, Kennard C, Scholtz CL *et al.* (1987). Omnipause neurons in two cases of opsoclonus associated with oat cell carcinoma of the lung. *Brain* **110**: 1699–1709.
Rootman J (1988). *Diseases of the Orbit*. Philadelphia: JB Lippincott.
Rootman J and Nugent R (1982). The classification and management of acute orbital pseudotumors. *Ophthalmology* **89**: 1040–1048.
Rootman J, Hay E, Graeb D *et al.* (1986). Orbital-adnexal lymphangiomas: A spectrum of hemodynamically isolated vascular hamartomas. *Ophthalmology* **93**: 1558–1570.
Rosenberg M, Sharpe J and Hoyt WF (1975). Absent vestibulo-ocular reflexes and acute supratentorial lesions. *J Neurol Neurosurg Psychiat* **38**: 6–10.
Rowland LP (1988). Controversies about the treatment of myasthenia gravis. *J Neurol Neurosurg Psychiat* **43**: 644.
Ruben ST, Lee JP, O'Neil D *et al.* (1994). The use of botulinum toxin for the treatment of acquired nystagmus and oscillopsia. *Ophthalmology* **101**: 783–787.
Saad N and Lee J. Medial rectus electromyographic abnormalities in Duane syndrome. *J Paed Ophthalmol Strab* **20**: 88–91.

Sanders MD and Brown P (1986). Acute presentation of thyroid ophthalmopathy. *Trans Ophthalmol Soc UK* **105**: 720–722.

Sanders MD, Hoyt WF and Daroff RB (1968). Lid nystagmus evoked by ocular convergence: an ocular EMG study. *J Neurol Neurosurg Psychiat* **31**: 368–371.

Savino PJ, Hiliker JK, Casell GH and Schatz NJ (1982). Chronic sixth nerve palsies: Are they really harbingers of serious disease? *Arch Ophthalmol* **100**: 1442–1444.

Schatz NJ, Savino PJ and Corbett JC (1977). Primary aberrant oculomotor regeneration: A sign of intracavernous meningioma. *Arch Neurol* **34**: 29–32.

Schiller PH, Sandell JH and Maunsell JHR (1987). The effect in frontal eye field and superior colliculus lesions on saccadic latencies in the rhesus monkey. *J Physiol* **57**: 1033–1049.

Scott AB, Kraft SP (1985). Botulinum toxin injection in the management of lateral rectus paresis. *Ophthalmology* **92**: 676–683.

Sergott RC and Glaser JS (1981). Grave's ophthalmopathy. A clinical and immunologic review. *Surv Ophthalmol* **26**: 1–21.

Sevel D (1981). Brown's syndrome — A possible etiology explained embryologically. *J Pediat Ophthalmol Strab* **18**: 26–31.

Sharpe JA and Morrow MJ (1991). Cerebral hemispheric smooth pursuit disorders. *Neuro-Ophthalmology* **11**: 87–98.

Sharpe JA, Rosenberg MA, Hoyt WF *et al.* (1974). Paralytic pontine exotropia: *Neurology* **24**: 1076–1081.

Sharpe JA, Bondar RL and Fletcher WA (1985). Contralateral gaze deviation after frontal lobe haemorrhage. *J Neurol Neurosurg Psychiatr* **48**: 86.

Shorr N and Sieff SR (1986)
. The four stages of surgical rehabilitation of the patient with dysthyroid ophthalmopathy. *Ophthalmology* **93**: 476–483.

Shults WT, Hoyt WF, Behrens M *et al.* (1986). Ocular neuromyotonia. *Arch Ophthalmol* **104**: 1028–1034.

Soliven BD, Lange DJ and Penn AS (1988). Seronegative myasthenia gravis. *Neurology* **38**: 514–517.

Spector RH (1993). Vertical diplopia. *Surv Ophthalmol* **38**: 31–62.

Stern RM and Tomsak RL (1986). Magnetic resonance images in a case of 'divergence paralysis.' *Surv Ophthalmol* **30**: 397.

Stern BJ, Krumholz A, Johns C *et al.* (1985). Sarcoidosis and its neurological manifestations. *Arch Neurol* **49**: 909–917.

Striph GG and Burde RM (1988). Abducens nerve palsy and Horner's syndrome revisited. *J Clin Neuro-Ophthalmol* **8**: 13–17.

Susac JO, Hoyt WF, Daroff RB and Lawrence W (1970). Clinical spectrum of ocular bobbing. *J Neurol Neurosurg Psychiat* **33**: 771–775.

Ter Bruggen JP, Tijessen CC and Bastiaensen LAK (1993). Myotonic dystrophy: the natural history of eye movement disorders. *Neuro-Ophthalmology* **13**: 85–88.

Thomas R, Mathai A, Gieser SC and Ratmannal J (1993). Bilateral synergistic divergence. *J Pediat Ophthalmol Strab* **30**: 122–123.

Tomsak RL, Remler BF, Averbuch-Heller L *et al.* Unsatisfactory treatment of acquired nystagmus with retrobulbar injection of botulinum toxin. *Am J Ophthalmol* **119**: 489–496.

Towfighi J, Marks K, Palmer E and Vannucci R (1979). Möbius syndrome. Neuropathologic observations. *Acta Neuropathol* **48**: 11–17.

Traboulsi EI and Maumenee IH (1986). Extraoclar muscle aplasia in Moebius syndrome. *J Pediat Ophthalmol Strab* **23**: 126–127.

Trobe JD (1984). Cyclodeviation in acquired vertical strabismus. *Arch Ophthalmol* **102**: 717–720.

Troost BT (1989). Nystagmus: a clinical review. *Rev Neurol (Paris)* **45**: 417–428.

Troost BT and Daroff RB (1977). The ocular motor defects in progressive supranuclear palsy (PSP). *Ann Neurol* **2**: 397–403.

Tusa RJ, Zee DS, Hain TC and Simonsz HJ (1992). Voluntary control of congenital nystagmus. *Clin Vision* Sci **7**: 195–210.

Uyama J, Mimura O, Ikeda N and Shimo-Oku M (1993). Single fibre electromyography of extraocular muscles in myasthenia gravis. *Neuro-Ophthalmology* **13**: 253–261.

Van Dalen JTW, Van Mourek-Noordenbos AM (1984). Isolated inferior rectus paresis: A report of six cases. *Neurol-Ophthalmology* **4**: 89.

Victor DI (1976). The diagnosis of congenital unilateral third-nerve palsy. *Brain* **99**: 711–718.

Volpe NJ and Lessell S (1993). Remitting sixth nerve palsy in skull base tumours. *Arch Ophthalmol* **111**: 1391–1395.

Wall M and Wray SH (1983). The one-and-a-half syndrome — A unilateral disorder of the pontine tegmentum: A study of 20 cases and review of the literature. *Neurology* **33**: 971–980.

Waterson JA, Barnes GR and Grealy MA (1992). A quantitative study of eye and head movements during smooth pursuit in patients with cerebellar disease. *Brain* **115**: 1343–1358.

Weinberg DA, Lesser RL and Vollmer TL (1994). Ocular myasthenia: A protean disorder. *Surv Ophthalmol* **39**: 169–210.

Weiss A and Biersdorf WR (1989). Visual sensory disorders in congenital nystagmus. *Ophthalmology* **96**: 517–523.

White OB, Saint-Cyr JA and Tomlinson RD *et al.* (1988). Ocular motor deficits in Parkinson's disease. III. Coordination of eye and head movements. *Brain* **111**: 115–129.

Williams CS and Hoyt CS (1989). Acute concomitant esotropia in children with brain tumours. *Arch Ophthalmol* **107**: 376–378.

Wright JE (1988). Doyne Lecture: Current concepts in orbital disease. *Eye* **2**: 1–11.

Zee DS (1989). Adaptation to vestibular disturbances. *Neuro-Ophthalmology* **11**: 111–116.

Zee DS and Levi L (1989). Neurological aspects of vergence eye movements. *Rev Neurol* **145**: 613–620.

Zimmerman CF, Roach ES and Troost BT (1986). See-saw nystagmus associated with Chiari I malformation. *Arch Neurol* **43**: 299–300.

9

Disorders of facial nerve and eyelid function

FACIAL NERVE

SYNOPSIS OF ANATOMY

The neural pathways for the muscles of facial expression arise in the motor cortex, and are relayed via the facial nucleus in the pons to the facial (VIIth cranial) nerve. The peripheral facial nerve passes through the subarachnoid space (in the cerebellopontine angle), and the temporal bone before forming an extracranial segment to reach the face.

Supranuclear pathways
The cortical control for voluntary facial movements lies in the precentral gyrus of the frontal cerebral cortex. Supranuclear fibres are carried by the corticobulbar tract to the genu of the internal capsule and then to the facial nucleus in the pons via the cerebral peduncles. The portion of the facial nucleus supplying the muscles of the upper face (frontalis, orbicularis, oculi) receives corticobular fibres from both cerebral hemispheres, but those supplying the lower face are all crossed. Thus a unilateral hemisphere lesion will tend to cause a contralateral weakness of the lower face only, while a lower motor neuron facial weakness will involve the entire face on the same side. Exceptions to this principle do sometimes arise and selective involvement of facial musculature in peripheral lesions may be seen.

Reflex and automatic facial movements are regulated by the extrapyramidal system with the result that patients with this group of disorders demonstrate either a lack of facial expression as in Parkinson's disease, or the involuntary facial movements which characterize Meige's syndrome of blepharospasm and orofacial dystonia among other conditions.

Pons
In the pons, the facial nucleus is located in the ventrolateral angle of the tegmentum under the facial colliculus. Four separate subnuclei can be identified:

1) dorsomedial (auricular and occipital muscle)
2) intermediate (frontalis and orbicularis oculi)
3) ventromedial (platysma)
4) lateral (buccinator and buccolabial).

The motor axons pass dorsally, looping around the abducens nerve to form the pontine genu in the floor of the fourth ventricle before exiting the brain stem laterally together with the vestibulo-acoustic (VIIIth) nerve and the nervus intermedius. The nervus intermedius comprises visceral efferent fibres passing from the superior salivary nucleus to the sublingual, submandibular and lacrimal glands, together with special visceral afferent fibres serving taste sensation in the anterior two-thirds of the tongue and somatic sensory afferents from the posterior wall of the external auditory meatus.

Cerebellar pontine angle

The facial nerve, nervus intermedius and the VIIIth cranial nerve share a meningeal covering on exit from the pons before entering the lateral pontine cistern. The fibres of the nervus intermedius are loosely joined to the motor facial nerve near the entry to the internal acoustic meatus in the cerebellopontine angle, and the anterior inferior cerebellar artery may loop between the VIIth and VIIIth nerves at this point. In addition to causing facial weakness, mass lesions in the cerebellar pontine angle frequently impair function of the nervus intermedius resulting in abnormalities of tearing, taste and submandibular saliva flow, and of the vestibulo-acoustic nerve to impair hearing and balance. Large tumours also cause defects of the Vth, IXth and Xth nerves (for example cholesteatoma, vestibular schwannoma, meningioma). In addition, hyperkinetic disorders may be attributed to vascular compression to the facial nerve root as it crosses the subarachnoid space.

Temporal bone

In a Z-shaped course through the temporal bone, the facial nerve incorporates labyrinthine, tympanic and mastoid segments. The labyrinthine segment includes the geniculate ganglion, serving the afferent fibres of the nervus intermedius. The greater superficial petrosal nerve leaves the facial nerve at this point to synapse at the sphenopalatine ganglion and eventually reach the lacrimal gland via the zygomaticotemporal branch of the Vth nerve (V2) and the lacrimal nerve (V1). Lacrimal fibres also reach their destination via branches of the Vth and IXth cranial nerves. Turning a right angle posteriorly at the genu, the facial nerve passes through the middle ear (tympanic segment) giving off a branch to the stapedius muscle and then turns inferiorly (mastoid segment) to exit the temporal bone at the stylomastoid foramen. The chorda tympani is the terminal branch of the nervus intermedius and usually arises from the mastoid segment to convey secretor motor fibres to the sublingual and submandibular glands, special sensory afferents from the anterior tongue, and somatic sensory afferents from the posterior wall of the external auditory meatus.

Extracranial segment

After giving off branches to muscles of the anterior triangle of the neck, the main trunk of the facial nerve enters the parotid gland, bifurcates and then divides again in a variety of patterns to form temporal, zygomatic, buccal, mandibular and cervical branches. Intercommunications between these branches and fibres to the salivary glands accounts for the aberrant regeneration syndromes of facial synkinesis and crocodile tears which may follow facial nerve injury.

FACIAL WEAKNESS

Clinical assessment

Careful observation of the patient at rest often reveals a subtle facial weakness resulting in a flattened nasolabial fold and a wider palpebral aperture on the affected side. In supranuclear lesions, preservation of forehead frontalis function is typical due to bilateral cortical representation of these muscles. In other supranuclear disorders, there may be a dissociation between normal involuntary facial movements such as grimacing or blinking at a bright light and inability to perform voluntary movements. In infranuclear lesions, weakness of the orbicularis oculi muscle group becomes especially obvious on attempted eyelid closure, because the eye may stay open (lagophthalmos) and the palpebraloculogyricreflex (Bell's phenomenom) is preserved driving the eye upwards and outwards (Francis and Loughhead, 1984).

Impaired ipsilateral taste function and tear secretion indicates that the lesion is peripheral to the facial nucleus. Tear secretion is important clinically not only because of the localizing value of noting loss of function in fibres to the lacrimal gland via the greater superficial petrosal nerve and nervus intermedius, but also because of the increased risk of corneal ulceration and visual loss in facial palsy which results from incomplete lid closure when combined with deficient lubrication. Many patients with facial weakness may in fact have epiphora because orbicularis weakness leads to poor tear drainage either from paralytic ectropion or functional loss of the lacrimal pump which accompanies a normal blink. This epiphora may not reduce the risk of corneal ulceration because reflex tear secretion rates will still be impaired. The Schirmer's test of tear production is helpful, but slit lamp assessment of the precorneal tear film and corneal epithelial health is much more useful when available. Corneal health is further imperilled by defective function of the ophthalmic division of the trigeminal nerve as neuropathic changes can damage the epithelium even without the exposure and lubrication deficits associated with a facial nerve paresis. The combination of both Vth and VIth nerve lesions is therefore particularly dangerous for the eye.

Causes of peripheral facial palsy

Table 9.1 Causes of facial nerve disorders

Cause	Number (%)
Bell's palsy (idiopathic)	1272 (53)
Trauma	502 (21)
Accidental	
Iatrogenic and surgical	
Herpes zoster (Ramsay–Hunt syndrome)	173 (8)
Tumours	155 (7)
Acoustic neuroma	
Facial neuroma	
Non-Hodgkin's lymphoma	
Carcinomatous meningitis	
Infections and inflammation	88 (4)
Polyradiculopathy	
Infectious mononucleosis	
Lyme disease	
Middle ear infection	
Basal meningitis	
Sarcoidosis	
Melkersson-Rosenthal syndrome	
Birth (congenital and acquired)	78 (3)
Hemifacial spasm	54 (2)
CNS disease (axial lesions)	27 (1)
Other	57 (2)
Acute porphyrias	
Myasthenia gravis	
Botulism	
Myotonic dystrophy	
Progressive hemifacial atrophy	

From May and Galetta (1990).

Intra-axial lesions

The facial nerve is involved in the dorsolateral pontine syndrome of Foville, comprising ipsilateral paralysis of abduction (or gaze palsy), lower motor neuron facial palsy, loss of taste in the anterior two-thirds of the tongue, Horner's syndrome, facial analgesia and peripheral deafness. Partial forms are more frequent than the full syndrome. Facial weakness is also seen in paramedian and basal pontine lesions (Millard-Gubler syndrome) with additional ipsilateral abducens palsy and contralateral hemiplegia. Intrinsic pontine lesions are usually the result of infarction, haemorrhage, tumour or demyelination. Congenital facial palsy often arises at the level of the brain stem, referred to as the Möbius syndrome (see Chapter 8).

Peripheral lesions

Peripheral causes of facial palsy include herpes zoster cephalicus (geniculate herpes or Ramsay-Hunt syndrome) in which there is severe pain in and around the ear together with the appearance of vessicle in the ear, neck, face and mouth in a distribution which reflects the degree of involvement of nerves with communicating branches to the facial nerve (nerves V, IX, X, and C2–4), and the appearance of a facial palsy. Other infectious and immune-related neuropathies which cause facial weakness include postinfectious polyradiculopathy (Guillain-Barré syndrome), infectious mononucleosis, Lyme disease, complicated otitis media (Gradinego's syndrome), leprosy and syphilis.

Additional causes include trauma (basal skull fractures, neurosurgery), tumours in the cerebellopontine angle and facial neuromas, metastatic deposits or carcinomatous meningitis, and sarcoidosis.

Finally, metabolic diseases (acute porphyria) and myopathic processes (myasthenia gravis, myotonic dystrophy, botulism) need to be excluded before a diagnosis of idiopathic acute facial palsy (Bell's palsy) can be made. In Bell's palsy, subjective complaints of pain and facial numbness are frequent, as are recurrent episodes. Dysacusis and abnormalities of taste and salivary secretion indicate a lesion of the tympanomastoid portion of the facial nerve within the temporal bone. There is an association between Bell's palsy and both diabetes and pregnancy, and a positive family history may be present.

Ophthalmic aspects of the management of facial palsy

Undoubtedly the most pressing aspect of the care of a patient with facial palsy is protection of the eye (Table 9.2). Lagophthalmos results in corneal drying and epithelial

Table 9.2 The House classification system for reporting results of recovery from facial palsy (House, 1983)

Degree of injury	Grade	Definition
Normal	I	No abnormality
Mild dysfunction	II	Complete eyelid closure without effort; slight smile asymmetry
Moderate dysfunction	III	Obvious weakness on resting; brow ptosis; eyelid closure on effort; mouth movement with effort
Moderate-severe dysfunction	IV	Disfiguring weakness; incomplete eyelid closure; mouth asymmetry on maximal effort; synkinesis and mass movement
Severe dysfunction	V	Motion barely perceptible; synkinesis and mass movement absent
Total paralysis	VI	No movement and complete loss of tone

ulceration with the risk of blindness from infective keratitis and corneal vascularization. The risk is increased because of concomitant tear film insufficiency, and most of all when there is additional loss of function in the ophthalmic division of the trigeminal nerve causing loss of sensation and neurotrophic corneal changes. The use of ocular lubricants alone is often inadequate and lid taping is mandatory when the patient is asleep or unconscious. When the corneal epithelium ulcerates in spite of these measures, a temporary ptosis induced by botulinum toxin levator chemodenervation may be valuable to allow time for spontaneous recovery of facial function or the planning of some form of tarsorraphy. Nowadays oculoplastic surgery can be used to achieve some degree of palpebral symmetry in unrecovered facial palsy, as well as to provide corneal protection. Available techniques include medial and lateral tarsorraphy, canthal slings and procedures to lower the upper lid by retractor recession or by weighting the tarsus with gold implants. Facial nerve anastomosis, facial–hypoglossal nerve transfer and temporalis transfer may all play an additional role in rehabilitation.

Hyperkinetic facial syndromes

Spontaneous anomalous facial movements may frequently present as an ophthalmic complaint. These include primary and secondary blepharosplasm, hemifacial spasm, facial synkinesis following recovery from facial palsy, tonic contracture and myokymia.

Blepharospasm

Essential (idiopathic) blepharospasm is form of focal dystonia typically affecting patients in their sixth and seventh decades, more frequently women than men, which is characterized by involuntary and repetitive eyelid closure due to spasmodic contraction of the the orbicularis oculi muscles in the absence of significant ocular pathology (Elston *et al.*, 1988). Eyebrow depression is a characteristic finding during spasms. It is usually bilateral and often progressive in severity (Table 9.3). In many patients the movement disorder includes both blepharospasm and oromandibular dystonia (Breughel's syndrome or Meige's disease) (Beradelli *et al.*, 1985). In others blepharospasm arises as part of a generalized or secondary dystonia of which the causes include basal ganglia infarction, Wilsons's disease, neuroleptic drugs, progressive supranuclear palsy, encephalitis lethargica, Parkinson's disease, Huntingdon's disease and Shy Drager syndrome.

The intensity of spasms may range from increased blinking caused by external stimuli (bright lights, wind), to mild noticeable inappropriate eyelid closure through to moderate spasms and severe, functionally incapacitating spasms. Whilst formerly considered a functional disorder requiring psychological therapies, it is now evident that blepharospasm has an organic basis. The neuronal arc of the facial reflexes mediated by the Vth and VIIth nerves are normal, but there appears to be an abnormal excitatory drive,

Table 9.3 Assessment of visual disability in blepharospasm (Elston *et al.*, 1988)

Category / description	Visual function
1. Blind	No effective function
2. Dependent	Needs assistance to move outside familiar environment
3. Independent (poor function)	Able to walk independently; unable to drive, read, watch television; severe photophobia
4. Independent (moderate function)	Limited practical functions; unable to read or work
5. Inconvenienced	Intermittent interference; unable to drive; can work
6. Normal	

perhaps from the basal ganglia, to the facial motor neurons and the interneurons which mediate the facial reflexes in the brain stem (Beradelli *et al.*, 1985). Use of EMG recordings of the orbicularis oculi (OO) during involuntary closure shows dystonic activities lasting from 200ms to several minutes. This is associated with prolonged periods of involuntary inhibition of the levator palpebrae (LP) making it impossible for the patient to open their eyes.

In some individuals LP inhibition is the dominant abnormality (atypical blepharospasm) due to disturbed reciprocal innervation of LP and OO (Aramideh *et al.*, 1994; Elston, 1992b), especially those with extrapyramidal syndromes. Lid elevation may be accomplished after backward head thrusts, extensive frontalis action or by digital rubbing of the the frontalis. This is often termed apraxia of eyelid opening (Goldstein and Cogan, 1965) although because movements can be voluntarily achieved, albeit intermittently, this term is not entirely appropriate.

Pharmacological and biofeedback therapies are usually disappointing and surgical treatments including orbicularis stripping and facial nerve avulsion are only indicated in the last resort. However, injections of the presynaptic blocking agent botulinum ('a gift from Ophthalmology to Neurology' — Alan Scott) is undoubtedly efficaceous. Botulinum is injected subcutaneously into the orbicularis oculi muscles with the result that most patients enjoy a significant reduction in facial spasms within a few days of injection and lasting for an average of 3 months. Longer term benefit is limited by axonal respouting resulting in reinervation of injected muscles but repeated injections are well tolerated (Savino *et al.*, 1984; Elston *et al.*, 1988; Osako and Keltner, 1991). Patients with typical blepharospasm including depressed eyebrows and with obvious orbital orbicularis contraction respond better to botulinum toxin injections than those with no obvious contracture of the orbicularis. Injection of botulinum into multiple sites in the orbicularis, especially the pretarsal portion may be associated with better and less variable responses to treatment (Aramideh *et al.*, 1994).

Hemifacial spasm

In hemifacial spasm unilateral periodic tonic and clonic facial contractions usually start around the eye and then as the condition progresses, spasms may involve the whole face including the platysma muscle. In contrast to idiopathic blepharospasm, the involuntary movements occur in sleep as well as when the patient is awake. The differential diagnosis includes focal epilepsy, facial neuromyotonia, myokymia and facial synkinesia. Imaging of the posterior fossa by MR may reveal extramedullary compressive lesions of the facial nerve including basilar aneurysm and tumours in the cerebellopontine angle (Moller and Janetta, 1984). When there is no mass, neurosurgical microvascular decompression of a tortuous or ectatic anterior inferior cerebellar, posterior inferior cerebellar or basilar artery (Fig. 9.1) itself may be beneficial but the patient is exposed to a risk of permanent facial weakness and the possibility of more general complications (Barker *et al.*, 1995). Many patients can be satisfactorily managed by using botulinum toxin injections to the affected muscles with repeated treatments as required: others find that night-time use of carbamazepine is adequate (Osako and Keltner, 1991; Neilsen, 1984; Elston *et al.*, 1988; Boglan and May, 1986).

Facial synkinesis

Following a VIIth nerve paresis, a patient may demonstrate ipsilateral involuntary narrowing of the palpebral apperture when other facial muscle groups are voluntarily moved. In a typical instance, mouth movements (orbicularis oris) whilst eating or smiling are associated with unwanted eye closure (Putterman, 1990). Botulinum toxin injections may offer temporary relief, given on the same basis as for the treatment of hemifacial spasm.

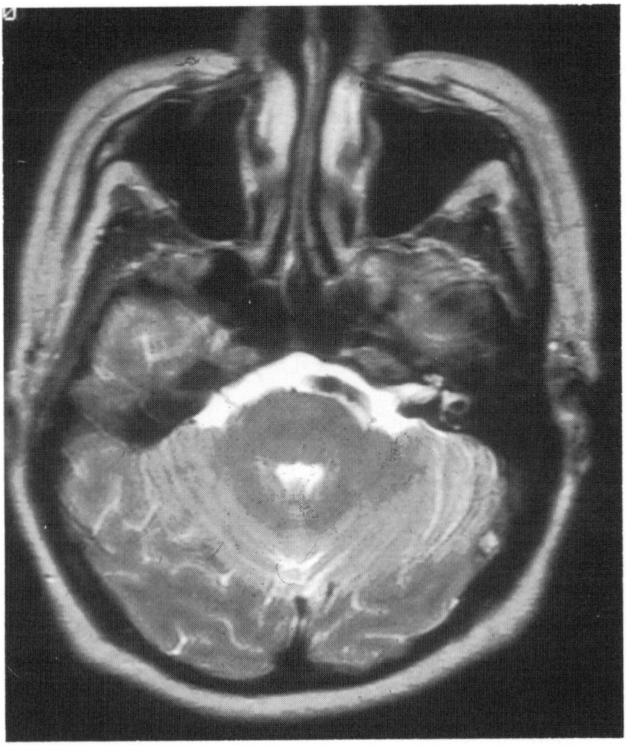

Figure 9.1 MRI scan of basilar artery ectasia in a patient with hemifacial spasm.

A clear distinction can be made between synkinesis due to aberrant regeneration syndromes and the rare congenital inverse jaw-winking (Marcus–Gunn) phenomenon. In this entity, there is congenital inhibition of the levator muscle giving rise to a resting ptosis which is released on stimulation of the trigeminal nerve motor supply to the medial or lateral pterygoid muscles resulting in the upper lid moving up and down on jaw movement. Electromyography shows that orbicularis oculi involvement is not part of the jaw-winking phenomenon, in distinction to the facial nerve synkinetic syndromes.

A further aberrant regeneration syndrome following facial nerve injury at or above the level of the geniculate ganglion is gustatory tearing (crocodile tears) where parasympathetic fibres supplying the salivary glands via the chorda tympani become misrouted with the result that the stimulus to salivate (food or the prospect of food) is inappropriately accompanied by ipsilateral tearing. A variety of anatomical mechanisms have been proposed: misrouting of visceromotor fibres from the chorda tympani to the greater superfical petrosal nerve and thence to the lacrimal gland, anomalous collateral sprouting of fibres from the glossopharyngeal nerve to the greater superficial petrosal nerve at the tympanic plexus, and proximal misrouting at the site of afferent and visceromotor fibres in the nervus intermedius. Transtympanic division of the tympanic branch of the glossopharyngeal nerve may offer a surgical solution to an acquired gustolacrimal reflex following facial palsy. Vidian neurectomy in the pteygopalatine fossa may also help.

Facial myokymia

Facial myokymia is characterized by a fine fibrillary movement of the facial muscles in a unilateral intermittent pattern. A benign form is common, limited to the eyelids in a transient manner which is apparently exacerbated by anxiety or fatigue. More generalized involvement is associated with intrinsic brain stem lesions and with extramedullary compression, requiring formal evaluation. Occasionally there is additional facial contracture and paresis indicating an intrinsic pontine lesion rostral to the facial nucleus.

EYELIDS

SYNOPSIS OF ANATOMY AND PHYSIOLOGY

The levator palpebrae superioris is the principle muscle involved in opening the upper lid and maintaining normal lid position — accessory roles are played by the frontalis and Müller's muscles. The origin of the levator is blended with the superior rectus the lesser wing of the sphenoid bone at the orbital apex. About 1cm behind the orbital septum it ends as a membranous expansion, or aponeurosis which spreads out to attach to the tarsal plate, the orbital septum and the suspensory ligaments. Müller's muscle is composed of a thin band of smooth muscle fibres lying on the inferior surface of the levator and inserts onto the tarsal plate. The frontalis muscle acts as an indirect lid elevator by means of attachments to the orbicularis oculi muscle.

The tone of the levator palpebrae muscle is governed by both the corticobulbar and extrapyramidal systems which synapse with neurons of the levator nucleus in the oculomotor complex via the periaqueductal grey. Although the LP motor nucleus is unpaired, the premotor control of the LP is lateralized in part in the cortex, extrapyramidal system and rostral brain stem. The diffuse projections of the reticular activating system also influence eyelid opening and lid position reflects arousal levels. Within the oculomotor complex in the mesencephalon, the levator nucleus lies in the midline, caudally and dorsally sending fibres to join the other axons of each oculomotor nerve. The principle of equal innervation of yoked extraocular muscles (Hering's law) applies to the eyelids so that if one eyelid is ptotic, the other will retract as extra innervation flows to both sides. During normal fast and slow vertical eye movements the tonus of the levator is directly linked to that of the superior rectus so that the upper lids accurately follow the movements of the globe. During sleep and forced eyelid closure, however, the levator is inhibited as the superior rectus contracts (Bell's phenomenon).

PRINCIPLES OF EXAMINATION AND TOPICAL DIAGNOSIS

Ptosis

Neuropathic ptosis is usually the result of loss of function of the oculomotor nerve or the oculosympathetic pathway (infranuclear ptosis) but both supranuclear and nuclear forms are also seen.

Both unilateral and bilateral ptosis may occur in hemispheric lesions, usually following a stroke (cerebral ptosis). One characteristic variant is the failure of initiation of eyelid opening which results from a transient failure to overcome levator inhibitory pathways. This is known as 'apraxia of eyelid opening' and frequently full elevation of the upper lids can only be accomplished by a special manoeuvre such as thrusting the head backwards, or by massaging the brow. Apraxia of eyelid opening is also a frequent feature of dystonic blepharospasm (see above).

Dysfunction of voluntary lid control can also manifest as an inability to initiate or sustain lid closure ('apraxia of lid closure or closing impersistence'). This has been observed in patients with focal or diffuse hemispheric damage (encephalitis, stroke, Creutzfeldt-Jakob disease, progressive supranuclear palsy, and may also be unilateral (Russell, 1980).

Mesencephalic ptosis results from destructive or congenital lesions of the upper brain stem which involve the caudal portion of the oculomotor complex, or the floor of the third ventricle or rostral midbrain (Büttner-Ennever *et al.*, 1989) and infranuclear ptosis may result from fascicular and peripheral lesions of the oculomotor nerve. Pupillary and extraocular muscle involvement is usual, but an isolated unilateral ptosis may arise in patients with intracranial aneurysm and intracavernous meningioma. In ptosis due to oculosympathetic paresis (Horner's syndrome) the abnormality is usually mild, there is an 'upside down' ptosis of the lower lid due to involvement of the lower lid Müller's muscle and ipsilateral miosis (see Chapter 2).

Ptosis arising from abnormalities at the neuromuscular junction and from myopathies may be congenital or acquired. Congenital ptosis occurs frequently and is usually due to maldevelopment of the levator muscle or its tendon. Unilateral and bilateral involvement may be seen: typically in addition to limitation of lid elevation on upgaze, there is limited depression on downgaze reflecting abnormal muscle relaxation. Acquired ptosis is seen in the mitochondrial cytopathies which cause chronic progressive external ophthalmoplegia, in myotonic dystrophy, in myasthenia and other neuromuscular junction diseases, and also following trauma, inflammation or infiltration of the levator or its tendon.

Disinsertion of the levator tendon results in involutional ptosis in the elderly, in long-term contact lens wearers and following various types of elective ocular surgery. In such cases the range of levator function is typically full, and the skin is indistinct and elevated. Diagnostic confusion is also caused by 'pseudoptosis' arising when one eye is deviated downwards (hypotropic) or in enophthalmos and microphthalmos.

Inappropriate elevation of the upper lid

Congenital causes of lid retraction include the Marcus–Gunn phenomenon in which there is paradoxic eyelid retraction evoked by jaw movement or swallowing. This is thought to represent a trigemino-oculomotor synkinesis, and is subdivided into internal pterygoid and external pterygoid forms. The external pterygoid form is the most frequent, in which there is a unilateral ptosis followed by lid elevation in association with the jaw moving to the opposite side or projecting forward. In the internal pterygoid form the lid elevates on closing the mouth or clenching the teeth.

Acquired eyelid retraction may arise in supranuclear lesions of the periaqueductal and dorsal midbrain regions. This is referred to as Collier's sign and may be seen in isolation or in association with the other features of Parinaud's syndrome (pupillary light-near dissociation, vertical gaze abnormalities, convergence-retraction nystagmus). Eyelid retraction is also seen in aberrant regeneration of the oculomotor nerve, when the lid elevates in association with elevation, depression or adduction of the involved eye. Primary aberrant regeneration of the IIIrd nerve is said to be a characteristic feature of intracavernous aneurysms and meningiomas. The commonest pattern observed is retraction of the lid on depression of the eye (pseudo-von Graefe's sign) but medial rectus contraction and adduction may also generate the same effect. When the fellow eye is ptotic, the upper lid may show abnormal retraction as a result of equal innervation flowing to each lid in an attempt to overcome a peripheral weakness on one side.

Myopathic processes cause abnormal lid elevation: maternal hyperthyroidism causes transient congenital lid retraction. In established dysthyroid eye disease, lid retraction may reflect hyperthyroidism with potentiation of the action of Müller's muscle, pathologic shortening of the levator muscle or overaction of the superior rectus–levator muscle complex in an attempt to overcome a pathologically shortened inferior rectus muscle.

The upper lids may be involved in nystagmus. Eyelid nystagmus on attempted convergence is associated with ill-defined cerebellar or brain stem damage (Sanders *et al.*, 1968).

REFERENCES

Adams CG and Kirkness JP (1987). Botulinum toxin A induced protective ptosis. *Eye* **1**: 603–608.

Aramideh M, Ongeboer de Vosser, Devriese PP *et al.* (1994). Electromyographic features of levator palpebrae superioris and orbicularis oculi muscles in blepharospasm. *Brain* **117**: 27–38.

Barker FG II, Janetta PJ, Bissonette DJ *et al.* (1995). Microvascular decompression for hemifacial spasm. *J Neurosurg* **82**: 201–210.

Beradelli A, Rothwell JC, Day BL and Marsden CD (1985). Pathophysiology of blepharospasm and oromandibular dystonia. *Brain* **108**: 593–608.

Boglan AW and May M (1986). Treatment of facial spasm with oculinum. *J Paed Ophthalmol Strab* **23**: 216–221.

Büttner-Ennever JA, Acheson JF, Buttner U *et al.* (1989). Ptosis and supranuclear downgaze palsy. *Neurology* **39**: 385–389.

Dutton JJ and Buckley E (1986). Botulinum toxin in the management of blepharospasm. *Arch Neurol* **43**: 380–382.

Elston JS (1988). The clinical use of botulinum toxin. *Sem Ophthalmol* **III**: 249–260.

Elston JS (1992a). The management of blepharospasm and hemifacial spasm. *J Neurol* **239**: 5–8.

Elston JS (1992b). A new variant of blepharospasm. *J Neurol Neurosurg Psychiat* **55**: 369–371.

Elston JS, Marsden CD, Grandas F and Quinn NP (1988). The significance of ophthalmological symptoms in idiopathic blepharospasm. *Eye* **2**: 435–439.

Francis IL and Loughhead JA (1984). Bell's phenomenon. A study of 508 patients. *Aust J Ophthalmol* **12**: 15–21.

Goldstein JE and Cogan DG (1965). Apraxia of lid opening. *Arch Ophthalmol* **73**: 155.

House JW (1983). Facial nerve grading system. *Laryngoscope* **93**: 1056–1069.

Jordan DR, Anderson RL and Thiese SM (1989). Intractable orbicularis myokymia: treatment alternatives. *Ophthal Surg* **20**: 280–283.

Keane JR and Young JA (1985). Blepharospasm with bilateral basal ganglia infarction. *Arch Neurol* **42**: 1206–1208.

Lepore F (1987). Bilateral cerebral ptosis. *Neurology* **37**: 1043–1046.

May M and Galetta S (1990). Causes of facial nerve disorders. In *The Facial Nerve and Related Disorders of the Face*. (ed. JS Glaser), pp. 255. Philadelphia: JP Lippincott.

Moller AR and Jenetta PJ (1984) On the origin of synkinesis in hemifacial spasm: results of intracranial recordings. *J Neurosurg* **61**: 569–576.

Nielsen VK (1984). I. Pathophysiology of hemifacial spasm: A reversible pathophysiologic state. *Neurology* **34**: 418–426.

Osako M and Keltner JL (1991). Botulinum A toxin in Ophthalmology. *Surv Ophthalmol* **36**: 28–45.

Putterman AN (1990). Botulinum toxin injection in the treatment of VIIth nerve misdirection. *Am J Ophthalmol* **110**: 205–206.

Russell RW (1980). Supranuclear palsy of eyelid closure. *Brain* **103**: 71–82.

Sanders MD, Hoyt WF and Daroff RB (1968). Lid nystagmus evoked by ocular convergence: an ocular EMG study. *J Neurol Neurosurg Psychiat* **31**: 368–371.

Savino PJ, Stern M, Hurtig H *et al.* (1984). Pharmacologic therapy versus botulinum in the treatment of blepharospasm: A preliminary report. *Ann Neurol* **16**: 125.

Schmidtke K and Büttner-Ennever A (1992). Nervous control of eyelid function. *Brain* **115**: 227–247.

Scott AB, Rosenbaum A and Collins CC (1973). Pharmacological weakening of the extraocular muscles. *Invest Ophthalmol Vis Sci* **12**: 924–927.

10

Neuro-ophthalmic aspects of migraine and other headaches

MIGRAINE

Migraine is a periodic paroxysmal disorder of the central nervous system affecting up to 10% of the healthy population; 80% of migraine sufferers experience their first attack before the age of 30 years (Table 10.1).

The typical headache of migraine lasts for 4–72 hours, has a unilateral location, a pulsating quality, is of moderate or severe intensity so as to inhibit or prohibit normal activities, is aggravated by physical exertion, and is associated with nausea, vomiting, photophobia or phonophobia. The pain experienced in both migraine with aura (classic migraine) and migraine without aura (common migraine) is the same and represents activation of the same nociceptive pathway. Migraine can produce visual disturbances involving both the afferent and efferent visual system, the best known of which is the aura of classic migraine in which a visual field defect surrounded by positive phenomena develops and expands from a central paracentral abnormality to a luminous crescent of moving, coloured angles. This is known as a fortification spectrum, or teichopsia. Although migraine rarely causes a stroke, it is a common cause of stroke in young otherwise healthy adults and accounts for up to 25% of cases of stroke in patients under the age of 50. Some patients with migraine-related stroke also have mitral valve prolapse, but the significance of this association is uncertain. In other patients there are elevated concentrations of antiphospholipid antibodies which may cross-react with platelets to produce cerebral or retinal thrombosis (Bogousslavsky *et al.*, 1988; Hupp *et al.*, 1989).

Table 10.1 Classification of migraine

Common migraine
Classic migraine
Complicated migraine
Cerebral and basilar
Ophthalmoplegic
Ocular
Migrainous neuralgia (cluster headaches)

COMMON MIGRAINE

In common migraine, the chief features are headache and a variety of autonomic disturbances including nausea. During a prodrome lasting between hours and days there may be vague mood changes followed by headache which may be focal or unilateral initially and which then becomes generalized and which lasts for a few hours. Nausea and vomiting accompany the acute attack, and regression of symptoms is normally associated with a diuresis. Ocular signs and symptoms of classic migraine include conjunctival injection, lid swelling and photophobia – these are more marked however in migrainous neuralgia (see below). Often the pain is retro-orbital and may be mistaken for eye or sinus disease.

CLASSIC MIGRAINE

In classic migraine, episodes are marked by a distinct prodrome or aura when visual symptoms are prominent and this usually lasts for about 20 minutes. This is followed in typical cases by headaches in a stereotyped pattern for the affected individual. Sometimes the headache and the aura have their onset at the same time. The visual sensations can be dramatic and intense starting in a localized part of the visual field and spreading slowly outwards (spreading depression). Typically there is a negative scotoma surrounded by scintillations forming highly defined geometrical zig-zag patterns known as fortification spectra (Woods *et al.*, 1994). This characteristic build-up and march of scintillating scotoma only occurs in some 10% of migraine patients, but some form of scintillating positive scotoma occurs in about 80% of all classic migraine sufferers. Additional visual disturbances include metamorphopsia, diplopia, polyopia and transient visual loss. In distinction to the flashing, flickering or bright moving spots of occipital epilepsy, migrainous visual phenomena last for minutes rather than seconds.

COMPLICATED MIGRAINE

In complicated migraine, a variety of transient paroxysmal neurological phenomena accompany a migrainous episode. Three categories with visual features are cerebral migraine, ophthalmoplegic migraine and ocular migraine.

Cerebral migraine

A variety of abnormalities arise during the migrainous aura, including homonymous field defects, paraestheia, hemiplegia and dysphasia, followed by headache. In some cases cortical dysfunction includes disturbances of colour vision, facial recognition, reading, transient global amnesia or acute confusion or psychosis. In others the prodrome encompasses alterations of time sense and body image, as well as distortion of vision such as illusions of enlargement, shrinking and elongation ('the Alice in Wonderland syndrome'). Children in particular may develop paroxysmal neurological symptoms referrable to brain stem and posterior cerebral artery ischaemia as a component of the migrainous episode (basilar migraine). These symptoms include bilateral visual loss, ataxia, vertigo, and dysarthria, followed by severe headache, usually in the occipital region (Hupp, 1989).

In some migraineurs, negative visual phenomena are prominent: these include homonymous, central, altitudinal or tunnel scotomas accompanied by scintillations. The entire visual field may appear faded, blurred or appear as though seen through water.

Sometimes the episodic migrainous dysfunction may occur without any headache, and further diagnostic difficulty is presented by the variety of diseases which may mimic migrainous visual disturbances. Uniocular phosphenes and photopsia may reflect posterior vitreous or retinal detachment, inflammation or infection of the retina or choroid, or optic neuritis. A scintillating scotoma may be an occipital cortex seizure focus due to a tumour or arteriovenous malformation (AVM) but in such cases the headache is not typically migrainous. Posterior cerebral hemisphere transient ischaemic attacks may also cause scintillations, but the onset is typically instantaneous without any build-up and other features of vertebrobasilar insufficiency such as syncope, vertigo and diplopia are common.

Ophthalmoplegic migraine

In ophthalmoplegic migraine an episodic ocular motor nerve palsy occurs which is usually associated with severe ipsilateral hemicranial headache (Stommel *et al.*, 1993; Bailey *et al.*, 1984). Typically the IIIrd cranial nerve is involved, often but not always including the pupil, and function can be permanently lost following repeated episodes. Normally the paresis resolves days or weeks after the cessation of headache. With the advent of modern neuroimaging and angiography, many cases formerly described as ophthalmoplegic migraine in fact turn out be due to aneurysm, cavernous sinus inflammatory disease and tumours. Ophthalmoplegic migraine affects children or young adults (a younger age group than that normally presenting with a painful IIIrd nerve palsy due to intracranial aneurysm). The IVth and VIth nerves are less frequently involved. On occasion, incomplete IIIrd nerve pasy is seen, adding to diagnostic difficulties. Unilateral cyclical pupillary mydriasis has been ascribed to migraine in some individuals, but when there is absolutely no abnormality of extraocular movements or a ptosis, it is vital to exclude intermittent angle closure glaucoma. Ophthalmoplegic migraine probably arises as a result of vasospasm and microvascular insuffiency of the blood supply to the peripheral oculomotor nerve, although direct evidence for this is lacking (Sarkies *et al.*, 1985; Edelson and Levy, 1974; Woods *et al.*, 1984).

Ocular migraine

Ocular migraine affects only the anterior visual pathways causing monocular visual loss arising either in association with a migraine attack or in an individual with a strong history of either classic or common migraine. The visual loss may reflect vasospasm in the retinal or posterior ciliary circulations resulting in ischaemia of either neurosensory retina, or choroid, or optic nerve. The term 'retinal' or 'choroidal' migraine is sometimes used (O'Sullivan, *et al.*, 1992). A choroidal pattern of vascular involvement is suggested when small irregular patchy scotomas within the monocular field progress to complete blindness. Most attacks of partial or complete loss of vision that originate in the eye as part of a migraine syndrome are transient, but permanent monocular or binocular loss or acuity, field or both may develop. This may be the result of ischaemic optic neuropathy, central and branch retinal artery occlusion, central serous retinopathy, cotton wool spot formation, or retinal or vitreous haemorrhage. The retinal vessels may appear markedly constricted if examined during an attack, but more commonly the diagnosis is made only after exhaustive studies to exclude an occult source of embolism or other cause of amaurosis fugax in a patient with a strong history of migraine. Features of amaurosis fugax which make a diagnosis of ocular migraine more likely include onset before the age of 40, headache over the symptomatic eye, and a history of full recovery after prolonged periods of visual loss (Katz, 1986; McDonald and Sanders, 1971; Coppeto *et al.*, 1986).

CLUSTER HEADACHE (MIGRAINOUS NEURALGIA)

Patients develop severe unilateral face or head pain associated with ipsilateral tearing, conjunctival injection, nasal congestion and facial flushing. There is transient oculosympathetic paresis (Horner's syndrome) of ptosis and pupillary miosis which may persist after the attack. In cluster headaches, the pain is centred around the eye, and unlike all other migraine variants, is much commoner in men than women and frequently affects individuals in their fourth and fifth decade with no previous headache history. Unlike typical migraineurs who retire to a quiet dark room at the onset of an attack, cluster headaches frequently induce restless behaviour with the individual pacing the room and holding on to his face. To make a diagnosis there should be at least five attacks of pain each lasting for between 15 and 120 minutes with a frequency of between one every alternate day to 8 per day. When the pain is persistent and unremitting with a Horner's syndrome (Raeder's paratrigeminal neuralgia) or external ophthalmoplegia, stuctural abnormalities of the middle cranial fossa floor such as an internal carotid aneurysm must be excluded by appropriate investigations (Waldenlind *et al.*, 1993).

PATHOGENESIS OF MIGRAINE

Multiple phenomena are responsible for the aura and the headache that occurs as part of the migraine syndrome. The process of spreading cortical depression produces the aura. Vasoconstriction followed by vasodilation of extracerebral cranial arteries, with inflammation of these vessels related to neurotransmitter release and activity of trigeminovascular fibres, and a reduction in pain threshold are responsible for the headache. A number of factors may precipitate an attack of migraine and avoidance of these factors is a vital part of effective treatment (Tansey *et al.*, 1993). These include stress or emotional upset, endocrine changes including the normal menstrual cycle and pregnancy, foods containing tyramine, monosodium glutamate, nitrates, aspartame, and phenylalanine (e.g. chocolate). Minor head trauma and non-specific stimuli including exertion, fatigue, mild hypoglycaemia and bright or flickering lights are additional triggers in some individuals (Goadsby and Edvinsson, 1993; Lauritzen, 1987; Zwelsloot *et al.*, 1993).

OTHER HEADACHES

In addition to migraine, many other entities encompass both headache and pain around the face and eye. These include trigeminal neuralgia, temporal arteritis, muscle tension, intracranial tumours, vascular diseases and depression. The temporal course of symptoms is a very helpful guide to the likely diagnosis: sudden onset of pain may reflect trauma, or meningeal irritation from blood or infection, or a mass due to raised intracranial pressure. Headache of increasing (crescendo) intensity may suggest an ocular, dental or sinus related cause, in addition to raised intracranial pressure. Chronic,

Table 10.2 An overview of common headaches at different ages

Age: 3–16 years	17–60 years	60 plus years
Migraine Tension Psychogenic Post-traumatic	Migraine Tension Cluster Post-traumatic	Referred from neck Giant cell arteritis Acute glaucoma Tumours: cranial, dural and cerebral
Raised intracranial pressure	Tumours: cranial, dural and cerebral Depression	Post-herpetic neuralgia Continuing migraine Continuing tension

or intermittent headache, with no signs of neurological dysfunction, suggests ocular, dental or sinus disease, tension (when constant), migraine (when intermittent), neuralgia and giant cell arteritis (Dalessio, 1980; Raskin, 1988). The age of the patient is also important when considering a likely cause as summarized in Table 10.2.

GIANT CELL (CRANIAL) ARTERITIS – CLINICAL FEATURES

Giant cell (cranial or temporal arteritis) is a systemic disorder featuring an inflammatory arteritis of medium sized, elastin containing vessels, particularly involving the extradural branches of the external and internal carotid arteries. The most prominent clinical feature is headache. This is felt in the scalp, usually in the territory of inflamed vessels along the course of the superficial temporal and occipital arteries and their branches. The patient may notice localized swelling and redness in these areas. Palpation may confirm redness and localized oedema with loss of pulsation and tenderness. Many patients complain spontaneously of scalp tenderness, such as when resting their head on the pillow, or on brushing or combing hair. In addition, there may be muscular ache affecting the hips and shoulder (polymyalgia rheumatica) which may precede the onset of headache by a period of several months. Polymyalgia may be associated with weight loss, sweating and low grade pyrexia. Jaw claudication may also be reported where there is pain on mastication which is relieved on resting (Meadows, 1966; Bengstsson and Malmvall, 1981).

Involvement of the ophthalmic artery leads to visual loss from ischaemic optic neuropathy often combined with cotton wool spots in the peripapillary area though sometimes there is a central retinal artery occlusion (Chapter 5). Cranial arteritis is also a cause of amaurosis fugax arising as a premonitory symptom (Chapter 4). Visual loss may be posturally dependent with symptoms on standing or sitting up which are relieved on lying down. Occasionally visual loss may occur in the absence of headache. Less commonly, vertebrobasilar ischaemia may be prominent, and there may be an external ophthalmoplegia as a result of involvement of the extraocular muscles or the intraorbital portion of the ocular motor nerves (III, IV and VI) or both. As a general rule the intracranial arteries are spared – however, cerebral or brain stem infarction may result from complete inflammatory occlusion of the extracranial vessels or from embolism from mural thrombus in inflamed arteries. Cranial arteritis is a systemic disease and in some patients the granulomatous arteritis produces prominent vascular occlusion away from the head and neck, involving the aortic arch, subclavian and coronary vessels, or causes mononeuritis multiplex (Wilkinson and Ross Russell, 1972; Butt *et al.*, 1991).

DIAGNOSIS AND MANAGEMENT

In addition to a normochromic normocytic anaemia, the erythrocyte sedimentation rate (ESR) is regularly and markedly elevated in 90% of untreated patients with established disease. Acute phase proteins (C-reactive protein, fibrinogen, alpha-2 and gama-globulins) are also elevated. Autoantibodies are negative. Histology shows a subacute granulomatous arteritis with thickening of the vessel wall and occasional obliteration of the lumen. Because up to 10% of patients may have an ESR of less than 40mm/h (Biller *et al.*, 1982), biopsy is indicated in most cases. Foreign body giant cells are found in relation to focal necrosis of the media and elastic lamina. However, false negative biopsies also arise in up to one-third of cases because of the presence of skip lesions and serial sections of a long (2 cm) length of artery should be undertaken to maximize the chances of histological confirmation of the diagnosis. The external carotid and vertebral arteries are consistently involved, but intradural vessels are spared — this has been ascribed to the small amount of elastic tissue in these vessels. In the orbit, arteritis may involve the main trunk and all the branches of the ophthalmic artery including the short posterior ciliary vessels and the central retinal artery within the dural sheath. Arteries within the optic nerve and retina are spared.

In view of the serious risk of visual loss, steroids are started immediately on suspicion of the diagnosis, without awaiting the result of a biopsy. Nevertheless, because the management of the condition may extend over many years, histological confirmation is invaluable. Biopsy is best perfomed within 48 hours of initiating steroid treatment. Following the introduction of steroids (oral prednisolone 60–80 mg daily, or i.v. methylprednisolone 500mg-1g daily for 3 days), relief of headache, malaise and polymyalgia is usually dramatic. Salvage of vision in established optic nerve or retinal ischemia is exceptional, but general supportive measures such as lowering the intraocular pressure with oral acetazolamide to improve optic nerve head perfusion, and lying the patient down in bed may help. Low doses of subcutaneous heparin can also be used when there is second eye involvement at presentation. Over the following weeks and months a tapering dose of steroids is then given, titrated against the clinical symptoms and the ESR (Faarvang *et al.*, 1989).

INTRACRANIAL MASS LESIONS

It has been estimated that almost two-thirds of patients with a brain tumour complain of headache, and in up to half, the headache may be the primary complaint. The pain may arise as a result of pressure on the meninges or dural venus sinuses and is typically worsened by exertion and postural changes. Intracranial pressure is often elevated, but is not essential for the development of headache in the presence of a brain tumour. The headache of raised intracranial pressure without an intracranial mass (idiopathic intracranial hypertension) and is relieved either following lumbar puncture, or after treatment with acetazolamide. Cough headache is a sudden diffuse severe headache triggered by the Valsalva manoeuvre, sneezing, bending or lifting. About 10% of patients with a cough headache have an intracranial abnormality, frequently a Chiari-1 malformation at the craniocervical junction.

POST-TRAUMATIC SYNDROME

Following a head injury, headaches are a frequent symptom and form part of the post-traumatic or postconcussion syndrome which follows both severe and mild trauma. Unconsciousness at the time of impact need not occur. Other symptoms include impairment of memory and concentration and emotional instability. The onset of post-traumatic syndrome may be immediately after the injury, or, delayed for weeks. Both classic and common migraine are exacerbated by head injury and there may be some overlap between the two symptom complexes.

ANEURYSM AND ARTERIOVENOUS MALFORMATION

Unruptured aneurysms can produce headache. In the days preceding subarachnoid haemorrhage from a ruptured berry aneurysm, up to 50% of patients may experience a sentinel headache which may be severe, perhaps representing partial rupture. A sudden severe excruciating headache together with neck stiffness and vomiting and confusion are the classic features of a ruptured aneurysm. The immediate appearance of a homonymous hemianopia indicates intracerebral bleeding often from an arteriovenous malformation.

OCULAR CAUSES OF HEADACHE

Several ocular diseases may present with generalized headache, although more commonly each is a cause of local symptoms only. These include acute glaucoma, iritis, corneal lesions, orbital pseudotumour, optic neuritis, scleritis, refractive errors and muscle imbalance. Usually the ophthalmic physical signs are obvious if the eye is responsible for a headache.

CAROTID DISSECTION

Pain in the angle of the jaw, ipsilateral headache, Horner's syndrome and atypical facial pain may suggest spontaneous dissection of the carotid or vertebral arteries. Intraluminal dissection may occur spontaneously in fibrous dysplasia, or following neck injuries ('whiplash injury').

FACIAL PAIN

Trigeminal neuralgia, or tic doloureux, is characterized by repetitive attacks of lightning jabs of lancinating pain in the maxillary and mandibular divisions of the trigeminal nerve. When the ophthalmic division is involved, this is usually together with the lower face. The onset is in the sixth or seventh decade and women are more frequently affected than men. Symptoms are often triggered by touch, cold, eating or drinking. The possible cause is vascular compression at the entry of the sensory root of the trigeminal nerve to the brain stem, but cerebellopontine angle tumours and multiple sclerosis may cause the same syndrome, especially in younger patients. Medical treatment includes carbamazepine, baclofen or clonazepam either alone or in combination. Surgical measures for refractory cases include posterior fossa vascular decompression or selective percutaneous radiofrequency ablation of the trigeminal ganglion in the middle cranial fossa. In contrast, atypical facial pain is less clearly defined and responds less well to specific medical treatment. Organic causes include dental and temporomandibular joint abnormalities and skull base tumours. Often depression is a prominent feature.

REFERENCES

Bailey TD, O'Connor PS, Tredici TJ and Shakett DE (1984). Ophthalmoplegic migraine. *J Clin Neuro-Ophthalmol* **4**: 225–228.

Bengtsson B-A and Malmvall B-E (1981). The epidemiology of giant cell arteritis including temporal arteritis and polymyalgia rheumatica. Incidences of different clinical presentations and eye complications. *Arthritis Rheum* **24**: 899–904.

Biller J, Asconape J, Weinblatt ME *et al.* (1982). Temporal arteritis associated with a normal sedimentation rate. *J Am Med Assoc* **247**: 486–487.

Bogousslavsky J, Regli F, Van Melle G *et al.* (1988). Migraine stroke. *Neurology* **38**: 223–227.

Butt Z, Cullen JF and Mutlakan E (1991). Pattern of arterial involvement of the head, neck and eyes in giant cell arteritis: three case reports. *Br J Ophthalmol* **75**: 368–371.

Coppeto JR, Lessell S, Sciarca R and Bear L (1986). Vascular retinopathy in migraine. *Neurology* **36**: 267–270.

Dalessio DJ (1980). *Wolff's Headaches and Other Head Pain* 4th edn New York: Oxford University Press.

Edelson RN and Levy DE (1974). Transient benign unilateral pupillary dilatation in young adults. *Arch Neurol* **31**: 12–14.

Faaryang FM, Williams JK, Breese KR *et al.* (1989). Giant cell arteritis: loss of vision during corticosteroid therapy. *J Int Med* **225**: 215–216.

Goadsby PJ and Edvinsson L (1993). The trigeminovascular system and migraine; studies characterizing cerebrovascular and neuropeptide changes seen in humans and cats. *Ann Neurol* **33**: 48–56.

Hallet M and Cogan DG (1970). Episodic unilateral mydriasis in otherwise normal patients. *Arch Ophthalmol* **84**: 130–136.

Hupp SL, Kline LB and Corbett JJ (1989). Visual disturbances of migraine. *Survey Ophthalmol* **33**: 221–236.

Katz B (1986). Migrainous central retinal artery occlusion. *J Clin Neuro-Ophthalmol* **6**: 69–71.

Lauritzen M (1987). Cortical spreading depression as a putative migraine mechanism. *Trends Neurosci* **10**: 8–13.
McDonald WI and Sanders MD (1971). Migraine complicated by ischaemic papillopathy. *Lancet* **ii**: 521.
Meadows SP (1966). Temporal or giant cell arteritis. *Proc R Soc Med* **59**: 329–333.
O'Sullivan F, Rossor M and Elston JS (1992) Amaurosis fugax in young people. *Br J Ophthalmol* **76**: 660–662.
Raskin NH (1988). *Headache* 2nd edn. New York: Churchill Livingstone.
Sarkies NJC, Sanders MD and Gautier-Smith PC (1985). Letter: Episodic unilateral mydriasis and migraine. *Am J Ophthalmol* **99**: 217–218.
Stommel EW, Ward TN and Harris RD (1993). MRI findings in a case of ophthalmoplegic migraine. *Headache* **33**: 234–237.
Tansey MJB, Pilgrim AJ and Lloyd K (1993). Sumatriptan in the acute treatment of migraine. *J Neurol Sci* **114**: 109–116.
Waldenlind E, Ekbom K and Torhall J (1993). MR-angiography during spontaneous attacks of cluster headaches. *Headache* **33**: 291–295.
Wilkinson IMS and Ross Russell RW (1972). Arteries of the head and neck in giant cell arteritis. A pathological study to show the pattern of arterial involvement. *Arch Neurol* **27**: 378–391.
Woods D, O'Connor PS and Fleming R (1984). Episodic unilateral mydriasis and migraine. *Am J Ophthalmol* **98**: 229–234.
Woods RP, Iacoboni M, Mazziotta JC and Gomez CR (1994). Brief report: Bilateral spreading cerebral hypoperfusion during spontaneous migaine headache. *New Engl J Med* **331**: 1689–1692.
Zwelsloot CP, Caerbeke JFV and Ferrari MD (1993). Lack of asymmetry of middle cerebral artery blood velocity in unilateral migraine. *Stroke* **24**: 1335–1338.

Index